Statistical Models in
Epidemiology

Statistical Models in

Epidemiology

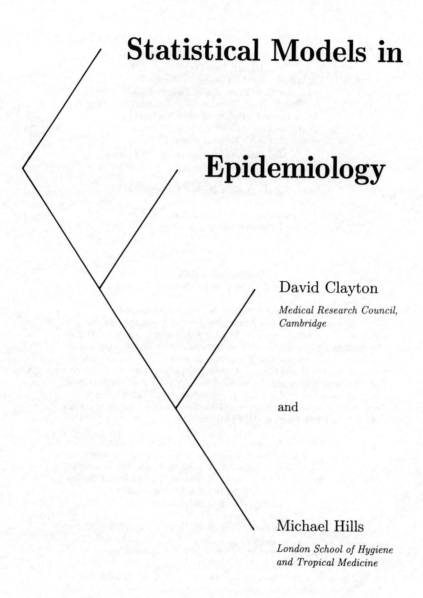

David Clayton

Medical Research Council,
Cambridge

and

Michael Hills

London School of Hygiene
and Tropical Medicine

OXFORD · NEW YORK · TOKYO
OXFORD UNIVERSITY PRESS

Oxford University Press, Walton Street, Oxford OX2 6DP

Oxford New York
Athens Auckland Bangkok Bombay
Calcutta Cape Town Dar es Salaam Delhi
Florence Hong Kong Istanbul Karachi
Kuala Lumpur Madras Madrid Melbourne
Mexico City Nairobi Paris Singapore
Taipei Tokyo Toronto
and associated companies in
Berlin Ibadan

Oxford is a trade mark of Oxford University Press

Published in the United States by
Oxford University Press Inc., New York

First published 1993
Reprinted 1994 (twice), 1995, 1996

A catalogue record for this book is available from the British Library

Library of Congress Cataloging in Publication Data
Clayton, David, statistician.
Statistical models in epidemiology/David Clayton and Michael Hills.
Includes bibliographical references and index.
1. Epidemiology—Statistical methods. I. Hills, Michael. II. Title.
[DNLM: 1. Epidemiology. 2. Models, Statistical. WA 105 C622s 1993]
RA652.2M3C53 1993 614.4'072—dc20 93–19448
ISBN 0 19 852221 5

Printed in Great Britain on acid-free paper by
Biddles Ltd, Guildford and King's Lynn

Preface

The aim of this book is to give a self-contained account of the statistical basis of epidemiology. The book is intended primarily for students enrolled for a masters degree in epidemiology, clinical epidemiology, or biostatistics, and should be suitable both as the basis for a taught course and for private study.

Although we anticipate that most readers will have taken a first course in statistics, no previous knowledge is assumed, and the mathematical level of the book has been chosen to suit readers whose basic training is in biology. Some of the material in the book could be omitted at first reading, either because it is rather more demanding of mathematical skills or because it deals with rather specialized points. We have been careful to gather such material either into complete chapters or complete sections and to indicate these with a marginal symbol, as here.

$\boxed{\star}$

Epidemiologists today have ready access to computer programs of great generality, but to use these sensibly and productively it is necessary to understand the ideas which lie behind them. The most important of these is the idea of a *probability model*. All statistical analysis of data is based on probability models, even though the models may not be explicit. Only by fully understanding the model can one fully understand the analysis.

Models depend on parameters, and values must be chosen for these parameters in order to match the model to the data. In showing how this is done we have chosen to emphasize the role of likelihood because this offers an approach to statistics which is both simple and intuitively satisfying. An additional advantage of this approach is that it requires the model and its parameters to be made explicit, even in the simplest situations. More complex problems can then be tackled by natural extensions of simple methods and do not require a whole new way of looking at things.

Most of the material in this book was developed during successive residential summer courses in epidemiology and statistics, held in Florence under the auspices of the European Educational Programme in Epidemiology. We are grateful to the International Agency for Cancer Research, the Regional Office for Europe of the World Health Organization, the Commission of the European Communities, and the Tuscany Regional Government, for sponsoring the program, and to Walter Davies, Organizing Secretary, and Rodolfo Saracci, Course Director, whose respective skills ensured that the course took place each year. We also acknowledge with thanks helpful comments on earlier drafts from Damien Jolley, Bendix Carstensen, Dave Leon, and Nick Hills.

Cambridge   David Clayton
London   Michael Hills
February 1993

Dedication

To the students of the Florence course, 1988 – 92, without whose help and encouragement this book would never have appeared.

Contents

⋆   Denotes a chapter which could be omitted from a first course.

Part I

Probability models and likelihood

1
Probability models

1.1 Observation, experiments and models

Science proceeds by endless repetition of a three-stage process,

1. observation;
2. building a model to describe (or 'explain') the observations; and
3. using the model to predict future observations. If future observations are not in accord with the predictions, the model must be replaced or refined.

In quantitative science, the models used are mathematical models. They fall into two main groups, *deterministic* models and probability (or *stochastic*) models. It is the latter which are appropriate in epidemiology, but the former are more familiar to most scientists and serve to introduce some important ideas.

DETERMINISTIC MODELS

The most familiar examples of deterministic models are the laws of classical physics. We choose as a familiar example *Ohm's law*, which applies to the relationship between electrical potential (or voltage), V, applied across a conductor and the current flowing, I. The law holds that there is a strict proportionality between the two — if the potential is doubled then the current will double. This relationship is represented graphically in Fig. 1.1.

Ohm's law holds for a wide range of conductors, and simply states that the line in Fig. 1.1 is straight; it says nothing about the gradient of the line. This will differ from one conductor to another and depends on the resistance of the conductor. Without knowing the resistance it will not be possible to predict the current which will flow in any *particular* conductor. Physicists normally denote the resistance by R and write the relationship as

$$I = \frac{V}{R}.$$

However, R is a different sort of quantity from V or I. It is a *parameter* — a number which we must fix in order to apply the general law to a specific case. Statisticians are careful to differentiate between observable variables

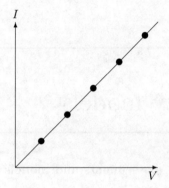

Fig. 1.1. A deterministic model: Ohm's law.

(such as V and I) and parameters (such as R) and use Greek letters for the latter. Thus, if Ohm were a modern statistician he would write his law as

$$I = \frac{V}{\rho}$$

In this form it is now clear that ρ, the resistance, is a parameter of a simple mathematical model which relates current to potential. Alternatively, he could write the law as

$$I = \gamma V$$

where γ is the conductance (the inverse of the resistance). This is a simple example of a process called *reparametrization* — writing the model differently so that the parameters take on different meanings.

STOCHASTIC MODELS

Unfortunately the phenomena studied by scientists are rarely as predictable as is implied by Fig. 1.1. In the presence of measurement errors and un-controlled variability of experimental conditions it might be that real data look more like Fig. 1.2. In these circumstances we would not be in a position to predict a future observation with certainty, nor would we be able to give a definitive estimate of the resistance parameter. It is necessary to extend the deterministic model so that we can predict a range of more probable future observations, and indicate the uncertainty in the estimate of the resistance.

Problems such as this prompted the mathematician Gauss to develop his *theory of errors*, based on the Gaussian distribution (often also called the *Normal* distribution), which is the most important probability model for these problems. A very large part of statistical theory is concerned with this model and most elementary statistical texts reflect this. Epidemiology,

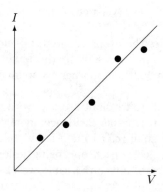

Fig. 1.2.   Experimental/observational errors.

however, is more concerned with the occurrence (or not) of certain events in the natural history of disease. Since these occurrences cannot be described purely deterministically, probability models are also necessary here, but it is the models of Bernoulli and Poisson which are more relevant. The remainder of this chapter discusses a particularly important type of data generated by epidemiological studies, and the nature of the models we use in its analysis.

1.2   Binary data

Many epidemiological studies generate data in which the response measurement for each subject may take one of only two possible values. Such a response is called a *binary* response. Two rather different types of study generate such data.

COHORT STUDIES WITH FIXED FOLLOW-UP TIME

In a *cohort* study a group of people are followed through some period of time in order to study the occurrence (or not) of a certain event of interest. The simplest case is a study of *mortality* (from any cause). Clearly, there are only two possible outcomes for a subject followed, say, for five years — death or survival.

More usually, it is only death from a specified cause or causes which is of interest. Although there are now three possible outcomes for any subject — death from the cause of interest, death from another cause, or survival — such data are usually dealt with as binary data. The response is taken as death from cause of interest as against survival, death from other causes being treated as premature termination of follow-up. Premature termination of follow-up is a common feature of epidemiological and clinical follow-up studies and may occur for many reasons. It is called *censoring*, a word which reflects the fact that it is the underlying binary response which we would have liked to observe, were it not for the removal of the subject from observation.

In *incidence studies* the event of interest is new occurrence of a specified disease. Again our interest is in the binary response (whether the disease occurred or not) although other events may intervene to censor our observation of it.

For greater generality, we shall use the word *failure* as a generic term for the event of interest, whether incidence, mortality, or some other (undesirable) outcome. We shall refer to non-failure as *survival*. In the simplest case, we study N subjects, each one being followed for a fixed time interval, such as five years. Over this time we observe D failures, so that $N - D$ survive. We shall develop methods for dealing with censoring in later chapters.

CROSS-SECTIONAL PREVALENCE DATA

Prevalence studies have considerable importance in assessing needs for health services, and may also provide indirect evidence for differences in incidence. They have the considerable merit of being relatively cheap to carry out since there is no follow-up of the study group over time. Subjects are simply categorized as affected or not affected, according to agreed clinical criteria, at some fixed point in time. In a simple study, we might observe N subjects and classify D of them as affected. An important example is serological studies in infectious-disease epidemiology, in which subjects are classified as being seropositive or seronegative for a specified infection.

1.3   The binary probability model

The obvious analysis of our simple binary data consisting of D failures out of N subjects observed is to compute the proportion failing, D/N. However, knowing the proportion of a cohort which develops a disease, or dies from a given cause, is of little use unless it can be assumed to have a wider applicability beyond the cohort. It is in making this passage from the particular to the general that statistical models come in. One way of looking at the problem is as an attempt to predict the outcome for a new subject, similar to the subjects in the cohort, but whose outcome is unknown. Since the outcome for this new subject cannot be predicted with certainty the prediction must take the form of *probabilities* attached to the two possible outcomes. This is the *binary probability model*. It is the simplest of all probability models and, for the present, we need to know nothing of the properties of probability save that probabilities are numbers lying in the range 0 to 1, with 0 representing an impossible outcome and 1 representing a certain outcome, and that the probability of occurrence of either one of two distinct outcomes is the sum of their individual probabilities (the *additive* rule of probability).

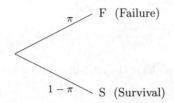

Fig. 1.3.   The binary probability model.

THE RISK PARAMETER

The binary probability model is illustrated in Figure 1.3. The two outcomes are labelled F (failure) and S (survival). The model has one *parameter*, π, the probability of failure. Because the subject must either fail or survive, the sum of the probabilities of these two outcomes must be 1, so the probability of survival is $1 - \pi$. In the context where π represents the probability of occurrence of an event in a specified time period, it is usually called the *risk*.

THE ODDS PARAMETER

An important alternative way of parametrizing the binary probability model is in terms of the *odds* of failure versus survival. These are

$$\pi : (1 - \pi),$$

which may also be written as

$$\frac{\pi}{1 - \pi} : 1.$$

It is convenient to omit the : 1 in the above expression and to measure the odds by the fraction

$$\frac{\pi}{1 - \pi}.$$

This explains why, although the word odds is plural, there is often only one number which measures the odds.

Exercise 1.1. Calculate the odds of F to S when the probability of failure is (a) 0.75, (b) 0.50, (c) 0.25.

In general the relationship between a probability π and the corresponding odds Ω is

$$\Omega = \frac{\pi}{(1 - \pi)}.$$

This can be inverted to give

$$\pi = \frac{\Omega}{1 + \Omega}, \quad 1 - \pi = \frac{1}{1 + \Omega}.$$

Exercise 1.2. Calculate the probability of failure when Ω, the odds of F to S is (a) 0.3, (b) 3.0.

RARE EVENTS

In this book we shall be particularly concerned with *rare events*, that is, events with a small probability, π, of occurrence in the time period of interest. In this case $(1 - \pi)$ is very close to 1 and the odds parameter and the risk parameter are nearly equal:

$$\Omega \approx \pi.$$

This approximation is often called the *rare disease assumption*, but this is a misleading term, since even the common cold has a small probability of occurrence within, say, a one-week time interval.

1.4   Parameter estimation

Without giving a value to the parameter π, this model is of no use for prediction. Our next problem is to use our observed data to estimate its value. It might seem obvious to the reader that we should estimate π by the proportion of failures, D/N. This corresponds to estimating the odds parameter Ω by $D/(N - D)$, the ratio of failures to survivors.

It might also seem obvious that we should place more reliance on our estimate (and upon any predictions based on it) if N is 1000 than if N is 10. The formal statistical theory which provides a quantitative justification for these intuitions will be discussed in later chapters.

1.5   Is the model true?

A model which states that every one of a group of patients has the same probability of surviving five years will seem implausible to most clinicians. Indeed, the use of such models by statisticians is a major reason why some practitioners, brought up to think of each patient as unique, part company with the subject!

The question of whether scientific models are *true* is not however, a sensible one. Instead, we should ask ourselves whether our model is *useful* in describing past observations and predicting future ones. Where there remains a choice of models, we must be guided by the criterion of *simplicity*. In epidemiology probability models are used to describe past observations of disease events in study cohorts and to make predictions for future individuals. If we have no further data which allows us to differentiate subjects in the cohort from one another or from a future individual, we have no option save to assign the same probability of failure to each subject. Further data allows elaboration of the model. For example, if we can identify subjects as exposed or unexposed to some environmental influence, the model can be extended to assign different probabilities to exposed and unexposed subjects. If additionally we know the level of exposure we can extend the model by letting the probability of failure be some increasing function of exposure.

In this book we shall demonstrate the manner in which more complicated models may be developed to deal with more detailed data. The binary model has been our starting point since it is the basic building brick from which more elaborate models are constructed.

Solutions to the exercises

1.1   (a) Odds $= 0.75/0.25 = 3$.
(b) Odds $= 0.50/0.50 = 1$.
(c) Odds $= 0.25/0.75 = 0.3333$.

1.2   (a) Probability $= 0.3/1.3 = 0.2308$.
(b) Probability $= 3/4 = 0.75$.

2
Conditional probability models

In this chapter we introduce the idea of *conditional probability*, which allows us to extend the binary model so that the probability of failure can depend on earlier events. The natural way of thinking about conditional probabilities is in terms of a tree diagram. These diagrams are used extensively throughout the book.

2.1 Conditional probability

Suppose a binary probability model assigns a probability to a subject's death during some future time period. It may be that this prediction would be better if we knew the subject's smoking habits. This would be the case if the probability of death for a smoker were 0.015 but only 0.005 for a non-smoker. These probabilities are called *conditional* probabilities; they are the probabilities of death conditional on being a smoker and a non-smoker respectively. Epidemiology is mainly concerned with conditional probability models that relate occurrence of some disease event, which we call failure, to events which precede it. These include potential causes, which we call *exposures*.

When subjects are classified as either exposed (E+) or not exposed (E−), the conditional probability model can be represented as a tree with 6 branches. The first two branches refer to E+ and E−; then there are two referring to failure and survival if the subject is exposed, and two referring to failure and survival if the subject is not exposed. An example is shown in Fig. 2.1. The tips of the tree correspond to the four possible combinations of exposure and outcome for any subject.

The probabilities on the first two branches of the tree refer to the probability that a subject is exposed and the probability that a subject is not exposed. Using the smoking example we have taken these to be 0.4 and 0.6. The probabilities in the next two pairs of branches are conditional probabilities. These are 0.015 (F) and 0.985 (S) if a subject is exposed (smokes), and 0.005 (F) and 0.995 (S) if a subject is not exposed (does not smoke).

The probability of any combination of exposure and outcome is obtained by multiplying the probabilities along the branches leading to the

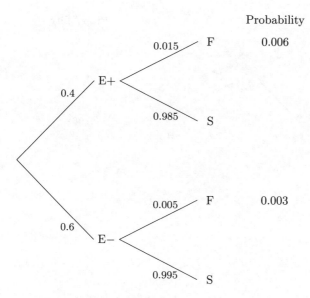

Fig. 2.1.   A conditional probability tree.

tip which corresponds to that combination. For example, the probability that a subject is exposed and fails is

$$0.4 \times 0.015 = 0.006,$$

and the probability that a subject is not exposed and fails is

$$0.6 \times 0.005 = 0.003.$$

This is called the multiplicative rule.

Exercise 2.1. Calculate the probabilities for each of the remaining 2 possibilities. What is the overall probability of failure regardless of exposure?

This overall probability is usually called the *marginal* probability of failure.

STATISTICAL DEPENDENCE AND INDEPENDENCE

Fig. 2.1 illustrates a model in which the probability of failure differs according to whether an individual was exposed or not. In this case, exposure and failure are said to be *statistically dependent*. If the probability of failure is the same, whether or not the subject is exposed, then exposure and failure are said to be *statistically independent*.

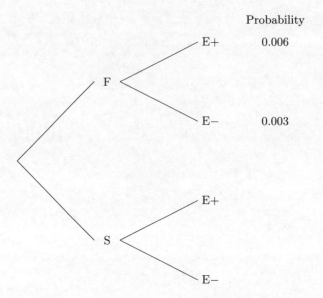

Fig. 2.2. Predicting exposure from the outcome.

2.2 Changing the conditioning: Bayes' rule

The additive and multiplicative rules are the basic building blocks of probability models. A simple application of these rules allows us to change the direction of prediction so that, for example, a model for the probability of failure given exposure can be transformed into a model for the probability of exposure given failure.

We shall demonstrate this by using the tree in Fig. 2.1, where the first level of branching refers to exposure and the second to outcome. This is turned round in Fig. 2.2, so that the first level of branching now refers to outcome and the second to exposure. The probabilities of the different combinations of exposure and outcome are the same whichever way the tree is written; our problem is to fill in the probabilities on the branches of this new tree.

Working backwards from the tips of the tree, the probability of failure regardless of exposure is $0.006 + 0.003 = 0.009$. This is the probability for the first branch of the tree to F. Since the probability corresponding to any tip of the tree is obtained by multiplying the probabilities in the branches that lead to the tip, it follows that the probability in the branch from F to E+, for example, is $0.006/0.009 = 0.667$. This is the conditional probability of being exposed given the outcome was failure. This process of reversing the order of the conditioning is called Bayes' rule, after Thomas Bayes.

Exercise 2.2. Calculate the remaining conditional probabilities.

The following exercise, inspired by problems in screening, demonstrates one of the many uses of Bayes' rule.

Exercise 2.3. A screening test has a probability of 0.90 of being positive in true cases of a disease (the *sensitivity*) and a probability of 0.995 of being negative in people without the disease (the *specificity*). The prevalence of the disease is 0.001 so before carrying out the test, the probability that a person has the disease is 0.001.
(a) Draw a probability tree in which the first level of branching refers to having the disease or not, and the second level to being positive or negative on the screening test. Fill in the probabilities for each of the branches and calculate the probabilities for the four possible combinations of disease and test.
(b) Draw the tree the other way, so that the first level of branching refers to being positive or negative on the screening test and the second level to having the disease or not. Fill in the probabilities for the branches of this tree. What is the probability of a person having the disease given that they have a positive test result? (This is called the *positive predictive value*.)

2.3 An example from genetics

Our next exercises illustrate a problem in genetic epidemiology. For a specified genetic system (such as the HLA system), each person's *genotype* consists of two *haplotypes*,* one inherited from the mother and one from the father. If a mother has haplotypes (a,b), then one of these is passed to the offspring with probability 0.5. Likewise for a father's haplotypes, (c,d) say. Fig. 2.3 shows the probability tree for the genotype of the offspring. The presence of haplotype (a) carries a probability of disease of 0.05 while, in its absence, the probability is only 0.01.

Exercise 2.4. Work out the probabilities for the four tips of the probability tree which end in disease (F). Hence work out the probabilities of the four possible genotypes conditional on the fact that the offspring is affected by disease (Fig. 2.4).

Exercise 2.5. In practice the probabilities of disease conditional upon genotype are not known constants but unknown parameters. Repeat the previous exercise *algebraically*, replacing the probabilities 0.01 and 0.05 by π and $\theta\pi$ respectively. How are the conditional probabilities changed if the subject's father has genotype (c,c)?

The parameter θ, described in Exercise 2.5, is a *risk ratio*,

$$\theta = \frac{\text{Risk of disease if haplotype (a) present}}{\text{Risk of disease if haplotype (a) absent}}.$$

---

*The word haplotype refers to a group of genetic loci which are closely linked and therefore inherited together.

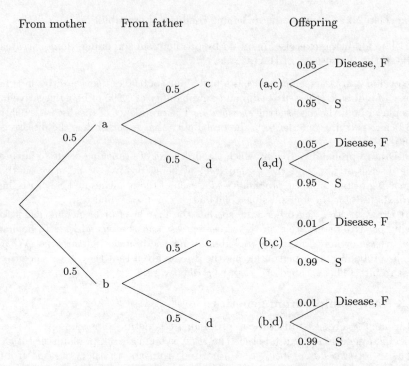

Fig. 2.3. Disease conditional upon inheritance.

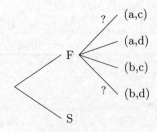

Fig. 2.4. Inheritance conditional upon disease.

It measures the strength of statistical dependence (or *association*) between the presence of haplotype (a) and occurrence of disease. The above exercise shows that the conditional probability of genotype given the presence of disease and parental genotypes depends only on this risk ratio.

Solutions to the exercises

2.1

$$Pr(E+ \text{ and } S) = 0.4 \times 0.985 = 0.394$$
$$Pr(E- \text{ and } S) = 0.6 \times 0.995 = 0.597$$

The overall probability of failure is $0.006 + 0.003 = 0.009$.

2.2 See Fig. 2.5. The conditional probabilities of E+ and E− given survival are

$$\frac{0.394}{0.991} = 0.3976, \qquad \frac{0.597}{0.991} = 0.6024.$$

2.3 (a) See Fig. 2.6.
(b) See Fig. 2.7. The probability of disease given a positive test result is

$$\frac{0.0009}{0.005895} = 0.1527.$$

Note that this is much lower than 0.90, the sensitivity of the test. The remaining conditional probabilities are calculated in a similar manner.

2.4 The probabilities for each of the four tips are obtained by multiplying along the branches of the tree. The sum of the four probabilities is 0.0300. The *conditional* probabilities sum to 1.0.

Genotype	Disease	Probability	Conditional prob.
(a,c)	F	$0.5 \times 0.5 \times 0.05 = 0.0125$	$0.0125/0.03 = 0.417$
(a,d)	F	$0.5 \times 0.5 \times 0.05 = 0.0125$	0.417
(b,c)	F	$0.5 \times 0.5 \times 0.01 = 0.0025$	$0.0025/0.03 = 0.083$
(b,d)	F	$0.5 \times 0.5 \times 0.01 = 0.0025$	0.083
Total		0.0300	1.0

2.5 Repeating the above calculations algebraically yields:

Genotype	Disease	Probability	Conditional Prob.
(a,c)	F	$0.5 \times 0.5 \times \theta\pi = 0.25\theta\pi$	$\theta/(2\theta + 2)$
(a,d)	F	$0.5 \times 0.5 \times \theta\pi = 0.25\theta\pi$	$\theta/(2\theta + 2)$
(b,c)	F	$0.5 \times 0.5 \times \pi = 0.25\pi$	$1/(2\theta + 2)$
(b,d)	F	$0.5 \times 0.5 \times \pi = 0.25\pi$	$1/(2\theta + 2)$
Total		$0.25\pi(2\theta + 2)$	1.0

If the father has genotype (c,c) then he can only pass on (c) and the possible genotypes of offspring are (a,c) and (b,c). Prior to observation of disease presence, these both have probabilities 0.5. Thus, for a subject known to have disease, we have

Genotype	Disease	Probability	Conditional Prob.
(a,c)	F	$0.5 \times \theta\pi = 0.5\theta\pi$	$\theta/(\theta+1)$
(b,c)	F	$0.5 \times \pi = 0.5\pi$	$1/(\theta+1)$
Total		$0.5\pi(\theta+1)$	1.0

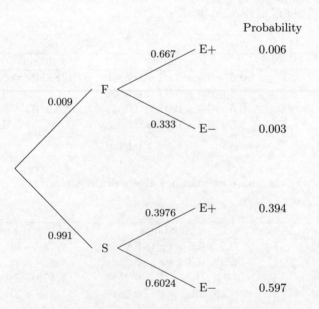

Fig. 2.5. Probability tree for exposure given outcome.

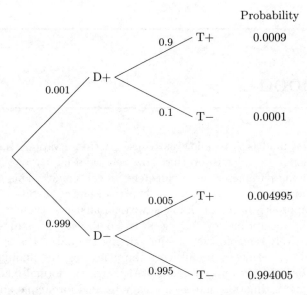

Fig. 2.6. Test results, T, given disease status, D.

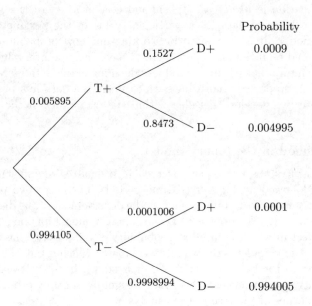

Fig. 2.7. Disease status given test results.

3
Likelihood

The purpose of models is to allow us to use past observations (*data*) to make predictions. In order to do this, however, we need a way of choosing a value of the parameter (or parameters) of the model. This process is called parameter *estimation* and this chapter discusses the most important general approach to it. In simple statistical analyses, these stages of model building and estimation may seem to be absent, the analysis just being an intuitively sensible way of summarizing the data. However, the analysis is only scientifically useful if we can generalize the findings, and such generalization must imply a model. Although the formal machinery of modelling and estimation may seem heavy handed for simple analyses, an understanding of it is essential to the development of methods for more difficult problems.

In modern statistics the concept which is central to the process of parameter estimation is *likelihood*. Likelihood is a measure of the *support* provided by a body of data for a particular value of the parameter of a probability model. It is calculated by working out how probable our observations would be if the parameter were to have the assumed value. The main idea is simply that parameter values which make the data more probable are better supported than values which make the data less probable. In this chapter we develop this idea within the framework of the binary model.

3.1 Likelihood in the binary model .

Fig. 3.1 illustrates the outcomes observed in a small study in which 10 subjects are followed up for a fixed time period. There are two possible outcomes for each subject: *failure*, such as the development of the disease of interest, or *survival*. We adopt a binary probability model for the outcome for each subject in which failure has probability π and survival has probability $1 - \pi$. The complete tree would have many branches but only those corresponding to the observed study result is shown in full. To calculate the probability of occurrence of this result we simply multiply probabilities along the branches of the tree in the usual way:

$$\pi \times \pi \times (1 - \pi) \times \cdots \times (1 - \pi) = (\pi)^4(1 - \pi)^6.$$

Subject

(1)   (2)   (3)   (4)   (5)   (6)   (7)   (8)   (9)   (10)

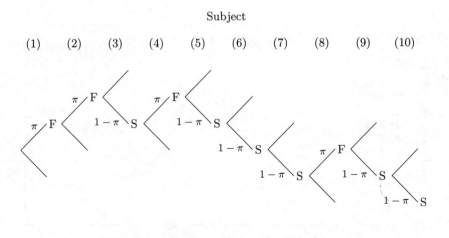

Fig. 3.1.   Study outcomes for 10 subjects.

This expression can be used to calculate the probability of the observed study result for any specified value of π. For example, when $\pi = 0.1$ the probability is

$$(0.1)^4 \times (0.9)^6 = 5.31 \times 10^{-5}$$

and when $\pi = 0.5$ it is

$$(0.5)^4 \times (0.5)^6 = 9.77 \times 10^{-4}.$$

The results of these calculations show that the probability of the observed data is greater for $\pi = 0.5$ than for $\pi = 0.1$. In statistics this is often expressed by saying that $\pi = 0.5$ is more *likely* than $\pi = 0.1$, meaning that the former value is better supported by the data. In everyday use the words probable and likely mean the same thing, but in statistics the word likely is used in this more specialized sense.

Exercise 3.1. Is $\pi = 0.4$ more likely than $\pi = 0.5$?

The result of the expression

$$(\pi)^4(1 - \pi)^6,$$

is a probability, but when we use it to assess the amount of support for different values of π it is called a *likelihood*. More generally, if we observed D failures in N subjects, the likelihood for π would be

$$(\pi)^D(1 - \pi)^{N-D},$$

and we shall call this expression the *Bernoulli* likelihood, after the Swiss mathematician. Because there are so many possible outcomes to the study,

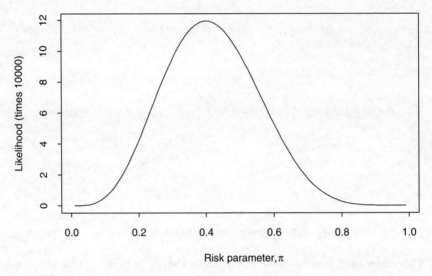

Fig. 3.2. The likelihood for π.

the likelihood (which is the probability of just one of these) is a small number. However, it is not the *absolute* value of the likelihood which should concern us, but its *relative* value for different choices of π.

Returning to our numerical example, Fig. 3.2 shows how the likelihood varies as a function of π. The value $\pi = 0.4$ gives a likelihood of 11.9×10^{-4}, which is the largest which can be achieved. This value of π is called the *most likely value* or, more formally, the *maximum likelihood estimate* of π. It coincides with the observed proportion of failures in the study, $4/10$.

3.2 The supported range for π

The most likely value for π is 0.4, with likelihood 11.9×10^{-4}. The likelihood for any other value of π will be less than this. How much less is measured by the *likelihood ratio*, which takes the value 1 when $\pi = 0.4$ and values less than 1 for any other values of π. This provides a more convenient measure of the degree of support than the likelihood itself. It can be used to classify values of π as either supported or not according to some critical value of the likelihood ratio. Values of π with likelihood ratios above the critical value are reported as 'supported', and values with likelihood ratios below this critical value as 'not supported'. The *supported range* for π is the set of values of π with likelihood ratios above the critical value. The choice of the critical value is a matter of convention.

For our observation of 4 failures and 6 survivors, the likelihood ratio as a function of π is shown in Figure 3.3. We have used the number 0.258

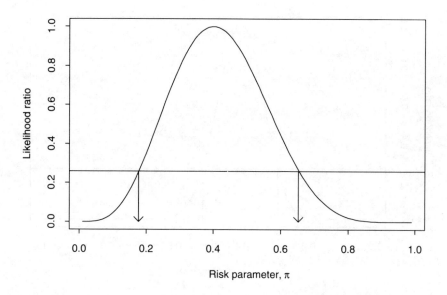

Fig. 3.3.   The likelihood ratio for π.

for the critical value of the likelihood ratio and indicated the limits of the supported range with the two arrows. The range of supported values for π is rather wide in this case: from 0.17 to 0.65.* For any choice of critical value the width of the supported range reflects the uncertainty in our knowledge about π. The main thing which determines this is the quantity of data used in calculating the likelihood. For example, if we were to observe 20 failures in 50 subjects, the most likely value of π would still be 0.4, but the supported range would be narrower (see Figure 3.4).

Although the concept of a supported range based on likelihood ratios is intuitively simple, it requires some consensus about the choice of critical value. The achievement of this has not proved easy, since many scientists lack an intuitive feel for the amount of uncertainty corresponding to a stated numerical value for the likelihood ratio. As a result, statistical theorists have tried to find ways to measure the uncertainty about the value of a parameter in terms of *probability* which, it is argued, is more easily interpreted. The way of doing this which is most widely accepted in the scientific community is by imagining a large number of repetitions of the study. This approach is known as the *frequentist* theory of statistics and leads to a *confidence interval* for π rather than a supported range. Another approach, often favoured by mathematicians, is based on a probability measure for the subjective 'degree of belief' that the parameter value lies in a stated *credible*

---

*These values were obtained from the graph, as illustrated. We shall be describing more convenient approximate methods for their computation in Chapter 9.

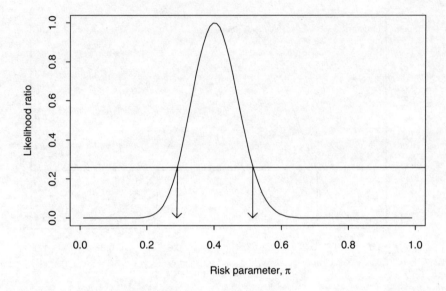

Fig. 3.4.   The likelihood ratio based on 20 failures in 50 subjects.

interval. This is the *Bayesian* theory of statistics.

Luckily for applied scientists, these philosophical differences can be resolved, at least for the analysis of moderately large studies. In this case, we will show in Chapter 10 that the supported range based on a likelihood ratio criterion of 0.258 coincides approximately with a 90% confidence interval in the frequentist theory of statistics and a 90% credible interval in the Bayesian theory. We shall, therefore, set aside these difficulties for the present and continue to develop the idea of likelihood, which holds a central place in both theories of statistics and from which most of the statistical methods of modern epidemiology can be derived.

3.3   The log likelihood

The likelihood, when evaluated for a particular value of the parameter, can turn out to be a very small number, and it is generally more convenient to use the (natural) logarithm of the likelihood in place of the likelihood itself.[†] When combining log likelihoods from independent sets of data the separate log likelihoods are added to form the combined likelihood. This is because the likelihoods themselves, being the probabilities of independent sets of data, are combined by multiplication. The log likelihood for π, in

---

[†]Readers not completely familiar with the logarithmic function, $\log(x)$ and its inverse, the exponential function, $\exp(x)$, are referred to Appendix A.

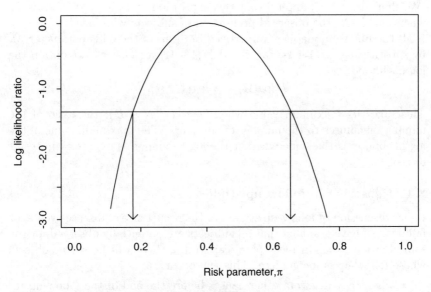

Fig. 3.5.   The log likelihood ratio for π.

this example, is
$$4\log(\pi) + 6\log(1-\pi).$$

Exercise 3.2. Calculate the log likelihood when $\pi = 0.5$ and when $\pi = 0.1$.

The log likelihood takes its maximum at the same value of π as the likelihood, namely $\pi = 0.4$, so its maximum is

$$4\log(0.4) + 6\log(0.6) = -6.730.$$

To obtain the log likelihood *ratio*, this maximum must be *subtracted* from the log likelihood. A graph of the log likelihood ratio is shown in Fig. 3.5. The supported range for π can be found from this graph in the same way as from the likelihood ratio graph, by finding those values of π for which the log likelihood ratio is greater than

$$\log(0.258) = -1.353.$$

Exercise 3.3. Calculate the log likelihood ratios for $\pi = 0.1$ and $\pi = 0.5$. Are these values of π in the supported range?

In general, the log likelihood for π, when D subjects fail and $N - D$ survive, is
$$D\log(\pi) + (N - D)\log(1-\pi).$$

We shall show in Chapter 9 that this expression takes its maximum value when $\pi = D/N$, the observed proportion of subjects who failed.

If the binary model is parametrized in terms of the odds parameter, Ω, by substituting $\Omega/(1 + \Omega)$ for π and $1/(1 + \Omega)$ for $(1 - \pi)$, we obtain the log likelihood

$$D \log(\Omega) - N \log(1 + \Omega).$$

This takes its maximum value when $\Omega = D/(N - D)$, the ratio of the number or failures to the number of survivors. The maximum value of the log likelihood is the same whether the log likelihood is expressed in terms of π or Ω.

3.4 Censoring in follow-up studies

In our discussion of follow-up studies of the occurrence of disease events, or failures, we have assumed that all subjects are potentially observed for the same fixed period. In most practical studies there will be some subjects whose follow-up is incomplete. This will occur

- when they die from other causes before the end of the follow-up interval;
- when they migrate and are no longer covered by the record system which registers failures;
- when they join the cohort too late to complete the follow-up period.

In all three cases the observation time for the subject is said to be censored. In fact, the first type of loss to follow-up, failure due to a *competing cause*, is rather different from the remaining two, but they are usually grouped together and dealt with in the same way. In Chapter 7 we shall discuss the justification for this practice. For the moment, we assume it to be reasonable.

Censoring puts our argument in some difficulty. The model allows for only two outcomes, failure and survival, while our data contains three, failure, survival, and censoring. For the present we shall avoid this difficulty with a simple pretence. As an illustration, suppose we have followed 1000 men for five years, during which 28 suffered myocardial infarction and 972 did not, but observation of 15 men was censored before completion of five years follow-up. If all 15 men were withdrawn from study on the *first* day of the follow up period, the size of the cohort would be 985 rather than 1000. Conversely, if they were all withdrawn on the *last* day, censoring could be ignored and the cohort size treated as a full 1000. When censoring is evenly spread over the study interval, we would expect an answer which lies somewhere in between these two extreme assumptions. This suggests treating the effective cohort size as 992.5 — mid-way between 985 and 1000. This convention is equivalent to the assumption that 7.5 subjects are censored on the first day of follow up and 7.5 on the last day.

Table 3.1.   Genotypes of 7 probands and their parents

Proband's genotype	Parents' genotypes Mother	Father	Number
(a,c)	(a,b)	(c,d)	4
(b,d)	(a,b)	(c,d)	1
(a,c)	(a,b)	(c,c)	2

With only 15 subjects lost to follow up through censoring, this crude strategy for dealing with censoring is quite satisfactory, but if 150 were censored it could be seriously misleading. In Chapter 4 we shall see how this problem can be dealt with by extending the model.

3.5   Applications in genetics

The use of the log likelihood as a measure of support is of considerable importance in genetics. However, in that field it is conventional to use logarithms to the base 10 rather than natural logarithms. Since the two systems of logarithms differ only by a constant multiple (see Appendix A), this is only a trivial modification of the idea.

As an illustration of the use of log likelihood in genetics, we continue the example introduced in Exercises 2.4 and 2.5. Table 3.1 shows some hypothetical data which might have formed part of that collected in a study of an association between disease risk and presence of a certain HLA haplotype. If we were to observe a set of families over time, in order to relate the genotype to the eventual occurrence or non-occurrence of disease, then we could calculate a likelihood based on the probability of disease conditional upon genotype. However, such studies are logistically very difficult and are rarely done. Instead it is more usual to obtain, usually from clinicians, a collection of known cases of disease (*probands*) and their relatives, and to compare the genotypes of probands with the predictions from the model.

As in Exercise 2.5, we shall consider the model in which presence of a given haplotype, (a) say, leads to a risk of disease θ times as high as in its absence. Table 3.1 shows data concerning 7 probands and their parents. For each of the genetic configurations shown in the table, we derived the conditional probability of the genotype of a proband conditional on the genotypes of parents in Exercise 2.5 and we showed that these probabilities depend only on the risk ratio parameter θ.

Exercise 3.4. Write down the expression for the log likelihood as a function of the unknown risk ratio, θ, associated with presence of haplotype (a). What is the log likelihood ratio for the value $\theta = 1$ (corresponding to there being no increase in risk) as compared with $\theta = 6.0$ (which is the most likely value of θ in this case). Is the value $\theta = 1$ supported?

Solutions to the exercises

3.1   The probability of the observed data when $\pi = 0.4$ is

$$0.4^4 \times 0.6^6 = 1.19 \times 10^{-3}.$$

which is more than the probability when $\pi = 0.5$. It follows that $\pi = 0.4$ is more likely than $\pi = 0.5$.

3.2   The log likelihood when $\pi = 0.5$ is

$$4\log(0.5) + 6\log(0.5) = -6.93.$$

The log likelihood when $\pi = 0.1$ is

$$4\log(0.1) + 6\log(0.9) = -9.84.$$

3.3   The maximum log likelihood, occurring at $\pi = 0.4$, is

$$4\log(0.4) + 6\log(0.6) = -6.73$$

so that the log likelihood ratio for $\pi = 0.5$ is $-6.93 - (-6.73) = -0.20$. For $\pi = 0.1$ it is $-9.84 - (-6.73) = -3.11$. Thus 0.5 lies within the supported range and 0.1 does not.

3.4   From the solution to Exercise 2.5, the conditional probabilities for each of the three genetic configurations are $\theta/(2\theta + 2)$, $1/(2\theta + 2)$, and $\theta/(\theta + 1)$. Thus, the log likelihood is

$$4\log\left(\frac{\theta}{2\theta + 2}\right) + 1\log\left(\frac{1}{2\theta + 2}\right) + 2\log\left(\frac{\theta}{\theta + 1}\right).$$

At $\theta = 1.0$ this takes the value

$$4\log\left(\frac{1}{4}\right) + 1\log\left(\frac{1}{4}\right) + 2\log\left(\frac{1}{2}\right) = -8.318,$$

and at $\theta = 6.0$ (the most likely value) it is

$$4\log\left(\frac{6}{14}\right) + 1\log\left(\frac{1}{14}\right) + 2\log\left(\frac{6}{7}\right) = -6.337.$$

The log likelihood ratio for $\theta = 1$ is the difference between these, -1.981. Thus the parameter value $\theta = 1$ lies outside the limits of support we have suggested in this chapter.

4
Consecutive follow-up intervals

In the last chapter we touched on the difficulty of estimating the probability of failure during a fixed follow-up period when the observation times for some subjects are censored. A second problem with fixed follow-up periods is that it may be difficult to compare the results from different studies; a five-year probability of failure can only be compared with other five-year probabilities of failure, and so on. Finally, by ignoring *when* the failures took place, all information about possible changes in the probability of failure during follow-up is lost.

The way round these difficulties is to break down the total follow-up period into a number of shorter consecutive intervals of time. We shall refer to these intervals of time as *bands*. The experience of the cohort during each of these bands can then be used to build up the experience over any desired period of time. This is known as the *life table* or *actuarial* method. Instead of a single binary probability model there is now a sequence of binary models, one for each band. This sequence can be represented by a conditional probability tree.

4.1 A sequence of binary models

Consider an example in which a three-year follow-up interval has been divided into three one-year bands. The experience of a subject during the three years may now be described by a sequence of binary probability models, one for each year, as shown by the probability tree in Fig.4.1. The four possible outcomes for this subject, corresponding to the tips of the tree, are

1. failure during the first year;
2. failure during the second year;
3. failure during the third year;
4. survival for the full three-year period.

The parameter of the first binary model in the sequence is π^1, the probability of failure during the first year; the parameter of the second binary model is π^2, the probability of failure during the second year, given the subject has not failed before the start of this year, and so on. These are

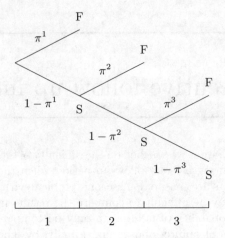

Fig. 4.1. A sequence of binary probability models.

all conditional probabilities — conditional on not having failed before the start of the year in question. The reason the probabilities are written with superscripts is that we have adopted the convention that a superscript is used to index *time*, and a subscript is used to index subjects or groups of subjects. It is important to distinguish these two situations, and using subscripts for both can be confusing.[*]

Suppose, for illustration, that the probability of failure is 0.3 in the first year; 0.2 in the second year, given the subject survives the first year without failure; and 0.1 in the third year, given the subject survives the first two years without failure. These illustrative values for the three conditional probabilities are shown on the conditional probability tree in Fig.4.2.

In this tree, the four final outcomes listed above correspond to the tips of the tree, and their probabilities can be calculated by multiplying conditional probabilities along the branches of the tree in the usual way. For example, the probability of the second outcome is made up from the probability that the subject survives the first year (0.7), multiplied by the probability that the subject fails during the second year (0.2). Using this rule, the four possible outcomes for any subject occur with probabilities:

$$0.3$$
$$0.7 \times 0.2$$
$$0.7 \times 0.8 \times 0.1$$
$$0.7 \times 0.8 \times 0.9$$

---

[*]Note that π^2 does not refer to $\pi \times \pi$. To avoid confusion we shall always use brackets when taking powers; for example, the square of π will be written $(\pi)^2$.

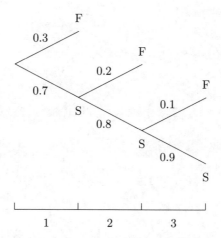

Fig. 4.2. Illustrative values for the conditional probabilities.

These probabilities work out to be 0.3, 0.14, 0.056, and 0.504, and these add to 1, as they should, since there are no other possible outcomes. The probability of failing at *some* stage is

$$0.3 + 0.14 + 0.056 = 0.496.$$

More conveniently this probability can be found by subtracting from 1 the probability of surviving the three years without failing, giving

$$1 - 0.504 = 0.496.$$

The probabilities of surviving one, two, and three years without failing are called the *cumulative survival probabilities* for the cohort. They are calculated by multiplying the conditional probabilities of surviving each year, and in this case are:

$$0.7$$
$$0.7 \times 0.8$$
$$0.7 \times 0.8 \times 0.9.$$

which work out to be 0.7, 0.56, and 0.504.

Exercise 4.1. In a three-year follow-up study the conditional probabilities of failure during the first, second, and third years are 0.05, 0.09, and 0.12 respectively. Draw a probability tree for the possible outcomes for a new subject, and label the branches of the tree with the appropriate conditional probabilities. Calculate the probability of each of the outcomes, and the probabilities of surviving

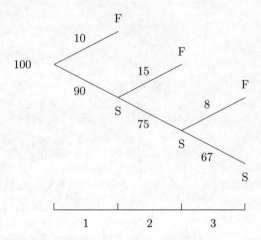

Fig. 4.3.   Survival of 100 subjects through three time bands.

one, two, and three years without failing. Calculate also the probability of failing at some time during the three-year follow-up.

4.2   Estimating the conditional probabilities of failure

Suppose that 100 subjects join the cohort at the start of the three-year interval and that 10 fail during the first year, 15 during the second, and 8 during the third, leaving 67 who survive until the end of three years (see Fig.4.3). Assuming the same conditional probabilities of failure for each of the 100 subjects, these data can be used to estimate their most likely values.

Intuitively it seems sensible to use the experience of those subjects who are observed in each year to estimate the conditional probability of failure during that year. The most likely values of the three conditional probabilities would then be

$$\frac{10}{100}, \frac{15}{90}, \frac{8}{75},$$

but is this a legitimate thing to do? It corresponds to regarding the three-year follow-up study as equivalent to three separate and independent one-year follow-up studies in which the subjects come from the survivors of the previous year. In fact this is a legitimate thing to do because the likelihood for π^1, π^2, and π^3 is the same whether the data are regarded as coming from one three-year study or from three one-year studies. This may be shown algebraically as follows.

The probabilities of the four possible outcomes in the three-year study are

$$\pi^1$$
$$(1 - \pi^1)\pi^2$$
$$(1 - \pi^1)(1 - \pi^2)\pi^3$$
$$(1 - \pi^1)(1 - \pi^2)(1 - \pi^3)$$

A subject who fails during the first year therefore contributes

$$\log(\pi^1)$$

to the log likelihood. A subject who fails during the second year contributes

$$\log(1 - \pi^1) + \log(\pi^2),$$

a subject who fails during the third year contributes

$$\log(1 - \pi^1) + \log(1 - \pi^2) + \log(\pi^3),$$

and a subject who survives all three years contributes

$$\log(1 - \pi^1) + \log(1 - \pi^2) + \log(1 - \pi^3).$$

Multiplying these by the numbers of subjects with each outcome, that is 10, 15, 8, and 67 respectively, and adding, gives a total log likelihood of

$$10 \log(\pi^1) + 90 \log(1 - \pi^1)$$
$$+15 \log(\pi^2) + 75 \log(1 - \pi^2)$$
$$+8 \log(\pi^3) + 67 \log(1 - \pi^3).$$

This is the same as the log likelihood obtained by regarding the data as from three separate and independent one-year studies; the first based on 10 failures and 90 survivors, the second on 15 failures and 75 survivors, and the third on 8 failures and 67 survivors.

Exercise 4.2. If we were to adopt the more restrictive model that π^1, π^2, π^3 are all equal with common value π, what would be the most likely value of π?

This exercise makes it clear that, in the analysis of such studies, the basic atom of data is not the subject, but the observation of one subject through one time band.

4.3   A cohort life table

In cohorts where subjects are examined at yearly intervals, the data are often presented in the form of numbers of failures and censorings occurring each year. An example is given in Table 4.1, which refers to survival of a

Table 4.1. Survival by stage at diagnosis

	Stage I			Stage II		
Year	N	D	L	N	D	L
1	110	5	5	234	24	3
2	100	7	7	207	27	11
3	86	7	7	169	31	9
4	72	3	8	129	17	7
5	61	0	7	105	7	13
6	54	2	10	85	6	6
7	42	3	6	73	5	6
8	33	0	5	62	3	10
9	28	0	4	49	2	13
10	24	1	8	34	4	6

group of women with cancer of the cervix diagnosed at either stage I or stage II. The women are examined annually, and censoring occurs if they cease attending the clinic; N is the number alive and still under observation at the start of each time band, D is the number who die during each band, and L is the number censored during each band.

The estimation of survival experience of the stage I women over the first four years is shown in Fig.4.4. Of the 110 subjects who started the first year, 5 die and 5 are censored. The effective size of the cohort in the first year is taken to be 107.5 and the probability of a subject dying during the first year, given the subject was alive at the start of the year, is estimated to be $5/107.5 = 0.0465$. The conditional probability of surviving the year is estimated to be

$$1 - 0.0465 = 0.9535.$$

The calculations of failure and survival probabilities are shown in Fig.4.4. The cumulative survival probabilities are found by multiplying the conditional survival probabilities for each year. For example, the cumulative probability of surviving 3 years is

$$0.9535 \times 0.9275 \times 0.9152 = 0.8093.$$

Exercise 4.3. Using Table 4.1, draw a tree showing the survival experience for stage II women over the first four years, and calculate the conditional survival probabilities for each of these years.

A table of cumulative survival probabilities by year is called a *life table*, and a plot of the cumulative survival probabilities against years survived is called a *survival curve*. The survival curves for both stage I and stage II

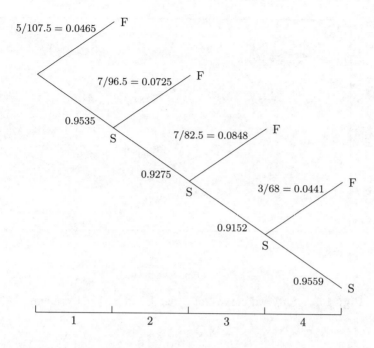

Fig. 4.4. Estimated conditional probabilities for stage 1 women.

women are shown in Fig.4.5. It is conventional to start survival curves at a probability of one for surviving at least zero years. These plots are useful for studying whether the probability of failure is changing with follow-up time, and for calculating survival probabilities for different periods of time.

Exercise 4.4. Use Fig.4.5 to read off the five-year survival probabilities in each of the two groups.

4.4   The use of exact times of failure and censoring

In the calculations described above, the conditional probability of failure during each time band has been estimated by assuming, as in Chapter 3, that half the losses during the band occurred at the start and half at the end. If the individual times at which failure (or censoring) occur are known then it is possible to avoid this assumptions by choosing the bands so short that each failure occupies a band by itself. Such a choice of bands is shown in Fig.4.6 for the early follow-up experience of 50 subjects. The horizontal line represents follow-up time, failures are marked as ●, and losses as ×. The bands are shown by vertical bars. Only the first few events are shown.

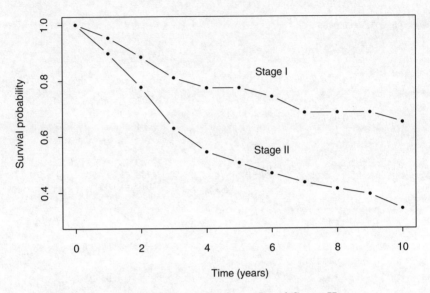

Fig. 4.5.   Survival curves for Stage I and Stage II women.

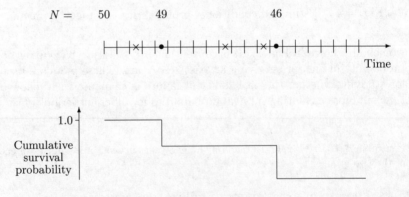

Fig. 4.6.   Early follow-up experience of 50 subjects.

For bands in which there are no failures the estimated survival probability
is 1. For bands which contain a failure the estimated survival probability
is $1 - 1/N$ where N is the number at risk just before the failure. Thus for
the band which contains the first failure $N = 49$ and the estimated survival
probability is $1 - 1/49 = 48/49$. The estimate of the cumulative survival
probability up to the end of this band is

$$1 \times 1 \times \cdots \times 48/49 = 0.9796.$$

For the band which contains the second failure $N = 46$, so the estimated survival probability for this band is $1-1/46 = 45/46$. The cumulative probability of survival up to the end of the fourth band is therefore estimated at

$$1 \times \cdots \times 48/49 \times 1 \times \cdots \times 45/46 = 0.9583.$$

These calculations continue until there are no more bands which contain failures.

The bands containing each failure can be made so short that they refer to the actual time of failure. When this is done the cumulative survival probability over time takes the value 1 until the first failure, when it drops to 0.9796; then it stays at 0.9796 until the second failure when it drops to 0.9583, and so on. The plot of cumulative survival probability versus time survived takes the stepped shape shown in Fig.4.6, where the steps occur at the failure times.

This method of estimating the cumulative survival probabilities is called the *Kaplan–Meier* method, after the authors of the paper which showed that this procedure yields the most likely value of the survival curve. It is widely used in clinical follow-up studies for which individual failure times are known. If the failure times are measured exactly the failures will all occur at separate times, but if they are measured to the nearest month (for example) then there may be several failures at the same time. In this case the probability of failure is estimated by dividing the number of failures at that failure time by the total number of subjects at risk just before the failure time. If losses also occur at this time then, by convention, they are included in the number at risk.

4.5   An example of the Kaplan–Meier method

Table 4.2 shows the time from diagnosis to death from melanoma, or loss to follow-up, for 50 subjects. Times are in complete months so that subjects dying during the first month are recorded as surviving one month, and so on. For two subjects diagnosis took place at death, so the time was recorded as zero.

Note that probabilities of failure are estimated only for times at which failures occurred. The first of these is at time zero; the number at risk is 50, with 2 failures, so the probability of failure at this time point is $2/50 = 0.04$, and the survival probability is $1 - 0.04 = 0.96$. The next time at which a failure occurs is one month; the number at risk is 48, with one failure, so the probability of failure at this time point is $1/48 = 0.0208$ and the probability of surviving is $1-0.0208 = 0.9792$. The next time at which a failure occurs is at 2 months, when there are two failures. The probability of failure is $2/47 = 0.0426$, and the survival probability is $1-0.0426 = 0.9574$. At three months there is one failure and one loss to follow-up. In fact this loss was a death from a cause other than melanoma, but when estimating survival

Table 4.2. Cumulative survival probabilities from the Kaplan–Meier method. Non-melanoma deaths (*) are counted as losses.

Month	N	D	L	Conditional probability of death	of survival	Cumulative prob. of survival
0	50	2		0.0400	0.9600	0.9600
1	48	1		0.0208	0.9792	0.9400
2	47	2		0.0426	0.9574	0.9000
3	45	1	1*	0.0222	0.9778	0.8800
8	43	1		0.0233	0.9767	0.8595
10	42	1		0.0238	0.9762	0.8391
12	41	1	1*	0.0244	0.9756	0.8186
13	39	1		0.0256	0.9744	0.7976
15	38	1		0.0263	0.9737	0.7766
18	37		1*			
19	36	1		0.0278	0.9722	0.7551
21	35		1			
27	34		2			
30	32		1			
33	31	1	1	0.0323	0.9677	0.7307
34	29	1		0.0345	0.9655	0.7055
38	28		1			
40	27		1			
41	26	1		0.0385	0.9615	0.6784
43	25		1			
44	24		1			
46	23		1			
54	22		1			
55	21	1		0.0476	0.9524	0.6461
56	20	1		0.0500	0.9500	0.6138
57	19		2			
60	17		1*			

probabilities from melanoma alone it is counted as a loss to follow-up. (We return to a fuller discussion of this point in Chapter 7.) The number at risk was 45, with one failure, so the probability of failure is $1/45 = 0.022$ and the probability of survival is $1 - 0.022 = 0.9778$, and so on. A plot of the cumulative survival probability against time is shown in Fig.4.7.

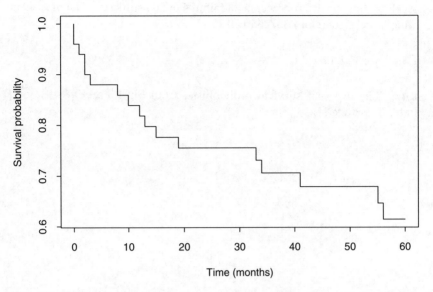

Fig. 4.7. Cumulative survival probability by the Kaplan–Meier method.

Solutions to the exercises

4.1 See Fig.4.8. The probabilities of failure during the first, second and third years are

$$0.05 \quad 0.95 \times 0.09 = 0.0855 \quad 0.95 \times 0.91 \times 0.12 = 0.1037.$$

The probability of surviving three years is

$$0.95 \times 0.91 \times 0.88 = 0.7608.$$

The survival probabilities for the three years are

$$0.95 \quad 0.8645 \quad 0.7608.$$

The probability of failure at some time during the three years is

$$0.05 + 0.0855 + 0.1037 = 0.2392$$

or

$$1 - 0.7608 = 0.2392.$$

4.2 The overall log likelihood is

$$33 \log(\pi) + 232 \log(1 - \pi),$$

which is equivalent to observing 33 failures in 265 subjects. The most likely value of π is, therefore $33/265 = 0.125$.

4.3   See Fig.4.9.

4.4   The five year survival probabilities from Fig.4.5 are 0.78 (Stage I) and 0.51 (Stage II).

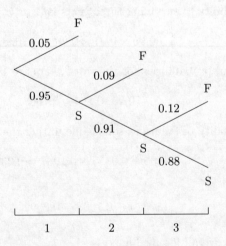

Fig. 4.8.   Solution to exercise 4.1.

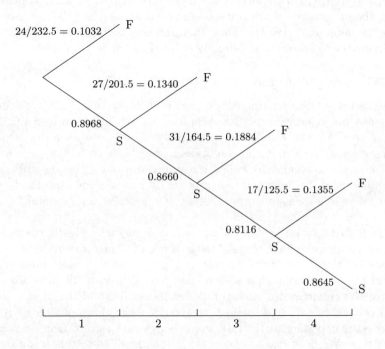

Fig. 4.9. Estimated conditional probabilities for stage II women.

5
Rates

We have shown how, by splitting the follow-up period into small enough bands, the importance of arbitrary assumptions about when the losses occur can be minimized. We now follow this argument to its logical conclusion and divide the follow-up into infinitely small time bands.

5.1 The probability rate

As the bands get shorter, the conditional probability that a subject fails during any one band gets smaller. When a band shrinks towards a single moment of time, the conditional probability of failure during the band shrinks towards zero, but the conditional probability of failure *per unit time* converges to a quantity called the *probability rate*. This quantity is sometimes called the *instantaneous* probability rate to emphasize the fact that it refers to a moment in time. Other names are *hazard* rate and *force of mortality*.

The probability rate refers to an *individual subject*. This is counter-intuitive to many epidemiologists, who think of a rate as an empirical summary of the frequency of failures in a group observed over time. We show in the next section that such a summary is, in fact, the most likely value of the common probability rate for the subjects in the group. It is general practice in epidemiology to refer to both the probability rate and its estimated value as the rate, even though this leads to many logical absurdities. We have tried to keep as close as possible to this tradition, while avoiding the logical contradictions, by referring to the probability rate as the rate parameter and its estimated value as the observed rate.

5.2 Estimating the rate parameter

Even though the rate parameter refers to a single individual it is not possible to estimate its value from the experience of that individual. The estimate must be based on the experience of a group of subjects assumed to have the same rate. Similarly, even though the rate parameter refers to a single moment of time, its estimated value is usually based on a period of follow-up over which the rate is assumed to be constant. The estimated rate for this period then refers to the constant value which the rate parameter

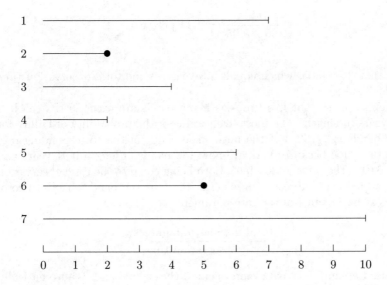

Fig. 5.1.   The follow-up experience of 7 subjects.

takes at all time points during the period.

The rate parameter over a follow-up period is estimated by dividing the period into a number of small time bands of equal length and estimating the *common* probability of failure for each of the bands. This is divided by the length of a band to get the rate per unit time. The process is illustrated using the follow-up experience of 7 subjects shown in Fig. 5.1, in which the follow-up experience of the subjects is shown as lines which end when follow-up ends. The lines for those subjects who fail end with a •, while those whose observation time is censored end with a short bar. The follow-up period has been divided into 10 short bands and for the present we shall assume that follow-up always stops at the end of a short band. From the figure we see that the follow-up of subject 1 stops after 7 bands due to censoring. For subject 6 the follow-up stops after 5 bands when the subject fails, and so on.

Exercise 5.1. How many observations of one subject through one time band are observed? How many of these ended in failure?

Assuming that the rate parameter is constant over the follow-up period, the conditional probability of failure is the same for all bands and its most likely value is 2/36. The most likely value of the corresponding rate parameter is 2/36 divided by the length of the bands. Suppose for illustration that each band has length 0.05 years. The most likely value of the rate parameter is then

$$\frac{2}{(36 \times 0.05)} = 1.11 \text{ per year.}$$

Note that 36×0.05, which equals 1.8 years, is the total observation time for the 7 subjects.

Now suppose that five times as many bands are used, so that each is 0.01 years in length. The most likely value of the probability of failure for these bands is 2/180, but the most likely value of the corresponding rate stays the same because there are now 180 bands of length 0.01 years and 180×0.01 is the same as 36×0.05, both being equal to the total observation time, added over subjects. In general, then, as the bands shrink to zero, the most likely value of the rate parameter is

$$\frac{\text{Total number of failures}}{\text{Total observation time}}.$$

Note that assumption that events occur at the end of bands is automatically true when the bands shrink to zero. This mathematical device of dividing the time scale into shorter and shorter bands is used frequently in this book, and we have found it useful to introduce the term *clicks* to describe these very short time bands.

Time can be measured in any convenient units, so that a rate of 1.11 per year is the same as a rate of 11.1 per 10 years, and so on. The total observation time added over subjects is known in epidemiology as the *person-time* of observation and is most commonly expressed as person-years. Because of the way they are calculated, estimates of rates are often given the units *per person-year* or *per 1000 person-years*.

The use of the general formula for the estimated value of a rate is now illustrated using data from a computer simulation of 30 subjects who are liable to only one disease (the failure) and the follow-up is indefinitely long, so that eventually all subjects develop the disease. The only variable in the outcome is how long it takes for the disease to develop, and these times are shown in Table 5.1.

Exercise 5.2. Using the time interval from the start of the study to the moment when the last subject develops the disease, find the total observation time for the 30 subjects and hence estimate the rate for this interval. Give your answer per 10^3 person-years as well.

Exercise 5.3. The previous exercise is rather unrealistic. Real follow-up studies are of limited duration and not all of the subjects will fail during the study period. Estimate the rate from a study in which the same subjects are observed only for the first five years.

Table 5.1.   Time until the disease develops, for 30 subjects

Subject	Years	Subject	Years
1	19.6	16	0.6
2	10.8	17	2.1
3	14.1	18	0.8
4	3.5	19	8.9
5	4.8	20	11.6
6	4.6	21	1.3
7	12.2	22	3.4
8	14.0	23	15.3
9	3.8	24	8.5
10	12.6	25	21.5
11	12.8	26	8.3
12	12.1	27	0.4
13	4.7	28	36.5
14	3.2	29	1.1
15	7.3	30	1.5

5.3   The likelihood for a rate

The argument of the last section, although leading to the most likely value of the rate parameter, does not allow us to explore the support for other values. In this section we shall obtain a formula for the likelihood for a rate parameter.

Consider a more general example in which D failures are observed for a total of N clicks of time, each of duration h years, where h is very small and N is very large. The total observation time in years is $Y = Nh$. Let π be the conditional probability of failure during a click. Then the likelihood for π is

$$(\pi)^D (1 - \pi)^{N-D}.$$

Let the corresponding rate parameter be λ, where, because h is small,

$$\lambda = \pi/h.$$

The likelihood for λ follows by replacing π by λh, and is

$$(\lambda h)^D (1 - \lambda h)^{N-D}.$$

The log likelihood for λ is therefore

$$D \log(\lambda) + D \log(h) + (N - D) \log(1 - \lambda h).$$

To see what happens when time is truly continuous, consider the behaviour of this expression as the click duration, h, becomes progressively
shorter. Since the total observation time Y remains unchanged it follows
that the number of clicks, N, must become progressively larger. As h becomes smaller and N becomes larger, eventually $N - D$ becomes nearly the
same as N, and λh becomes so small that

$$\log(1 - \lambda h) \approx -\lambda h.$$

(This property of the logarithmic function is discussed in Appendix A.)
Making these substitutions, the log likelihood becomes

$$D \log(\lambda) + D \log(h) - N \lambda h.$$

The term $D \log(h)$ does not depend on λ and is irrelevant since it cancels
out in log likelihood ratios. Omitting this term and noting that Nh is the
total observation time, Y, we obtain the following simplified expression for
the log likelihood:

$$D \log(\lambda) - \lambda Y.$$

The corresponding likelihood,

$$(\lambda)^D \exp(-\lambda Y),$$

is called the *Poisson likelihood* after the French mathematician. As we
would expect from the previous section it takes its maximum value when
$\lambda = D/Y$.

To illustrate the use of this likelihood, suppose 7 cases are observed and
the total observation time is 500 person-years. Then the log likelihood for
λ is

$$7 \log(\lambda) - 500\lambda.$$

A graph of the log likelihood ratio versus λ is shown in Fig. 5.2. The
maximum value of the log likelihood occurs at

$$\lambda = 7/500 = 0.014 \text{ per person-year.}$$

The supported range for λ may be found from the graph by reading off the
values of λ at which the log likelihood ratio has reduced to -1.353. In this
case the graph shows that the supported range for λ is from 7.0×10^{-3} to
24.6×10^{-3} per person-year.

Exercise 5.4. Calculate the value of the log likelihood at $\lambda = 0.01$, $\lambda = 0.014$,
and $\lambda = 0.02$. Using the fact that the log likelihood is at its maximum when
$\lambda = 0.014$ calculate the log likelihood ratio for $\lambda = 0.01$ and $\lambda = 0.02$.

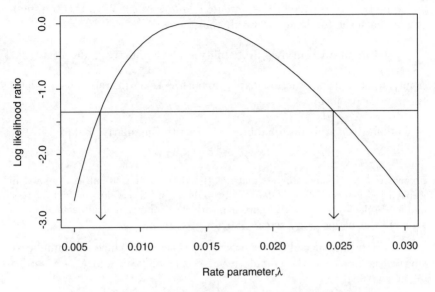

Fig. 5.2.   Log likelihood ratio for λ.

If we wish to estimate the rate over a restricted period of observation the argument requires only trivial modification; only the person-clicks falling in the period of interest contribute information so that D and Y refer to the number of events and the observation time which occur within the period.

5.4   Cumulative survival probability in terms of the rate

Suppose a subject experiences a constant rate λ with no possibility of loss during the follow-up. The cumulative probability that he or she will survive a given period of time, T, may be found from λ by dividing the period into N clicks, each of length h, so that $T = Nh$. The conditional probability of failure at each click is λh, so that the probability of surviving N such clicks is

$$(1 - \lambda h)^{N}.$$

The log of this cumulative survival probability is

$$N \log(1 - \lambda h)$$

and since $\log(1 - \lambda h)$ may be replaced by $-\lambda h$ when h is small this becomes

$$-\lambda Nh = -\lambda T.$$

The quantity λT is called the *cumulative failure rate*. With this terminology we have the fundamental result that

$$\log(\text{Cumulative survival probability}) = -\text{Cumulative failure rate}$$

Applying the antilog function, exp(), to both sides of this relationship yields the alternative form:

$$
\begin{aligned}
\text{Cumulative survival probability} \quad &= \quad \exp(-\text{Cumulative failure rate}) \\
&= \quad \exp(-\lambda T).
\end{aligned}
$$

Exercise 5.5. Using your estimate of the rate for the 30 subjects shown in Table 5.1 (Exercise 5.2), calculate the probability of survival for the first 5 years, and hence the 5-year risk. Compare this with the proportion of subjects observed to fail in this period (see Exercise 5.3).

An important special case concerns *rare events*, in which the cumulative survival is large and the cumulative risk is small. Since $\log(1 - x) \approx -x$ when x is small,

$$
\begin{aligned}
\log(\text{Cumulative survival probability}) \quad &= \quad \log(1 - \text{Cumulative risk}) \\
&\approx \quad -\text{Cumulative risk},
\end{aligned}
$$

so the cumulative risk and the cumulative failure rate are approximately equal for rare events.

5.5   Rates that vary with time

We have assumed that the rate parameter is constant over the follow-up period and this may be unrealistic over an extended follow-up. However, provided the rate parameter is not changing too quickly, the follow-up period can be divided into broad bands during which the rate can be assumed to be constant. This implies abrupt changes in the rate parameter from one band to the next, but even such a crude model proves useful in practice provided the changes are not too large.

Consider the first band and let D^1 be the number of failures Y^1 the total observation time and λ^1 the rate parameter. The log likelihood for λ^1 is

$$D^1 \log(\lambda^1) - \lambda^1 Y^1$$

and similarly for further bands. Thus once failures and total observation time have been partitioned between the time bands estimation of band-specific rates proceeds as before.

Exercise 5.6. Fig. 5.3 illustrates observation of three subjects across three time bands, showing the observation time (years) for each subject in each band. What are the estimated failure rates for each of the bands?

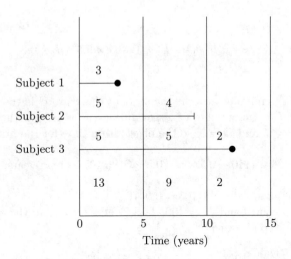

Fig. 5.3. Survival of three subjects across three time bands.

The relationship between the cumulative survival probability over several bands and the band-specific rates is also a simple generalization of our earlier result. For a time interval which has been divided into three bands of length T^1, T^2, and T^3, during which the rates are λ^1, λ^2, and λ^3, the log survival probabilities for each band are $-\lambda^1 T^1$, $-\lambda^2 T^2$, and $-\lambda^3 T^3$ respectively. The log of the cumulative survival probability over all three bands is therefore the sum of these, namely

$$-\lambda^1 T^1 - \lambda^2 T^2 - \lambda^3 T^3 = -(\lambda^1 T^1 + \lambda^2 T^2 + \lambda^3 T^3).$$

The quantity $(\lambda^1 T^1 + \lambda^2 T^2 + \lambda^3 T^3)$ is the cumulative failure rate over the whole interval. It follows that the relationship

$$\log(\text{Cumulative survival probability}) = -\text{Cumulative failure rate}$$

still holds when the rate varies from one band to the next.

The use of this relationship to calculate survival probabilities will be demonstrated using the data for the survival of women diagnosed with stage I cancer of the cervix, shown in Chapter 4. The time bands are one year in length and we shall assume that the rate is constant within a time band, but can vary between time bands. Since exact times of failure and loss are not given we shall assume that, on average, each failure contributes 0.5 years to the observation time in the band in which the failure takes place, and similarly for losses. The total observation time during any particular year of follow-up is then approximately

$$Y \approx (N - D - L) \times 1 + D \times 0.5 + L \times 0.5$$
$$= N - 0.5D - 0.5L,$$

where N is the number alive at the start of the year, D is the number of deaths, and L is the number of losses during the year. For the first band $N = 110$, $L = 5$, and $D = 5$, so the observation time for the first year is

$$Y^1 \approx (110 - 0.5 \times 5 - 0.5 \times 5) = 105 \text{ woman-years}$$

and the estimated rate is $5/105 = 0.0476$.

For the second band $N = 100$, $L = 7$, and $D = 7$, so the observation time for the second year is

$$Y^2 \approx (100 - 0.5 \times 7 - 0.5 \times 7) = 93 \text{ woman-years}$$

and the estimated rate is $7/93 = 0.0753$.

Exercise 5.7. Estimate the failure rate for stage I subjects during the third year.

The estimated cumulative failure rates for each year of the follow-up are shown in Table 5.2. The column headed 'cumulative survival probability' is obtained using the relationship

Cumulative survival probability = exp(−Cumulative failure rate).

A life table constructed in this way is sometimes referred to as a *modified life table*.

Exercise 5.8. Calculate the cumulative rate over the last five years only, and hence the probability that a woman survives for ten years *given* that she has survived the first five.

★ 5.6   Rates varying continuously in time

The assumption that the rate parameter is constant over broad bands of time, but changes abruptly from one band to the next, is widely used, but an alternative model, useful when exact times of failure and censoring are known, is to allow the rate parameter to vary from click to click. In Chapter 4 this kind of model led to the Kaplan–Meier estimate of the survival curve; when using rates it leads to the estimate known as the *Aalen–Nelson* estimate.

Fig. 5.4 shows the data that were used to describe the Kaplan–Meier estimate in Chapter 4, but the stepped graph now refers to the cumulative

Table 5.2. Modified life table for stage I women

Year	Rate	Cumulative rate	Cumulative survival probability
1	0.0476	0.0476	0.9535
2	0.0753	0.1229	0.8844
3	0.0886	0.2115	0.8094
4	0.0451	0.2566	0.7737
5	0.0000	0.2566	0.7737
6	0.0417	0.2983	0.7421
7	0.0800	0.3783	0.6850
8	0.0000	0.3783	0.6850
9	0.0000	0.3783	0.6850
10	0.0513	0.4296	0.6508

Number: 50   49   46

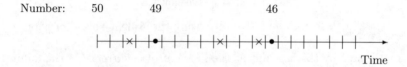

Time

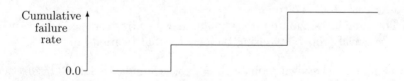

Cumulative failure rate

0.0

Fig. 5.4. Early follow-up of 50 subjects: the Aalen–Nelson estimate.

failure rate, not the cumulative survival probability. During the first of these clicks the estimated rate is $0/(50h)$. Similarly for all clicks which contain no failure the estimated rate is zero, so there is no addition to the cumulative rate at any of these points in time. The cumulative rate graph therefore remains horizontal during these clicks. For a click which contains a failure the rate is $1/(Nh)$, where N is the number in the study just before the click. Because this rate operates for a click of length h, the estimate of the cumulative rate increases by

$$\frac{1}{Nh} \times h = \frac{1}{N}.$$

Because the click can be thought of as being instantaneous, the cumulative

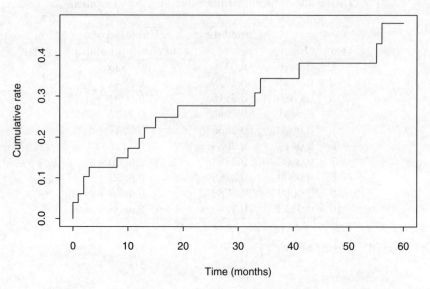

Fig. 5.5.   Cumulative rate using the Aalen–Nelson method.

rate jumps by this amount at the moment of occurrence of the failure. In our example, the first jump is of size $1/49$; the cumulative rate stays at this value until the click which contains the second failure when it jumps by a further $1/46$, and so on.

The cumulative failure rate estimate may also be expressed as a cumulative survival probability, using the now familiar relationship

Cumulative survival probability = exp(−Cumulative failure rate).

When this is done, the Aalen–Nelson estimate of the relationship of the cumulative survival probability with time looks very similar to the Kaplan–Meier estimate. Both have a stepped shape with steps at the times when failures occur. For most of the follow-up period, the two estimates are very close because of the approximate relationships,

$$\log(1 - 1/N) \approx -1/N$$
$$\exp(-1/N) \approx 1 - 1/N$$

for large N. At the end of the interval N is sometimes small and the two estimates may differ somewhat.

For reasons to be discussed in Chapter 7, it may be best to plot the cumulative failure rate and not the survival probability, even though the former is a little harder to interpret. One fairly clear message from the plot of cumulative failure rate is how the failure rate varies with time. If the failure rate is constant then the cumulative rate will rise linearly with time; if the rate is increasing the cumulative rate will rise non-linearly, showing an increase in gradient with time; if the rate decreases with time the cumulative rate will still rise, but now it will show a decrease in gradient with time.

The Aalen–Nelson plot of the cumulative rate for the melanoma data, introduced in Chapter 4, is shown in Fig. 5.5. This plot shows that the rate is higher during the first 20 months than during the period from 20 to 60 months.

Exercise 5.9. Use the plot in Fig. 5.5 to obtain a rough estimate of the rate during the first 20 months and during the period from 20 to 60 months

Solutions to the exercises

5.1   The total number of subjects observed through one band is

$$7 + 2 + 4 + 2 + 6 + 5 + 10 = 36,$$

and 2 of these end in failure.

5.2   The total observation time for the 30 subjects is $140.1 + 121.8 = 261.9$ years. The rate is $30/261.9 = 0.1145$ per year, or 114.5 per 10^3 person-years.

5.3   The total observation time is now

$$5 + 5 + 5 + 3.5 + 4.8 + 4.6 + 5 + \ldots + 1.5 = 115.8 \text{ years.}$$

The total number of failures is 14 so the rate is $14/115.8 = 0.1209$ per year, or 120.9 per 10^3 person-years.

5.4   The log likelihood at $\lambda = 0.01$ is

$$7 \log(0.01) - 500 \times 0.01 = -37.236.$$

Similarly the log likelihoods at $\lambda = 0.014$ and $\lambda = 0.02$ are -36.881 and -37.384. The log likelihood ratio at $\lambda = 0.01$ is

$$(-37.236) - (-36.881) = -0.3550.$$

Similarly the log likelihood ratio at $\lambda = 0.02$ is -0.5032.

5.5   When the rate is 0.1145 per year, the probability of surviving for 5 years is

$$\exp(-0.11452 \times 5) = 0.564$$

so that the mortality risk is 0.436. The proportion of subjects who failed in this period was, in fact, $14/30 = 0.467$.

5.6   The estimated failure rates for the three bands are $1/13$, $0/9$, and $1/2$ respectively.

5.7   The approximate person-years observation in year 3 is

$$Y^3 \approx 86 - 0.5 \times 7 - 0.5 \times 7 = 79$$

and the estimated rate is $7/79 = 0.0886$ per year.

5.8   The cumulative failure rate over the last five years is 0.173 so that the probability that a woman survives for 10 years given that she has survived the first 5 years is $\exp(-0.173) = 0.841$.

5.9   The gradient of the first part of the cumulative rate curve, from 0 to 20 months, is roughly $0.28/20 = 0.014$ per month, which is the rate over this period (assumed constant). For the second period, from 20 to 60, the gradient is roughly $(0.48 - 0.28)/(60 - 20) = 0.005$ per month, which is the rate over the second period (assumed constant).

6
Time

6.1 When do we start the clock?

In Chapter 5 we discussed the variation of rates with time. In that discussion, by assuming that all subjects entered the study at time zero, we implicitly interpreted time to mean time since entry into the study. However, there are many other ways of measuring time and some of these may be more relevant. For example, in epidemiology, it is usually important to consider the variation of rates with age, for which the origin is the date of birth, or with time since first exposure, for which the origin is the date of first exposure. Similarly, in clinical follow-up studies, time since diagnosis or start of treatment may be an important determinant of the failure rate. In different analyses, therefore, it may be relevant to start the clock at different points. Some possible choices for this starting point are described in Table 6.1.

6.2 Age-specific rates

Age is an extremely important variable in epidemiology, because the incidence and mortality rates of most diseases vary with age — often by several orders of magnitude. To ignore this variation runs the risk that comparisons between groups will be seriously distorted, or *confounded*, by differences in age structure.

The assumption that rates do not vary with age can be relaxed by dividing the age scale into bands and estimating a different *age-specific* rate in each band. If the follow-up period is short, so that the age of a

Table 6.1. Some time scales

Starting point	Time scale
Birth	Age
Any fixed date	Calendar time
First exposure	Time exposed
Entry into study	Time in study
Disease onset	Time since onset
Start of treatment	Time on treatment

Table 6.2.   Entry and exit dates for the cohort of four subjects

Subject	Born	Entry	Exit	Age at entry	Outcome
1	1904	1943	1952	39	Lost
2	1924	1948	1955	24	Failure
3	1914	1945	1961	31	Study ends
4	1920	1948	1956	28	Unrelated death

subject does not change appreciably during follow-up, age-specific rates can be estimated by classifying subjects into age *groups* by their age at entry. Each subject appears in only one age group and a separate rate is estimated for each group. For longer studies it will be necessary to take account of changing age during the study, and to treat age properly — as a time scale. This scale is then divided into *bands* and a separate estimate of the rate is made within each age band as described in Chapter 5. In this latter analysis, a subject can pass through several age bands during the course of the study.

To see how the failures and observation time are divided between age bands consider the cohort of four subjects, shown in Table 6.2. Subject 1 is lost to follow-up in 1952, subject 2 fails in 1955, subject 3 is still under observation when the study period ends, and subject 4 dies from an unrelated cause in 1956. The date when a subject joins the cohort is called the entry date and the date when observation stops, for whatever reason, is called the exit date. The time between the entry and exit dates is the observation time for the subject. To simplify the exercises, we give dates only as years and will assume that all events take place on the first day of the year. In practice, times would be worked out as accurately as the data allow.

Exercise 6.1. What are the observation times for the members of this cohort?

Figure 6.1 shows the observation of the subjects in calendar time, while Figure 6.2 shows it on a scale where time is measured from each subject's date of birth. To estimate a rate for a particular age band the failures are allocated to the bands in which they occurred, and the observation time is divided according to how long the subjects spend in each of the age bands. For example, the age band 30-34, which is from exact age 30 to just less than exact age 35, contains one failure and 10 person-years of observation time, so the estimated rate is 1/10 per person-year.

In this example the observation times in the different time bands have been obtained from the figure, but in practice the total observation time in an age band is obtained by using the dates when the subject changes age bands. For example, subject 1 is 39 years old on entry so he starts in the age band 35–39. He changes age band in 1944 (when he is 40), and again in 1949 (when he is 45), and he leaves the study in 1952 (when he

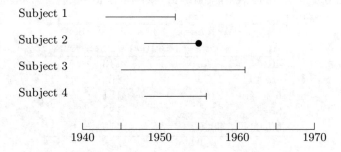

Fig. 6.1. Follow-up of four subjects by calendar time.

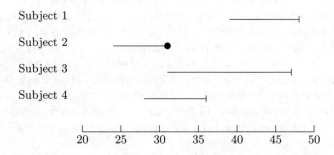

Fig. 6.2. Follow-up of four subjects by age.

emigrates). The observation time he spends in the different age bands is shown in Table 6.3.

As a check, the total observation time for subject 1 is from 1943 to 1952 which is 9 years, equal to the sum of the separate times spent in the different age bands.

Exercise 6.2. Subject 5 is born in 1931, joins the cohort in 1953, and is lost to follow-up in 1957. Divide the observation time for this subject between the five-year age bands shown in Figure 6.2.

Table 6.3. Time in each age band for subject 1

Age band	Date in	Date out	Time
35–39	1943	1944	1
40–44	1944	1949	5
45–49	1949	1952	3

Table 6.4. Woman-years and reference rates for a breast cancer study

Age	Woman-years	E & W rate per 100 000 woman-years
40–44	975	113
45–49	1079	162
50–54	2161	151
55–59	2793	183
60–64	3096	179

6.3   The expected number of failures

One reason for subdividing the total follow-up experience of a cohort into age bands is to determine whether the observed number of failures is more or less than we might have expected. Since mortality and incidence rates usually increase quite sharply with age, the distribution of person years observation between age bands is an extremely important determinant of the number of events we would expect to observe.

Table 6.4 shows the partition of woman-years between age bands for a cohort study of 974 women given a hormone treatment at menopause. During the follow-up period, 15 new cases of breast cancer occurred in the cohort. We might ask whether this is more or less than we would expect from national rates.

The third column of the table shows the age-specific incidence rates of breast cancer for England and Wales at the time the study was carried out. If the rates in the study population are the same as in the rest of England and Wales, the number of cases we would expect in each age band is simply the product of the woman-years observation and the rate. Thus, for the 40–44 age band, the expected number of cases is

$$975 \times \frac{113}{100\,000} = 1.10.$$

Exercise 6.3. Carry out these calculations for the remaining age groups and calculate the total expected number of cases of breast cancer.

This exercise shows that 16.77 cases are expected from national rates using the person years in the study. This expected number of cases is quite close to the observed 15, so that there is little suggestion that the rates in this cohort are unusual.

The expected number of cases, as calculated above, is not quite the same as the expected number in the usual statistical sense. The latter cannot depend upon the outcome of the study, but the former does, since the total person-time of observation in the study varies according to how many subjects fail and when. However, for the rare events studied by epidemiologists, this variation is small enough to be ignored.

6.4 Lexis diagrams

More than one time scale can be important in the same study. For example, mortality rates from cancer of the cervix depend upon age, as a result of the age-dependence of the incidence rate, and upon calendar time as a result of changes in treatment, population screening, and so on. The situation is further complicated by the strong dependence of the incidence of this disease upon sexual behaviour, which varies from one generation to the next.

The way to separate the effects of two time scales on a rate is to divide each scale into bands, usually of equal width, and to make a separate estimate of the rate for each pairing of bands. To see how this is done in practice it is best to show the subjects relative to the two scales simultaneously, in what is called a *Lexis diagram*.

The four subjects in Table 6.2 are shown relative to both age and calendar year simultaneously in the Lexis diagram in Figure 6.3. Each rectangular region in a Lexis diagram corresponds to a combination of two bands, one from each scale. To estimate rates for these combinations of bands the failures are allocated to the rectangles in which they occur and the observation time for each subject is divided between rectangles according to how long the subjects spends in each.

For example, subject 1 joins the cohort in 1943 aged 39. He changes age bands one year later in 1944 then 5 years later in 1949. He changes calendar periods in 1945 and 1950. Finally, observation stops in 1952. The subdivision of the observation time for this subject between different age and calendar period combinations is shown in Figure 6.4. Note that the times in the different bands add to 9 years, the total observation time for this subject. For each combination of age band and calendar period the rate is estimated by dividing the number of failures by the person-time of observation.

Exercise 6.4. Trace the progress of subject 1 through the squares in Figure 6.3 and verify the results given above. Divide the observation time for subject 2 between combinations of five-year bands of age and calendar time in the same way.

The same procedure can be used to separate the effect of age from the effect of time since entry, although there may not be enough data for some combinations of age and time since entry to estimate a rate. Figure 6.5 shows the four subjects in the cohort relative to age and time since entry. Five-year bands have again been chosen for both scales.

Exercise 6.5. Divide the observation time for subject 1 between different combinations of five-year bands of age and time since entry.

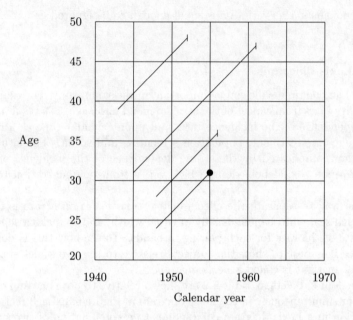

Fig. 6.3.   Lexis diagram showing age and calendar period.

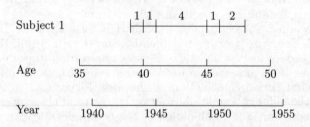

Fig. 6.4.   Follow-up of subject 1 by age and calendar time.

6.5   Reference rates by calendar period

Reference rates, used to calculate the expected numbers of failures, usually
come from national rates tabulated by age, sex, and calendar period. In the
UK these are calculated using an approximate figure for the person-years.
For example, the all-cause mortality rate for the age band 50–54 during
1983 is estimated by D/Y where D is the number of deaths during 1983
for which the subject's age at death was in the range 50–54, and Y is the
person-time lived during 1983 by that part of the population whose ages
were in the range 50–54 during 1983. Since the exact value of Y is not

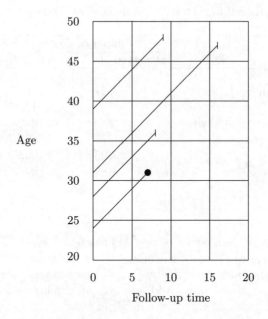

Fig. 6.5. Lexis diagram showing age and time since entry.

known an approximate value is obtained from

$$Y \approx \text{Population aged 50--54 in mid-1983} \times 1 \text{ year.}$$

For five-year calendar periods such as 1981–85,

$$Y \approx \text{Population aged 50--54 in mid-1983} \times 5 \text{ years.}$$

The population in the different age bands for any year is obtained from the census; directly for census years and indirectly for inter-census years by updating the last census by births, deaths, and migration.

Exercise 6.6. The total number of deaths from cancer of the lung in the SW region of England during the years 1981–88 were males: 14 751, females: 5420. The 1984 population of the region is estimated to be males: 2 154 900, females: 2 306 300. Calculate the mortality rate per 10^6 person-years for males and females separately.

When follow-up of a cohort takes place over an extended calendar period, the national age-specific rates will usually vary over this period, making it difficult to choose a single set of age-specific rates to use for comparison purposes. The solution is to compute the expected number of events by both age and calendar period, using the appropriate national rates for each calendar time period. To do this the person-years observation in the co-

Table 6.5.   Mortality following X-irradiation

Cause of	Number of deaths		Ratio
death	Observed, D	Expected, E	D/E
Cancers:			
Leukaemia	31	6.47	4.79
Colon	28	17.30	1.62
Heavily irradiated sites	259	167.50	1.55
Lightly irradiated sites	79	65.65	1.20
All neoplasms	397	256.92	1.55
Other causes	1362	804.68	1.69
All causes	1759	1061.61	1.66

hort study must be partitioned by age and calendar period. The expected number of failures can then be calculated for each combination of age and calendar period, as before, by multiplying the person-years observation by the appropriate national rate. Addition over all combinations of age and calendar period yields an expected number of cases which takes account of variation in national rates with both age and calendar time.

An example of this kind of calculation appears in Table 6.5, which shows some results taken from a study of cancer mortality in a cohort of ankylosing spondilitis patients who had been treated with a single course of X-irradiation of the spine.*   The follow-up of each patient started in the year of treatment (1935–1954) and continued until death, migration or 1970 (the date when this analysis was carried out). Follow-up was also terminated by a second course of treatment because the aim was to study the effect of a single course of X-rays and the time before this effect became apparent. The study was carried out in Great Britain and Northern Ireland, and the expected numbers of deaths calculated using the national rates for England and Wales, tabulated by five-year bands for both age and calendar time. It can be seen that mortality from all causes was higher in this cohort than in the reference population. Although accounting for relatively few excess deaths, the *ratio* of observed to expected deaths was particularly high for leukaemia. This ratio is an important index in epidemiology and is called the *standardized mortality ratio* (SMR). We shall discuss it further in Chapter 15.

Exercise 6.7.   Table 6.6 subdivides the observed and expected deaths from leukaemia according to time since X-ray treatment. How would this table have been calculated?

---

*From Smith, P.G. and Doll, R.(1982) *British Medical Journal*, **284**, 449–460.

Table 6.6. Leukaemia deaths by time since treatment

| | Time since treatment (years) | | | | | | | |
	0–2	3–5	6–8	9–11	12–14	15–17	18–20	>20
Observed	6	10	6	3	1	4	1	0
Expected	1.00	0.89	0.87	0.90	0.96	0.90	0.55	0.40
Ratio	6.00	11.24	6.90	3.33	1.04	4.44	1.82	0.00

Solutions to the exercises

6.1 The observation times for the four subjects are 9, 7, 16, and 8 years respectively.

6.2 Subject 5 is 22 years of age on joining the cohort and 26 when lost to follow-up. She contributes 3 years to the band 20–24, and 1 year to the band 25–29.

6.3 The expected numbers of cases in the five age bands are 1.10, 1.75, 3.26, 5.11, and 5.54. The sum of these values is 16.76, but working to full accuracy we obtain 16.77 for the total expected number of cases.

6.4 The Age×Period bands in which subject 2 was observed are as follows:

Age	Calendar period	Time in band
20–24	1945–49	1
25–29	1945–49	1
25–29	1950–54	4
30–34	1950–54	1

6.5 The Age×Follow-up bands in which subject 1 was observed are as follows:

Age	Follow-up time	Time in band
35–39	0–4	1
40–44	0–4	4
40–44	5–9	1
45–49	5–9	3

6.6 The estimated rate for males is

$$\frac{14\,751}{2\,154\,900 \times 8} = 856 \text{ per } 10^6 \text{ person-years}$$

and the estimated rate for females is

$$\frac{5\,420}{2\,306\,300 \times 8} = 294 \text{ per } 10^6 \text{ person-years.}$$

6.7   The follow-up of each subject can be represented by a line on a three-dimensional Lexis diagram with axes: age, period, and time since treatment. Age and period were divided into five-year bands and time since treatment into three-year bands. Observed deaths and person-years can be assigned to cells in the resulting three-dimensional table. Multiplication of person-years by national rates gives the expected number of deaths for each cell. Table 6.6 is formed by adding this table over age and period.

7
Competing risks and selection

7.1 Censoring in follow-up studies

Up to this point we have lumped all the different reasons for censoring together. In this chapter we look at this practice more carefully and make a distinction between censoring due to practical difficulties in maintaining follow-up (such as migration, refusal to participate further and so on), and censoring due to competing causes of failure.

The first class of events causes removal of a subject from observation, but after censoring the subject is still at risk of failure – a subject does not cease to run the risk of a myocardial infarction simply because he or she has ceased to participate in a follow-up study. Such observations are censored in the sense that this later experience is removed from our view. The second class of censoring events also causes removal of a subject from observation, but this time the subject is no longer at risk from the failure of interest. This is obviously true when a subject dies from a competing cause, but onset of a non-fatal competing disease can also remove a subject from the risk under study. For example, in a study of myocardial infarction in previously healthy subjects, a subject who suffers the onset of lung cancer would be considered as no longer at risk — although patients with lung cancer suffer myocardial infarctions quite frequently, the aetiology is so different as to be regarded as a different type of event.

7.2 Competing causes

The termination of follow-up by a competing cause is not due to imperfection of any one study, but is intrinsic to all imaginable studies. The binary model which underlies the measurement of disease frequency by rates and risks assumes only one type of failure. To allow for more than one type, the model must be extended. Fig. 7.1 illustrates a model with two causes of failure over a single study period of fixed duration. There are now three possible outcomes, labelled F1 and F2 for the two types of failure and S for survival. The probabilities of F1 and F2 are referred to as π_1 and π_2, so the probability of survival is $1 - \pi_1 - \pi_2$. In incidence studies, π_1 and π_2 represent *cause-specific* failure probabilities or risks.

It is easy to use likelihood to estimate the parameters π_1 and π_2. If N

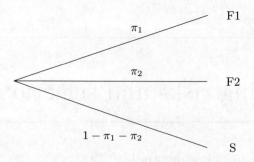

Fig. 7.1. Two causes of failure

subjects are studied and we observe D_1 failures of the first type and D_2 failures of the second type, the likelihood is

$$(\pi_1)^{D_1} (\pi_2)^{D_2} (1 - \pi_1 - \pi_2)^{N-D_1-D_2},$$

and the log likelihood is

$$D_1 \log(\pi_1) + D_2 \log(\pi_2) + (N - D_1 - D_2) \log(1 - \pi_1 - \pi_2).$$

This takes its maximum value when $\pi_1 = D_1/N$ and $\pi_2 = D_2/N$ so that the most likely values correspond with the intuitive measures — the *proportions* of subjects failing due to each cause.

Exercise 7.1. In a 5-year follow-up study of 1000 subjects, 27 suffered myocardial infarctions during the study period while 8 suffered strokes. (If any subject suffered both events, only the first was counted.) Estimate the cause-specific risks for these conditions. If myocardial infarctions and strokes are grouped together as 'cardiovascular events', what is the estimated risk of a cardiovascular event?

Fig. 7.2 illustrates the extension of this model to describe observation of a subject through several consecutive bands. Superscripts denote band and subscripts continue to indicate the type of failure. As in the case of a single cause, the π parameters are defined as *conditional probabilities*. For example, π_1^3 represents the probability of failure F1 during the third band, *conditional upon survival* through all preceding bands. The log likelihood behaves as if the time bands form separate studies involving different groups of subjects, so for each band the cause-specific failure probabilities are estimated by the proportion of those subjects at risk during the band, failing from the specified cause.

Exercise 7.2. The conditional probabilities of F1 and F2 remain constant at 0.1 and 0.2 respectively over three bands. List the 7 possible outcomes and calculate their probabilities.

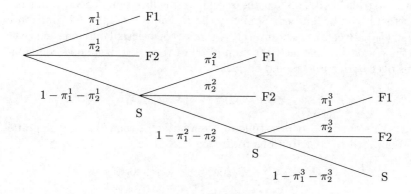

Fig. 7.2. Consecutive time bands

Table 7.1. Log likelihood contributions for a subject during one click

Outcome	Log likelihood
F1	$\log \lambda_1 + \log h$
F2	$\log \lambda_2 + \log h$
S	$-(\lambda_1 + \lambda_2)h$

7.3 Cause-specific rates

The same argument can be extended to rates by dividing the time scale into clicks. Fig. 7.1 now represents the possible outcomes for one subject during a single click. The conditional failure probabilities are

$$\pi_1 = \lambda_1 h, \qquad \pi_2 = \lambda_2 h,$$

where h is the duration of a click and λ_1 and λ_2 are cause-specific *rates* — conditional probabilities per unit time. Because the probabilities of failure are very small, we can make the approximation

$$\log(1 - \pi_1 - \pi_2) \approx -\pi_1 - \pi_2 = -(\lambda_1 + \lambda_2)h,$$

and the contributions to the log likelihood of a single subject during a single click are then those shown in Table 7.1. The total log likelihood is obtained by summing such terms over subjects and over clicks. There are D_1 clicks which result in failure of type F1 and these contribute a total of

$$D_1 \log(\lambda_1) + D_1 \log(h)$$

to the log likelihood. Since the second term does not depend upon parameters it can be ignored. Similarly the D_2 failures of type F2 contribute $D_2 \log(\lambda_2)$. Because every subject, regardless of eventual outcome, survives all the clicks save the last, the sum of all of these log likelihood contributions over both subjects and clicks is

$$\sum -(\lambda_1 + \lambda_2)h = -(\lambda_1 + \lambda_2)Y,$$

where Y is the total person-time of observation of the cohort. The grand total of all these contributions to the log likelihood is

$$D_1 \log(\lambda_1) + D_2 \log(\lambda_2) - (\lambda_1 + \lambda_2)Y.$$

A minor rearrangement of this expression leads to

$$D_1 \log(\lambda_1) - \lambda_1 Y \quad + \quad D_2 \log(\lambda_2) - \lambda_2 Y$$

so that the log likelihood is the sum of two parts, both Poisson in form, the first referring to F1 and the second to F2. The fact that the log likelihood falls into two distinct parts, one for each cause, justifies the standard practice of analyzing each cause separately, allowing for competing causes only in that they curtail further observation. The argument is easily generalized to allow for more than two causes.

7.4   Interpreting cause-specific rates

There has been some controversy as to whether the practice of estimating cause-specific rates in this way requires us to assume *independence* of causes – an assumption which might often not be justified. In fact, the split of the log likelihood into a sum of separate parts, one for each cause-specific rate, does not arise as a result of any assumption of independence of causes, but out of the way cause-specific rate parameters are defined. The rate for cause 1 is defined as the probability per unit time of failure due to cause 1, conditional upon the subject having previously survived *all* causes of failure. This quantity is not truly specific to one cause. Influences which directly influence one cause can, because of this, have an indirect affect on rates for another cause. The term *cause-specific* is misleading. For example, it is likely that myocardial infarction and stroke compete for the same high risk subgroup of the population: those with advanced atherosclerosis. A preventive measure which reduced the incidence rate of myocardial infarction without reducing the prevalence of atherosclerosis would result in an *increase* in the rate of stroke, since more of the atherosclerotic group would survive to be at risk from stroke.

It is a common practice to apply the formula

$$\log(\text{Cumulative survival probability}) = -\text{Cumulative rate}.$$

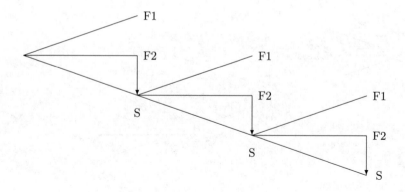

Fig. 7.3.   Elimination of cause F2

to the cumulative *cause-specific* rate to calculate a *cause-specific* survival probability, interpreted as the probability of survival which would be observed if all other causes of failure were eliminated. However, this interpretation *does* depend on the assumption that the different causes of failure are independent. This is illustrated in Fig. 7.3. If the causes are independent, subjects who would have failed failed due to F2 have exactly the same conditional probabilities of failure due to F1 as those who would not. Under these circumstances, elimination of cause F2 will have no effect on the subsequent rate for F1, and the exponential function of minus the cumulative cause-specific rate for F1 can be interpreted as a survival probability when cause F2 is eliminated. More generally we might expect elimination of other causes to have an effect on the rate for the remaining one and the cumulative cause-specific rate will then have no such interpretation. Since the independence of different causes is usually untestable, it is best to avoid such interpretations and to leave estimates of cumulative cause-specific failure rates, calculated by the modified life table or Aalen–Nelson method, without converting them to cumulative probabilities of survival. Conversely, if the actuarial life table and Kaplan–Meier methods of Chapter 4 are applied to cause-specific failure probabilities, the resulting 'survival probability' should be transformed to a cumulative rate by taking minus its logarithm.

7.5   Selection bias

We now turn to the other reasons for censoring in follow-up studies. The statistical theory is exactly the same as for competing causes – we simply relabel the two causes as failure and loss to follow-up (Fig. 7.4). However, the question of dependence between failure and censoring takes on a new significance, because censoring arises as a result of the imperfection of

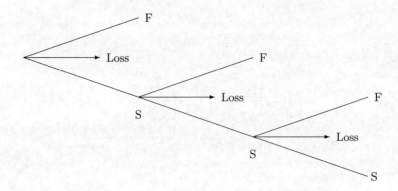

Fig. 7.4.   Loss to follow-up

real studies, rather than unavoidable biological realities. We would like to estimate what would have happened in an ideal study in which no censoring occurred, but in order to do this we need to assume that censoring and failure are independent. More precisely, this means that that those lost to follow-up due to censoring must have the same probabilities of failure in later bands as those remaining under observation. If this is the case, censoring is said to be *non-informative*. If not, the study results will be subject to *selection bias*.

A well known example of selection bias due to censoring arises in clinical trials when patients become so ill that their clinicians are unable ethically to maintain them on a randomized double blind protocol. The randomization code is then broken and the clinician is free to modify the treatment as necessary. If observation of such patients is regarded as censored at this point, the analysis is seriously biased, because these patients have a worse prognosis than those remaining in the trial. It will almost always be preferable to continue the follow-up of these patients and to analyze the data according to the initial treatment assigned. This is known as analysis by *intention to treat*.

Similar considerations apply when there is *late entry* to follow-up studies. Ideally, subjects should be recruited at the starting point for the failure process under study. This is usually the case in clinical epidemiology, where patients are recruited into the study at diagnosis, the natural starting point for a prognostic study. In many epidemiological studies, however, subjects are recruited some time after the natural starting point (see Fig. 7.5) This is known as *late entry*; it can introduce further selection bias if the new subjects have different subsequent probabilities of failure from the survivors they join. For example, clinical follow-up studies are frequently carried out in cohorts initially recruited from patients under treatment in a group

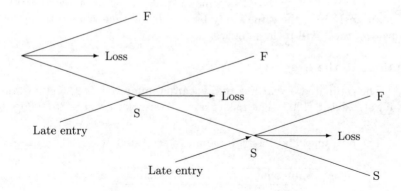

Fig. 7.5.   Selection due to loss and late entry

of participating hospitals when the study starts. These cohorts are then extended by addition of new patients as they are diagnosed. When carrying out analyses of survival times from diagnosis, the initial members of such a cohort are late entries, because their diagnosis preceded their entry into the study. This introduces possibilities for selection bias, because the initial cohort could include patients diagnosed elsewhere, but would omit patients diagnosed in the participating hospitals and referred elsewhere for treatment.

In epidemiological studies of the causes of disease, late entry is almost universal and we must be careful that it does not introduce bias. An example of bias arising this way is the *healthy worker* effect, so called because of the widespread empirical finding that occupationally recruited cohorts have lower mortality than general population rates would suggest. This arises partly because of selective recruitment into occupations but mainly because early retirement and job changes in response to ill health act to prevent entry of 'unhealthy' workers into the cohort. The ideal study would recruit subjects on entry to the occupation, but in practice the subjects actually recruited are those in employment on a particular date. Follow-up then starts on that date. Factors such as early retirement, and job changes in response to ill health, can operate in the period between joining the occupation and recruitment to prevent entry of unhealthy workers into the cohort.

The phenomenon of late entry is closely related to the distinction sometimes drawn between 'closed' cohorts (in which only failures and censoring can occur) and 'dynamic' cohorts, which can be refreshed by new entrants. This distinction implies that being closed or dynamic is a property of the cohort, but this is incorrect. The occurrence or non-occurrence of late entry is not a property of the cohort, but depends on the time scale chosen for analysis. If survival is analyzed by time in study there are no late entries, but in an analysis of the same study by age, or by time since entering an occupation, there will be late entries.

Solutions to the exercises

7.1   The estimated 5-year risk of myocardial infarction is 27/1000 while that for stroke is 8/1000. The risk of a cardiovascular event is 35/1000.

7.2   The outcomes and their probabilities are listed below.

Outcome	Probability
Band 1	
F1	0.1
F2	0.2
Band 2	
F1	$0.7 \times 0.1 = 0.07$
F2	$0.7 \times 0.2 = 0.14$
Band 3	
F1	$0.7 \times 0.7 \times 0.1 = 0.049$
F2	$0.7 \times 0.7 \times 0.2 = 0.098$
S	$0.7 \times 0.7 \times 0.7 = 0.343$

8
The Gaussian probability model

Until now we have been concerned only with the binary probability model. In this model there are two possible outcomes and the total probability of 1 is shared between them. It is an appropriate model when studying the occurrence of events, but not when studying a response for which there are many possible outcomes, such as blood pressure. For this the *Gaussian* or *normal* probability model is most commonly used.

In the Gaussian model the total probability of 1 is shared between many values. This is illustrated in the left panel of Fig. 8.1. When measurements are recorded to a fixed number of decimal places, there is a finite number of possible outcomes but, in principle, such measurements have infinitely many possible outcomes, so the probability attached to any one is effectively zero. For this reason it is the probability *density* per unit value which is specified by the model, not the probability of a given value. This is illustrated in the right panel of the figure. If π is the probability shared between values in a very narrow range, width h units, the probability density is π/h.

8.1 The standard Gaussian distribution

The standard Gaussian distribution has probability density centred at 0. The probability density at any value z (positive or negative) is given by

$$0.3989 \exp\left[-\frac{1}{2}(z)^2\right].$$

A graph of this probability density for different values of z is shown in Fig. 8.2. There is very little probability outside the range ± 3.

Tables of the standard Gaussian distribution are widely available, and these readily allow calculation of the probability associated with specified ranges of z. For our purposes it is necessary only to record that the probability corresponding to the range $(-1.645, +1.645)$ is 0.90 and that for the range $(-1.960, +1.960)$ is 0.95.

If the probability model for z is a standard Gaussian distribution then the probability model for $(z)^2$ is called the *chi-squared* distribution on one degree of freedom. Tables of chi-squared distributions can be used to find

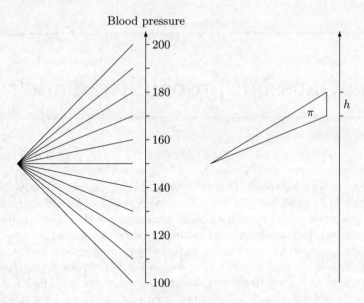

Fig. 8.1.   Probability shared between many outcomes.

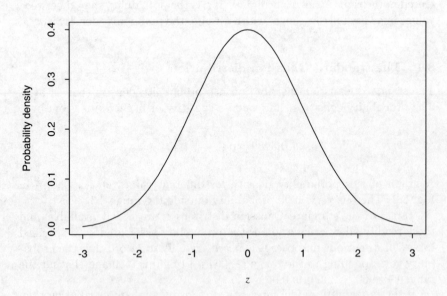

Fig. 8.2.   The standard Gaussian distribution.

the probabilities of exceeding specified values of $(z)^2$ in the same way as tables of the standard Gaussian distribution are used to find probabilities of exceeding specified values of z.

Exercise 8.1. Use the tables in Appendix D to find the probability of exceeding the value 2.706 in a chi-squared distribution on one degree of freedom.

Note that, for $(z)^2$ to exceed 2.706, z must lie outside the range ± 1.645 of the standard normal distribution.

8.2 The general Gaussian model

It would be remarkable if the data we are analysing fell into the range -3 to $+3$, so for modelling the variability of real data, it is necessary to generalize the model to incorporate two parameters, one for the central value or *location*, and one for the spread or *scale* of the distribution. These are called the *mean* parameter and *standard deviation* parameter and are usually denoted by μ and σ respectively. A variable with such a distribution is derived by multiplying z by the scale factor and adding the location parameter. Thus

$$x = \mu + \sigma z.$$

has a distribution of the same general shape as the standard Gaussian distribution but centred around μ with most of its probability between $\mu - 3\sigma$ and $\mu + 3\sigma$.

Exercise 8.2. If the mean and standard deviation of a general Gaussian distribution are 100 and 20 respectively, what ranges of values correspond to probabilities of 0.90 and 0.95 respectively?

Similarly, when x has a Gaussian distribution with mean μ and standard deviation σ then

$$z = \left(\frac{x - \mu}{\sigma} \right)$$

will have a *standard* Gaussian distribution. This fact can be used get the probability for a range of values of x using tables of z.

The probability density per unit of x when x has a Gaussian distribution with mean μ and standard deviation σ is

$$\frac{0.3989}{\sigma} \exp \left[-\frac{1}{2} \left(\frac{x - \mu}{\sigma} \right)^2 \right].$$

This expression is obtained by substituting $(x - \mu)/\sigma$ for z in the probability density of a standard Gaussian distribution to obtain the probability density per σ units of x, and then dividing by σ to obtain the probability density per unit of x. Sometimes the distribution is described in terms of the square of σ, which is called the *variance*.

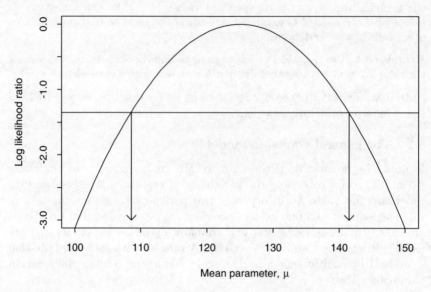

Fig. 8.3. The log likelihood ratio for the Gaussian mean, μ.

8.3   The Gaussian likelihood

Suppose a single value of x, say $x = 125$ is observed. Using the probability model that this is an observation from a Gaussian distribution with parameters μ and σ, the log likelihood for μ and σ is given by the log of the corresponding Gaussian probability density:

$$\log(0.3989) - \log(\sigma) - \frac{1}{2}\left(\frac{125 - \mu}{\sigma}\right)^2.$$

This log likelihood depends on two unknown parameters, but to keep things simple we shall assume that one of them, σ, is known from past experience to have the value 10. Omitting constant terms, the log likelihood for μ is then

$$-\frac{1}{2}\left(\frac{125 - \mu}{10}\right)^2.$$

The most likely value of μ is 125 and, since the above expression is zero at this point, this expression also gives the log likelihood *ratio* for μ. This is plotted in Fig. 8.3; curves with this shape are called *quadratic*.

We saw in Chapter 3 that we take the extremes of the supported range for a parameter to correspond to the value -1.353 for the log likelihood ratio. To find the limits of the supported range for μ we must therefore solve the simple equation

$$-\frac{1}{2}\left(\frac{125-\mu}{10}\right)^2 = -1.353.$$

This takes only a few lines:

$$\left(\frac{125-\mu}{10}\right)^2 = 2.706,$$

$$\left(\frac{125-\mu}{10}\right) = \pm 1.645,$$

$$\mu = 125 \pm 1.645 \times 10,$$

so that supported values of μ are those between 108.6 and 141.5. In general, the log likelihood ratio for μ is

$$-\frac{1}{2}\left(\frac{x-\mu}{\sigma}\right)^2,$$

the most likely value of μ is the observation x, and the supported range for μ is

$$x \pm 1.645\sigma,$$

where σ is the standard deviation (which we assume to be known).

We saw in Exercise 8.1 that the probability of exceeding 2.706 in a chi-squared distribution is 0.10, and the probability corresponding to the range ± 1.645 in the standard Gaussian distribution is 0.90. The fact that these numbers turn up in the above calculation is no accident and suggests that the log likelihood ratio criterion of -1.353 leads to supported ranges which have something to do with a probability of 0.90. This is indeed the case, but the relationship is not altogether straightforward and we shall defer this discussion to Chapter 10.

8.4 The likelihood with N observations

When there are N observations

$$x_1, x_2, \ldots, x_N,$$

the log likelihood for μ is obtained by adding the separate log likelihoods for each observation giving

$$\sum -\frac{1}{2}\left(\frac{x_i-\mu}{\sigma}\right)^2.$$

Let M refer to the mean of the observations,

$$M = \frac{x_1 + x_2 + \cdots + x_N}{N}.$$

It can be shown that the log likelihood can be rearranged as

$$-\frac{1}{2}\left(\frac{M-\mu}{S}\right)^2 + \sum -\frac{1}{2}\left(\frac{x_i - M}{\sigma}\right)^2$$

where $S = \sigma/\sqrt{N}$, sometimes called the *standard error of the mean*. This rearrangement involves only elementary algebra and the details are omitted. The second part of this new expression for the log likelihood does not depend on μ and cancels in the log likelihood ratio for μ which is

$$-\frac{1}{2}\left(\frac{M-\mu}{S}\right)^2,$$

The most likely value of μ is M, and setting the log likelihood ratio equal to -1.353 to obtain a supported range for μ gives

$$\mu = M \pm 1.645S.$$

As we would expect, with larger N, the value of S becomes smaller and the supported range narrower.

Exercise 8.3. The following measurements of systolic blood pressure were obtained from a sample of 20 men.

| 98 | 160 | 136 | 128 | 130 | 114 | 123 | 134 | 128 | 107 |
| 123 | 125 | 129 | 132 | 154 | 115 | 126 | 132 | 136 | 130 |

What is the most likely value for μ? Assuming that $\sigma = 14$, calculate the range of supported values for μ.

This exercise continues to make the unrealistic assumption, made throughout this chapter, that σ is *known*. In practice it must almost invariably be estimated from the data. We shall defer discussion of this until Chapter 34.

Solutions to the exercises

8.1 The probability of exceeding 2.706 in the chi-squared distribution with one degree of freedom is 0.10.

8.2 The range corresponding to a probability of 0.9 is

$$100 \pm 1.645 \times 20 = (67.1, 132.9)$$

and, for a probability of 0.95,

$$100 \pm 1.96 \times 20 = (60.8, 139.2).$$

8.3 The mean of the 20 measurements is 128.00 and this is the most likely value of μ. To calculate the supported range for μ, we first calculate

$$S = \frac{\sigma}{\sqrt{N}} = \frac{14}{\sqrt{20}} = 3.13$$

so that the range lies between

$$\mu = 128.00 \pm 1.645 \times 3.13$$

that is from 122.9 to 133.1 .

9
Approximate likelihoods

Because the Gaussian log likelihood for the mean parameter, μ, takes the simple form

$$-\frac{1}{2}\left(\frac{M-\mu}{S}\right)^2$$

the supported range for μ also takes a simple form, namely

$$M \pm 1.645S.$$

For log likelihoods such as the Bernouilli and Poisson there is no simple algebraic expression for the supported range, and the values of the parameters at which the log likelihood is exactly -1.353 must be found by systematic trial and error. However, the shapes of these log likelihoods are *approximately* quadratic, and this fact can be used to derive simple formulae for approximate supported ranges. Methods based on quadratic approximation of the log likelihood are particularly important because the quadratic approximation becomes closer to the true log likelihood as the amount of data increases.

9.1 Approximating the log likelihood

Consider a general likelihood for the parameter, θ, of a probability model and let M be the most likely value of θ. Since the quadratic expression

$$-\frac{1}{2}\left(\frac{M-\theta}{S}\right)^2$$

has a maximum value of zero when $\theta = M$ it can be used to to approximate the true log likelihood ratio, after an appropriate value of S has been chosen. Small values of S give quadratic curves with sharp peaks and large values of S give quadratic curves with broad peaks. We shall refer to S as the standard deviation of the estimate of θ. Alternatively, it is sometimes called the *standard error* of the estimate.

Once M has been found and S chosen, an approximate supported range for θ is found by solving the equation

$$-\frac{1}{2}\left(\frac{M-\theta}{S}\right)^2 = -1.353,$$

to give

$$\theta = M \pm 1.645S.$$

Full details of how S is chosen are given later in the chapter, but for the moment we shall give formulae for S, without justification, and concentrate on how to use these in practice.

THE RISK PARAMETER

The log likelihood for π, the probability of failure, based on D failures and $N - D$ survivors is

$$D\log(\pi) + (N - D)\log(1 - \pi).$$

The most likely value of π is D/N. To link with tradition we shall also refer to the most likely value of π as P (for proportion). The value of S which gives the best approximation to the log likelihood ratio is

$$S = \sqrt{\frac{P(1 - P)}{N}}.$$

For the example we worked through in Chapter 3, $D = 4$ and $N = 10$ so that the value of P is 0.4 and

$$S = \sqrt{\frac{0.4 \times 0.6}{10}} = 0.1549.$$

An approximate supported range for π is given by

$$0.4 \pm 1.645 \times 0.1549$$

which is from 0.15 to 0.65, while the supported range obtained from the true curve lies from 0.17 to 0.65. The true and approximate log likelihood curves are shown in Fig. 9.1. The curve shown as a solid line is the true log likelihood ratio curve, while the broken line indicates the Gaussian approximation.

THE RATE PARAMETER

The log likelihood for a rate λ based on D cases and Y person years is

$$D\log(\lambda) - \lambda Y.$$

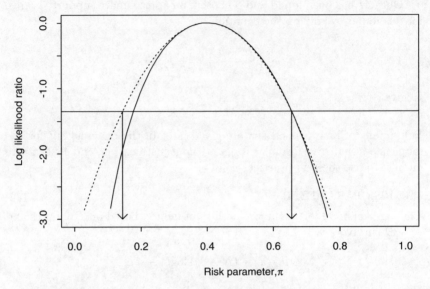

Fig. 9.1.   True and approximate Bernouilli log likelihoods.

The most likely value of λ is D/Y and the value of S which gives the best approximation to the log likelihood ratio is

$$S = \frac{\sqrt{D}}{Y}.$$

For the example in Chapter 5, $D = 7$ and $Y = 500$. The most likely value of λ is 0.014 and

$$S = \sqrt{7}/500 = 0.00529.$$

An approximate supported range for λ is therefore

$$0.014 \pm 1.645 \times 0.00529$$

which is from 5.3/1000 to 22.7/1000. The true (solid line) and approximate (broken line) log likelihood ratio curves are shown in Fig. 9.2. The range of support obtained from the true curve spans from 7.0 to 24.6 per 1000.

Exercise 9.1. Find the approximate supported range for π, the probability of failure, based 7 failures and 93 survivors. Find also the approximate supported range for λ, the rate of failure, based on 30 failures over 1018 person-years.

9.2   Transforming the parameter

The Gaussian log likelihood curve for μ is symmetric about M and extends *indefinitely* to either side. However, the parameters of some probability

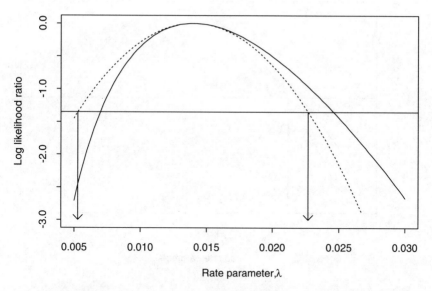

Fig. 9.2.   True and approximate Poisson log likelihoods.

models are not free to vary in this manner. For example, the rate parameter λ can take only positive values, and the risk parameter must lie between 0 and 1. Approximate supported ranges for such parameters calculated from the Gaussian approximation can, therefore, include impossible values.

The solution to this problem is to find some function (or *transformation*) of the parameter which is unrestricted and to first find an approximate supported range for the transformed parameter.

THE LOG RATE PARAMETER

The rate parameter λ can take only positive values, but its logarithm is unrestricted. To calculate an approximate supported range for λ it is better, therefore, to first calculate a range for $\log(\lambda)$, and then to convert this back to a range for λ. Note that the range for $\log(\lambda)$ will always convert back to positive values for λ. To find the approximate range for $\log(\lambda)$ we need a new value of S — that which gives the best Gaussian approximation to the log likelihood ratio curve when plotted against $\log(\lambda)$. When a rate λ is estimated from D failures over Y person-years, this value of S is given by

$$S = \sqrt{1/D}.$$

Fig. 9.3 illustrates this new approximation for our example in which $D = 7$ and $Y = 500$ person-years. Here,

$$S = \sqrt{1/7} = 0.3780,$$

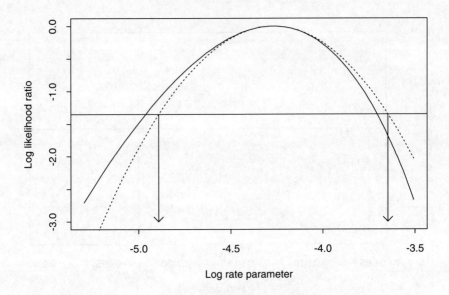

Fig. 9.3.   Approximating the log likelihood for $\log(\lambda)$.

and an approximate supported range for $\log(\lambda)$ is

$$\log(7/500) \pm 1.645 \times \sqrt{1/7},$$

which is from -4.890 to -3.647. The range for λ is therefore from $\exp(-4.890)$ to $\exp(-3.647)$ which spans from $7.5/1000$ to $26.1/1000$.

A more convenient way of carrying out this calculation is suggested by noting that the limits of the range for λ are given by

$$\frac{7}{500} \overset{\times}{\div} \exp\left(1.645\sqrt{\frac{1}{7}}\right) = 0.014 \overset{\times}{\div} 1.862.$$

The range is then from $0.014/1.862 = 7.5/1000$ to $0.014 \times 1.862 = 26.1/1000$, as before. We shall refer to the quantity

$$\exp\left(1.645 S\right)$$

as an *error factor*.

THE LOG ODDS PARAMETER

The same thing can be done when calculating a supported range for the risk parameter π based on D failures in N subjects. The value of π is restricted on both sides, by 0 on the left and by 1 on the right. The value of $\log(\pi)$ is still restricted on the right by zero because $\log(1) = 0$, but $\log(\Omega)$, where Ω is the odds corresponding to π, is not restricted at all. Hence we first find a range for $\log(\Omega)$ and then convert this back to a range for π. The most likely value of $\log(\Omega)$ is

$$M = \log\left(\frac{D}{N-D}\right)$$

and the value of S for approximating the log likelihood for $\log(\Omega)$ is

$$S = \sqrt{\frac{1}{D} + \frac{1}{N-D}}.$$

For the example where $D = 4$ and $N - D = 6$,

$$S = \sqrt{\frac{1}{4} + \frac{1}{6}} = 0.6455,$$

and an approximate supported range for $\log(\Omega)$ is given by

$$\log\left(\frac{4}{6}\right) \pm 1.645 \times 0.6455,$$

that is, from -1.4673 to 0.6564. This is a range for $\log(\Omega)$ and it is equivalent to a range for Ω from $\exp(-1.4673) = 0.231$ to $\exp(0.6564) = 1.928$. This can be calculated more easily by first calculating the error factor

$$\exp\left(1.645 \times 0.6455\right) = 2.892.$$

The most likely value of Ω is $4/6 = 0.667$, so that the supported range for Ω is

$$0.667 \overset{\times}{\div} 2.892$$

that is, from 0.231 to 1.928 as before. Finally, remembering that $\pi = \Omega/(1+\Omega)$, the range for π is given by

$$\frac{0.231}{1.231} \quad \text{to} \quad \frac{1.928}{2.928}$$

which is from 0.19 to 0.66.

Some of the more commonly used values of S obtained by approximating the log likelihood are gathered together in Table 9.1.

Exercise 9.2. Repeat Exercise 9.1 by first finding 90% intervals for $\log(\Omega)$ and $\log(\lambda)$ respectively, and then converting these to intervals for π and λ.

Exercise 9.3. Repeat the above exercise using error factors.

Table 9.1.   Some important Gaussian approximations

Parameter	M	S
π	$D/N = P$	$\sqrt{P(1-P)/N}$
λ	D/Y	$\sqrt{D}/Y$
$\log(\Omega)$	$\log[D/(N-D)]$	$\sqrt{1/D + 1/(N-D)}$
$\log(\lambda)$	$\log(D/Y)$	$\sqrt{1/D}$

★ **9.3   Finding the best quadratic approximation**

We now return to the problem of how to determine the values for M and
S. To do this we need some elementary ideas of calculus summarized
in Appendix B. In particular, we need to be able to find the *gradient*
(or *slope*) of the log-likelihood curve together with its *curvature*, which is
defined as the rate of change of the gradient. The mathematical terms for
these quantities are the first and second *derivatives* of the log likelihood
function.

The value of M can be found by a direct search for that value of of θ
which maximizes the log likelihood, but it is often easier to find the value
of θ for which the gradient of the log likelihood is zero; this occurs when
$\theta = M$.

The value of S is chosen to make the curvature of the quadratic approximation equal to that of the true log likelihood curve at M, thus ensuring
that the true and approximate log likelihoods are very close to each other
near $\theta = M$. The quadratic approximation to the log likelihood ratio is

$$-\frac{1}{2}\left(\frac{M-\theta}{S}\right)^2,$$

and the rules summarized in Appendix B show that the curvature of this
is constant and takes the value

$$-\frac{1}{(S)^2}.$$

We therefore choose the value of S to make $-1/(S)^2$ equal to the curvature
of the true log likelihood curve at its peak.

THE RATE PARAMETER

The log likelihood for a rate λ is

$$D\log(\lambda) - \lambda Y.$$

Using the rules of calculus given in Appendix B the gradient of $\log(\lambda)$ is $1/\lambda$ and the gradient of λ is 1. Hence the gradient of the log likelihood is

$$\frac{D}{\lambda} - Y.$$

The maximum value of the log likelihood occurs when the gradient is zero, that is, when $\lambda = D/Y$, so the most likely value of λ is D/Y. The curvature of a graph at a point is defined as the rate of change of the gradient of the curve at that point. The rules of calculus show this to be

$$-\frac{D}{(\lambda)^2}.$$

The peak of the log likelihood occurs at $\lambda = D/Y$ so the curvature at the peak is found by replacing λ by D/Y in this expression to obtain

$$-\frac{(Y)^2}{D}.$$

Setting this equal to $-1/(S)^2$ gives

$$S = \sqrt{D}/Y,$$

which is the formula quoted earlier.

THE RISK PARAMETER

The log likelihood for the probability π based on D positive subjects out of a total of N is

$$D\log(\pi) + (N - D)\log(1 - \pi).$$

The gradient of the log likelihood is

$$\frac{D}{\pi} - \frac{N - D}{1 - \pi}$$

which is zero at $\pi = D/N$, also referred to as P. The gradient of the gradient is

$$-\frac{D}{(\pi)^2} - \frac{N - D}{(1 - \pi)^2},$$

so the curvature at $\pi = P$ is

$$-\frac{D}{(P)^2} - \frac{N - D}{(1 - P)^2}.$$

Replacing D by NP and $N - D$ by $N(1 - P)$, this reduces to

$$-\frac{N}{P(1-P)}$$

so

$$S = \sqrt{\frac{P(1-P)}{N}}.$$

★ ## 9.4 Approximate likelihoods for transformed parameters

When the log likelihood for a parameter is plotted against the log of the parameter rather than the parameter itself, the curvature at the peak will be different. For example, the log likelihood for a rate parameter λ is

$$D \log(\lambda) - \lambda Y.$$

Plotting this against $\log(\lambda)$ is the same as expressing the log likelihood as a function of $\log(\lambda)$. To do this we introduce a new symbol β to stand for $\log(\lambda)$, so

$$\beta = \log(\lambda), \quad \lambda = \exp(\beta).$$

In terms of β the log likelihood is

$$D\beta - Y \exp(\beta).$$

The gradient of this with respect to β is

$$D - Y \exp(\beta)$$

and the curvature is

$$-Y \exp(\beta).$$

The most likely value of $\exp(\beta)$ (which equals λ) is D/Y, so the curvature at the peak is

$$-Y \times (D/Y) = -D.$$

It follows that

$$S = \sqrt{1/D}.$$

In general, derivations such as that above can be simplified considerably by using some further elementary calculus which provides a general rule for the relationship between the values of S on the two scales. In the case of the log transformation, this rule states that multiplying the value of S on the scale of λ by the gradient of $\log(\lambda)$ at $\lambda = M$ gives the value of S on the scale of $\log(\lambda)$. The rules of calculus tell us that, at $\lambda = M$, the gradient of the graph of $\log(\lambda)$ against λ is $1/M$. Since, on the λ scale, $M = D/Y$ and $S = \sqrt{D}/Y$, the rule tells us that the value of S for $\log(\lambda)$ is

$$\frac{\sqrt{D}}{Y} \times \frac{Y}{D} = \sqrt{\frac{1}{D}}.$$

This agrees with the expression obtained by the longer method.

A similar calculation shows that the curvature of the Bernouilli log likelihood, when plotted against $\log(\Omega)$, the log odds, is given by

$$S = \sqrt{\frac{1}{D} + \frac{1}{N-D}}.$$

Solutions to the exercises

9.1 An approximate supported range for π is given by

$$0.07 \pm 1.645S$$

where $S = \sqrt{0.07 \times 0.93/100}$. This gives a range from 0.028 to 0.112. An approximate supported range for λ is given by

$$30/1018 \pm 1.645S$$

where $S = \sqrt{30}/1018$. This gives a range from $21/1000$ to $38/1000$.

9.2 The approximate supported range for $\log(\Omega)$ is given by

$$\log(7/93) \pm 1.645S$$

where

$$S = \sqrt{\frac{1}{7} + \frac{1}{93}} = 0.3919.$$

This gives a range from -3.231 to -1.942. The range for Ω is from 0.040 to 0.143, and the range for π is from 0.038 to 0.125.
The approximate supported range for $\log(\lambda)$ is given by

$$\log(30/1018) \pm 1.645S$$

where

$$S = \sqrt{1/30} = 0.1826.$$

This gives a range from -3.825 to -3.224. The range for λ is from $22/1000$ to $40/1000$.

9.3   The error factor for Ω is

$$\exp(1.645 \times 0.3919) = 1.905.$$

The most likely value for Ω is $7/93 = 0.075$ and the range for Ω is from $0.075/1.905 = 0.040$ to $0.075 \times 1.905 = 0.143$.   The range for π is from 0.038 to 0.125.
The error factor for the rate is

$$\exp(1.645 \times 0.1826) = 1.350.$$

The most likely value of the rate is $29/1000$ with range from $29/1.350 = 22$ per 1000 to $29 \times 1.350 = 40$ per 1000.

10
Likelihood, probability, and confidence

The supported range for a parameter has so far been defined in terms of the cut-point -1.353 for the log likelihood ratio. Some have argued that the scientific community should accept the use of the log likelihood ratio to measure support as *axiomatic*, and that supported ranges should be reported as 1.353 unit supported ranges, or 2 unit supported ranges, with the choice of how many units of support left to the investigator. This notion has not met with widespread acceptance because of the lack of any intuitive feeling for the log likelihood ratio scale — it seems hard to justify the suggestion that a log likelihood ratio of -1 indicates that a value is supported while a log likelihood ratio of -2 indicates lack of support. Instead it is more generally felt that the reported plausible range of parameter values should be associated in some way with a *probability*. In this chapter we shall attempt to do this, and in the process we shall finally show why -1.353 was chosen as the cut-point in terms of the log likelihood ratio.

There are two radically different approaches to associating a probability with a range of parameter values, reflecting a deep philosophical division amongst mathematicians and scientists about the nature of probability. We shall start with the more orthodox view within biomedical science.

10.1 Coverage probability and confidence intervals

Our first argument is based on the frequentist interpretation of probability in terms of relative frequency of different outcomes in a very large number of repeated "experiments". With this viewpoint the statement that there is a probability of 0.9 that the parameter lies in a stated range does not make sense; there can only be one correct value of the parameter and it will either lie within the stated range or not, as the case my be. To associate a probability with the supported range we must imagine a very large number of repetitions of the study, and assume that the scientist would calculate the supported range in exactly the same way each time. Some of these ranges will include the true parameter value and some will not. The relative frequency with which the ranges include the true value is called the *coverage probability* for the range, although strictly speaking it is the coverage probability for the method of choosing the range.

We shall start with Gaussian probability model and consider the estimation of the mean μ, from a single observation x, when the standard deviation, σ, is known. The log likelihood ratio for μ is

$$-\frac{1}{2}\left(\frac{x-\mu}{\sigma}\right)^2.$$

We saw in Chapter 8 that the range of values for μ with log likelihood ratios above the cut-point of -1.353 is

$$x \pm 1.645\sigma.$$

We shall now show that the coverage probability of this range is 0.90 by imagining an endless series of repetitions of the study with the value of μ remaining unchanged at the true value. Each study will yield a different observation, X, and hence a different range (see Fig. 10.1). The range for any particular repetition will contain the true value of μ provided the true value is judged to be supported by the data X — in other words, provided that

$$-\frac{1}{2}\left(\frac{X-\mu}{\sigma}\right)^2 > -1.353,$$

where μ now refers to the true value. Writing

$$z = \left(\frac{X-\mu}{\sigma}\right)$$

this condition is equivalent to $(z)^2$ being less than 2.706, and since $(z)^2$ has a chi-squared distribution this occurs with probability 0.90. Hence the coverage probability is 0.90.

Exercise 10.1. In a computer simulation of repetitions of a study in which a single observation is made from a Gaussian distribution with $\mu = 100$ and $\sigma = 10$, the first four repetitions produced the observations 104, 115, 82, and 92. Calculate the log likelihood ratio for $\mu = 100$ for each of these four observations. In which repetitions would the true value of μ have been supported?

The idea of coverage probability has allowed us to attach a frequentist probability, such as 0.90, to a range of parameter values, but we cannot say that the probability of the true value lying within the stated range is 0.90, because the stated range either does or does not include the true value. To avoid having to say precisely what is meant every time the probability for a range is reported, statisticians took refuge in an alternative word and professed themselves 90% *confident* that the true value lies in the reported interval. Not surprisingly the distinction between probability and confidence is rarely appreciated by scientists.

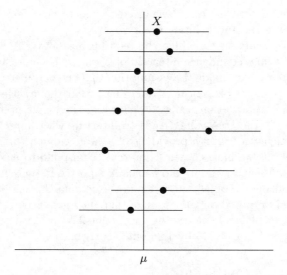

Fig. 10.1. Repeated studies and their supported ranges.

Exercise 10.2. Use tables of the chi-squared distribution to work out the cut-point for the log likelihood ratio which leads to a 95% coverage probability for the corresponding supported range, and give the formula for this range.

We have demonstrated the correspondence between the −1.353 cut-point for the log likelihood ratio and 90% coverage, but only for the case of the Gaussian log likelihood where the standard deviation is known. Fortunately the relationship also holds approximately for other log likelihoods such as the Bernoulli and Poisson. With increasing amounts of data these log likelihoods approach the quadratic shape of the Gaussian log likelihood and the coverage probability for the supported range based on the −1.353 cut-point is approximately 90%. In other words, if M is the most likely value of a parameter and S is the standard deviation of the Gaussian approximation to the likelihood, then the supported range

$$M \pm 1.645S$$

is also, at least approximately, a 90% confidence interval.

This raises the question of how much data is needed to use this approximate theory. For the Bernoulli likelihood, a reasonable guide is that the approximations are good if both D and $N - D$ are larger than 10, but can be misleading if either count is less than 5. In the Poisson case the observed number of events, D, should be larger than 10; there is no restriction on the number of person-years since this is irrelevant to the shape of the log likelihood curve. In Chapter 12 we discuss what to do when there are too few data to use the approximate theory.

The only likelihood for which the relationship between the supported range and the 90% confidence interval holds *exactly* is Gaussian likelihood, and even here we have made the assumption that the parameter σ is known. In the early years of this century it was shown that the practice of *estimating* the standard deviation using the data and thereafter pretending that this estimate is the true value, leads to intervals with *approximately* the correct coverage probability, providing N is large enough (more than 15).

The intervals we have chosen to present correspond to 90% confidence intervals but 95% intervals are more usually reported in the scientific literature. The routine use of 90% intervals in the epidemiological literature has recently been proposed on the grounds that they give a better impression of the range of plausible values. If you prefer 95% intervals these can be obtained by replacing 1.645 by 1.960 in the calculations.

⋆ 10.2 Subjective probability

The second approach to the problem of assigning a probability to a range of values for a parameter is based on the philosophical position that probability is a subjective measure of ignorance. The investigator uses probability as a measure of subjective *degree of belief* in the different values which the parameter might take. With this view it is perfectly logical to say that there is a probability of 0.9 that the parameter lies within a stated range.

Before observing the data, the investigator will have certain beliefs about the parameter value and these can be measured by *a priori* probabilities. Because they are subjective every scientist would be permitted to give different probabilities to different parameter values. However, the idea of scientific objectivity is not completely rejected. In this approach objectivity lies in the rule used to modify the *a priori* probabilities in the light of the data from the study. This is Bayes' rule and statisticians who take this philosophical position call themselves Bayesians.

Bayes' rule was described in Chapter 2, where it was used to calculate the probabilities of exposure given outcome from the probabilities of outcome given exposure. Once we are prepared to assign probabilities to parameter values, Bayes' rule can be used to calculate the probability of each value of a parameter (θ) given the data, from the probability of the data given the value of the parameter.

The argument is illustrated by two tree diagrams. Fig. 10.2 illustrates the direction in which probabilities are specified in the statistical model — given the choice of the value of the parameter, θ, the model tells us the probability of the data. The probability of any particular combination of data and parameter value is then the product of the probability of the parameter value and the probability of data given the parameter value. In

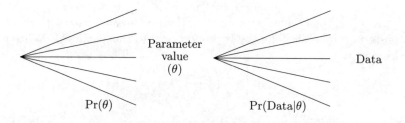

Fig. 10.2. From parameter value to data.

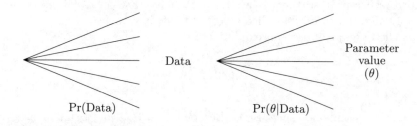

Fig. 10.3. From data to parameter value.

this product, the first term, $\Pr(\theta)$, represents the *a priori* degree of belief for the value of θ and the second term, $\Pr(\text{Data}|\theta)$, is the likelihood. Fig. 10.3 reverses the conditioning argument, and expresses the joint probability as the product of the overall probability of the data multiplied by the probability of the parameter given the data. This latter term, $\Pr(\theta|\text{Data})$, represents the *posterior* degree of belief in the parameter value once the data have been observed. Since the joint probability of data and parameter value is the same no matter which way we argue,

$$\Pr(\theta) \times \Pr(\text{Data}|\theta) = \Pr(\text{Data}) \times \Pr(\theta|\text{Data}),$$

so that

$$\Pr(\theta|\text{Data}) = \frac{\Pr(\theta) \times \Pr(\text{Data}|\theta)}{\Pr(\text{Data})}.$$

Thus elementary probability theory tells us how prior beliefs about the value of a parameter should be modified after the observation of data.

We shall now apply this idea to the problem of estimating the Gaussian mean, μ, given a single observation x. The likelihood for μ is

$$\exp\left[-\frac{1}{2}\left(\frac{x-\mu}{\sigma}\right)^2\right].$$

If prior to observing x we believe that no value of μ is any more probable than any other, then the prior probability density does not vary with μ and the posterior probability density is proportional to the likelihood. Writing the likelihood as

$$\exp\left[-\frac{1}{2}\left(\frac{\mu - x}{\sigma}\right)^2\right].$$

we see that after choosing the constant of proportionality to make the total probability for μ equal to 1, the posterior distribution for μ is a Gaussian distribution which has mean x and standard deviation σ. The 5 and 95 percentiles of the standard Gaussian distribution are -1.645 and 1.645 respectively so there is a 90% probability that μ lies in the range $x \pm 1.645\sigma$. This range is called a 90% credible interval.

When the quadratic approximation

$$-\frac{1}{2}\left(\frac{M - \theta}{S}\right)^2$$

is used for likelihoods such as the Bernoulli and Poisson, a similar argument shows that, provided the prior probability density for θ does not vary with θ, then the posterior distribution for θ is approximately Gaussian with mean M and standard deviation S. It follows that there is a 90% probability that θ lies in the range $M \pm 1.645S$.

It appears from this discussion that the frequentists and the Bayesians end up making very similar statements, differing only in their use of the words *confidence* and *probability*. But to achieve this agreement we have had to make the rather extreme assumption that *a priori* no one value of the parameter is more probable than any other. This is taking open mindedness too far and Bayesians would generally advocate the use of more realistic priors. When there is a large amount of data the posterior is more influenced by the likelihood than by the prior, and both approaches lead to similar answers regardless of the choice of prior. However, when the data are sparse, there can be serious differences between the two approaches. We shall return to this in Chapter 12.

Solutions to the exercises

10.1 When $x = 104$, the log likelihood ratio for $\mu = 100$ is

$$-\frac{1}{2}\left(\frac{104 - 100}{10}\right)^2 = -0.08.$$

For $x = 115, 82, 92$ the log likelihood ratio turns out to be $-1.125, -1.62$, and -0.32 respectively. Thus only for $x = 82$ is the support for the true value of μ less than the cut-off value of -1.353. In all other repetitions $\mu = 100$ is supported.

10.2 From tables of chi-squared, the value 3.841 is exceeded with probability 0.05, so

$$\left(\frac{x - \mu}{\sigma}\right)^2 > 3.841$$

with probability 0.05. The log likelihood ratio, which is minus one half of this quantity, is therefore less than

$$-0.5 \times 3.841 = -1.921$$

with probability 0.05. Thus the cut-point for the log likelihood ratio is -1.921.

11
Null hypotheses and p-values

11.1 The null value of a parameter

With most probability models there is one particular value of the parameter which corresponds to there being *no effect*. This value is called the *null* value, or *null hypothesis*. For a parameter θ we will denote this null value by $\theta_\oslash$. In classical statistical theory, considerable emphasis is placed on the need to disprove (or reject) the null hypothesis before claiming positive findings, and the procedures which are used to this end are called *statistical significance tests*. However, the emphasis in this theory on accepting or rejecting null hypotheses has led to widespread misunderstanding and misreporting in the medical research literature. In epidemiology, which is not an experimental science, the usefulness of the idea has been particularly questioned. Undoubtedly the idea of statistical significance testing has been overused, at the expense of the more useful procedures for *estimation* of parameters which we have discussed in previous chapters. However, it remains useful. A null hypotheses is a *simplifying* hypothesis and measuring the extent to which the data are in conflict with it remains a valuable part of scientific reasoning. In recent years there has been a trend away from a making a straight choice between accepting or rejecting the null hypothesis. Instead, the *degree* of support for the null hypothesis is measured, for example using the log likelihood ratio at the null value of the parameter.

EXAMPLE: GENETIC LINKAGE BY THE SIB PAIR METHOD

We shall illustrate the methods of this chapter with a simple statistical problem arising in the detection of *linkage* between a genetic marker and a gene which carries an increased susceptibility to a disease. At the marker locus each offspring receives one of two possible haplotypes from the mother and one of two possible haplotypes from the father. If there are many possible haplotypes we can safely assume that the mother and father together have four *different* marker haplotypes. The marker is then said to be highly *polymorphic*. If the mother has haplotypes (a,b) and the father (c,d), possible haplotype configurations for offspring are (a,c), (a,d), (b,c), and (b,d). If inheritance of the marker obeys Mendelian laws, the probability that

Table 11.1. Linkage of the HLA locus to nasopharyngeal cancer susceptibility

Haplotypes shared	Number of sib pairs	Probability (null value)
2	16	0.25
1	8	0.50
0	3	0.25

two siblings have completely different marker haplotypes (no haplotypes in common) is 0.25 and the probability that they have the same pair of haplotypes (two haplotypes in common) is also 0.25. The remaining possibility is that they have one marker haplotype in common, which has probability 0.50.

If we deliberately choose two siblings who are both affected by the disease, then these siblings will be more similar in that part of the genome surrounding the disease susceptibility gene than we would expect by chance. If the marker locus is in this vicinity, then the probabilities that two affected sibs will share 0, 1, or 2 marker haplotypes will depart from the (0.25, 0.5, 0.25) split indicated above. This way of looking for genetic linkage is called the *affected sib pair method*. If disease susceptibility is conferred by a *dominant* gene, it can be shown that the main effect of linkage is to reduce the probability of the affected sibs sharing no marker haplotypes and to increase the probability of their sharing both, while the probability of their sharing one marker haplotype is scarcely affected. A simple and reasonably efficient statistical analysis may therefore be carried out by disregarding the pairs sharing one marker haplotype.

Table 11.1 shows the frequency of shared HLA haplotypes amongst 27 pairs of sibs affected by nasopharyngeal carcinoma.* Assuming dominant inheritance of the disease susceptibility gene and ignoring the 8 sib pairs with only one marker gene in common leaves $N = 19$ pairs, 16 of which share both haplotypes, and 3 of which share no haplotypes. Let Ω be the odds that a pair shares both rather than no haplotypes. The log likelihood for Ω is

$$16 \log(\Omega) - 19 \log(1 + \Omega).$$

The most likely value of Ω is $16/3 = 5.33$, so that the maximum value of the log likelihood is

$$16 \log(5.33) - 19 \log(6.33) = -8.29$$

---

*From Day, N.E. and Simons, J. (1976) *Tissue Antigens*, **8**, 109–119.

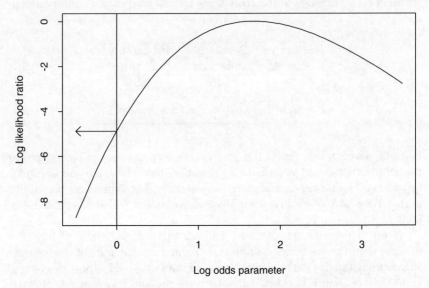

Fig. 11.1.   Log likelihood ratio for HLA linkage.

and the log likelihood ratio for any other value of Ω is

$$16 \log(\Omega) - 19 \log(1 + \Omega) - (-8.29).$$

Fig. 11.1 shows the log likelihood ratio plotted against $\log(\Omega)$.

Under the null hypothesis that there is no linkage, the two outcomes are equally probable, so the null value of Ω is 1.0 and the null value for $\log(\Omega)$ is 0. This is indicated in Fig. 11.1 by the vertical line. The log likelihood ratio for $\Omega = 1$ is

$$16 \log(1) - 19 \log(2) - (-8.29) = -4.88$$

(indicated on the graph with an arrow). The null value of Ω does not fall within the range which we have regarded as supported.

Whether the mode of inheritance of disease susceptibility is dominant or recessive must be established in studies of extended families. If it is dominant, the likelihood ratio test described above provides an efficient test of linkage. However, if the disease susceptibility gene is *recessive*, the probability that affected sibs will share one marker haplotype in common is also reduced and a more efficient test for linkage examines the 16:11 split between 2 and < 2 shared haplotypes. In this case the null value of the odds parameter Ω is $0.25/0.75 = 0.333$.

Exercise 11.1. If the evidence for Ω is based on the 16:11 split of sib pairs, find the log likelihood ratio for $\Omega = 0.333$.

11.2   Log likelihood ratios and p-values

As with the supported range for a parameter a general need is felt to measure support for the null hypothesis on the more familiar scale of probability. The way this is done in frequentist statistical theory is very similar to the way in which coverage probabilities are calculated for confidence intervals (see Chapter 10). We imagine a large number of repetitions of the study with the parameter equal to its null value and define the *p-value* as the proportion of these studies which provide less support for the null value than the data actually observed. If the p-value is small the data are at odds with the null hypothesis and the finding is said to be *statistically significant*. If the p-value is large, the finding is said to be *not statistically significant*. Traditionally the value $p = 0.05$ has been used to divide significant from non-significant results, but the modern practice is to report the actual p-value, particularly when it lies in the range 0.001 to 0.10. Outside this range it is enough to give the p-value as $p < 0.001$ or $p > 0.10$.

The argument which defines the p-value closely follows that used to define the coverage probability of a supported range in Chapter 10. As in that case, we shall start with the problem of drawing conclusions about the value of the Gaussian mean, μ, on the basis of a single observation, x. In this case, the value of the log likelihood ratio for a null value $\mu_\oslash$ is equal to

$$-\frac{1}{2}\left(\frac{x - \mu_\oslash}{\sigma}\right)^2.$$

Exercise 11.2. You observe a value $x = 116$ and wish to test the hypothesis that it was obtained from a Gaussian distribution with mean $\mu = 100$ (the null value). Assuming that σ is known to take the value 10, what is the value of the log likelihood ratio at the null value?

We imagine a large number of repetitions of the study when the null hypothesis is true. The p-value is the proportion of such repetitions with log likelihood ratios less than this observed value. One way that the p-value can be calculated is by computer simulation of such repetitions of the study.

Exercise 11.3. Such a simulation is envisaged in Exercise 10.1. Of the first four values generated, what proportion have log likelihood ratios at the null value less than that observed?

This is a very inaccurate estimate of the p-value. An accurate estimate would, of course, require several thousand repetitions to be generated.

The method of generating a p-value by computer simulation is known as a *Monte Carlo* test and it is quite widely used. However, in this case we do not need to resort to the computer as we can work out the p-value theoretically. If X represents the value obtained in such a repetition, the p-value is defined as the probability that this yields a smaller log likelihood ratio than that observed, that is,

$$\Pr\left[-\frac{1}{2}\left(\frac{X-\mu_\oslash}{\sigma}\right)^2 < \text{Observed log likelihood ratio}\right].$$

This is the same as

$$\Pr\left[\left(\frac{X-\mu_\oslash}{\sigma}\right)^2 > -2\times(\text{Observed log likelihood ratio})\right],$$

and since we are assuming that the null hypothesis is true in such repetitions, the above probability is obtained by referring

$$-2\times(\text{Observed log likelihood ratio})$$

to the chi-squared distribution on one degree of freedom.

Exercise 11.4. Use the table of the chi-squared distribution in Appendix D to find the p-value for the example of Exercise 11.2

For N observations from a Gaussian distribution, the same rule for obtaining the p-value holds, the value of minus twice the log likelihood ratio now being

$$\left(\frac{M-\mu_\oslash}{S}\right)^2$$

where M is the mean of the N observations and $S = \sigma/\sqrt{N}$.

This relationship between the log likelihood ratio and the p-value holds *approximately* for non-Gaussian log likelihoods. The approximation will be adequate providing there is a sufficient amount of data to ensure that the log likelihood curve is approximately quadratic.

In our example of testing for genetic linkage, using the method most appropriate for dominant inheritance, the log likelihood ratio at the null parameter value is -4.88 so that

$$-2\times(\text{log likelihood ratio}) = 9.76.$$

The probability of this being exceeded in a chi-squared distribution on one degree of freedom is 0.0018, so that the p-value is approximately 0.002. This is an example of a *log likelihood ratio test*.

Exercise 11.5. Use tables of the chi-squared distribution to find the p-value corresponding to the log likelihood ratio calculated in Exercise 11.1.

There are two other approximate methods of obtaining p-values which are widely used. These are called *Wald* tests and *score* tests, and both involve

quadratic approximations to the log likelihood curve. The problem of calculating exact p-values when these approximate methods cannot be used
will be discussed in Chapter 12.

11.3   Wald tests

The first quadratic approximation we shall consider is the same as that
used for approximate confidence intervals in Chapter 9. For a parameter,
θ, the log likelihood is approximated by the quadratic curve

$$-\frac{1}{2}\left(\frac{M-\theta}{S}\right)^2$$

where M is the most likely value of the parameter and S is the standard
deviation of the Gaussian approximation, calculated from the curvature of
log likelihood at its peak. This provides the closest possible approximation
in the region of the most likely value. Using this approximation, the approximate value of minus twice the log likelihood ratio at the null value,
$\theta_\oslash$, is

$$\left(\frac{M-\theta_\oslash}{S}\right)^2$$

For the log odds parameter of the Bernoulli likelihood, Ω, the values of
M and S are

$$M = \log\left(\frac{D}{N-D}\right)$$

$$S = \sqrt{\frac{1}{D}+\frac{1}{N-D}}.$$

For the log likelihood shown in Fig. 11.1,

$$M = \log\left(\frac{16}{3}\right) = 1.674$$

$$S = \sqrt{\frac{1}{16}+\frac{1}{3}} = 0.629.$$

The approximate log likelihood ratio curve corresponding to these values
is shown in Fig. 11.2 (broken lines). The arrow indicates the approximate
log likelihood ratio at the null value, $\log(\Omega) = 0.0$,

$$-\frac{1}{2}\left(\frac{1.674-0.0}{0.629}\right)^2 = -3.54$$

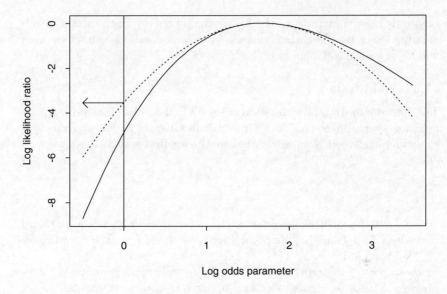

Fig. 11.2.   The Wald test.

The approximate value of minus twice the log likelihood ratio is

$$\left(\frac{1.674 - 0.0}{0.629}\right)^2 = 7.08$$

and referring this value to the chi-squared distribution yields an approximate p-value of 0.008. This method of obtaining an approximate p-value is called the *Wald test*.

Exercise 11.6. Carry out the Wald test which approximates the log likelihood ratio of Exercise 11.1.

11.4   Score tests

The second quadratic approximation to the log likelihood ratio which we consider is based on the gradient and curvature of the log likelihood curve at the null value of the parameter. This is the most accurate quadratic approximation *in the region of the null value*. This approximation to the log likelihood ratio of Fig. 11.1 is shown in Fig. 11.3. Here we have displaced the true log likelihood ratio curve upwards in order to demonstrate that the true and approximate curves are the same shape in the region of the null value.

If U is the gradient of the log likelihood at the null value of the parameter, $\theta_\oslash$, and V is minus the curvature (also at the null value), then this

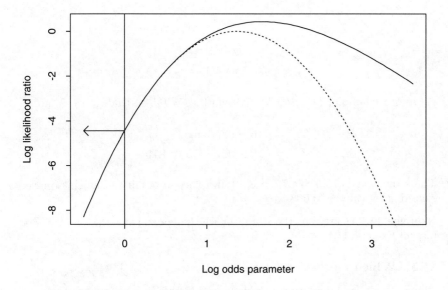

Fig. 11.3. The score test.

approximation to the log likelihood ratio is given by the formula

$$-\frac{V\left(\theta - \theta_\oslash - U/V\right)^2}{2}.$$

This approximate curve has its maximum value at $\theta_0 + U/V$ and minus twice the log likelihood ratio at $\theta = \theta_\oslash$ is

$$\frac{(U)^2}{V}.$$

The gradient, U, is called the *score* and we shall call V the *score variance*. The approximate score test is carried out by comparing $(U)^2/V$ with the chi-squared distribution with one degree of freedom.[†]

For the Bernoulli log likelihood in terms of the log odds parameter, $\log(\Omega)$, the score and score variance at the null value $\Omega_\oslash$ are most easily expressed in terms of the null value of the probability parameter,

$$\pi_\oslash = \frac{\Omega_\oslash}{1 + \Omega_\oslash}.$$

[†]The score test is usually carried out using the *expected value* of V (worked out assuming the null hypothesis to be true). In the applications discussed in this book this is not usually possible, and we have defined the score test in terms of the observed value of V.

They are

$$U = D - N\pi_\oslash,$$
$$V = N\pi_\oslash(1 - \pi_\oslash).$$

In our example, $D = 16$, $N = 19$, and $\pi_\oslash = 0.5$ so that

$$U = 16 - 9.5 = 6.5$$
$$V = 19 \times 0.5 \times 0.5 = 4.75$$

The score test is $(6.5)^2/4.75 = 8.89$ and the probability that chi-squared exceeds this value is 0.003.

Exercise 11.7. Carry out the score test which approximates the log likelihood ratio of Exercise 11.1.

11.5   Which method is best?

The methods for calculating p-values given in this chapter are approximate except for the special case of a Gaussian likelihood with known standard deviation σ, when the three methods coincide and yield exact p-values. In other cases, where the log likelihood is roughly quadratic, the approximations to the p-value are good and the three methods give similar answers. When the three methods give seriously different answers this means that the quadratic approximations are not sufficiently close to the true log likelihood curve over the region stretching from the null value of the parameter to the most likely value. Of course, if the most likely value and the null value are very far apart, the curve is very difficult to approximate. In this situation, all three methods will give very small p-values and although these may differ substantially from on another, the choice of statistical method would not affect our scientific conclusions. This is the case in our example in which the three methods gave p-values of 0.002, 0.008, and 0.003.

The log likelihood ratio test is the only one of the three tests which remains the same when the parameter is transformed, and is to be preferred in general. The approximate equivalence of the other two tests to the log likelihood ratio test depends on the quadratic approximation, and will be improved by choosing an appropriate scale for the parameter. In particular, for parameters such as the *odds*, or the *rate*, which can take only positive values, it is better to calculate Wald and score tests in terms of the log parameter. If the three methods differ seriously, even after choosing an appropriate scale for the parameter, it is usual to advise the use of exact p-values. Methods for calculating these will be discussed in Chapter 12, but these are not without their difficulties.

11.6   One-sided p-values

$\boxed{\star}$

We have defined the p-value as the probability that, when the null hypothesis is true, a repeated study will provide less support for the null value of the parameter than did the study actually observed. We have measured support for the null value of the parameter as the difference between the log likelihood at the null value and the log likelihood at the most likely value. This is satisfactory when the model allows the parameter to take any value within its natural range, but needs to be redefined if the model allows the parameter to vary only within a restricted range. In our HLA linkage example, if Ω is the odds that a sib pair shares both haplotypes rather than neither, the null value is $\Omega = 1$ and linkage is indicated by values in the range $\Omega > 1$. Values in the range $\Omega < 1$ are not allowed in a model for genetic linkage. In these circumstances, the value of Ω which is best supported by a study in which 5 sib pairs are found to share both haplotypes and 10 sib pairs to share neither is no longer 5/10, since this parameter value is not allowed by the model. The best supported value amongst *allowable* values is $\Omega = 1$. Thus only studies in which the split is in the expected direction would be regarded as providing evidence against the null hypothesis. The p-value calculated from this viewpoint is called a *one-sided* p-value, while the more usual p-value appropriate when the model allows the parameter to take values to both sides of the null value is called a *two-sided* p-value.

Approximate one-sided p-values can be obtained in most circumstances by simply halving the corresponding two-sided p-value. This follows from the fact that approximately half of the hypothetical repetitions of the study under the null hypothesis would lead to results in the wrong direction and, in a one-sided test, these would not be treated as evidence against the null value. In our example, the log likelihood ratio test for linkage gave $p \approx 0.0018$ and the approximate one-sided p-value is 0.0009.

The assumption that the probability model only allows its parameter to take on values to one side of the null value is a strong one and rarely justified in practice. Thus, one-sided p-values should only be used in exceptional circumstances. The genetic linkage example is one of these.

11.7   Tests for the rate parameter

We have described the three methods for obtaining approximate p-values using a null hypothesis which concerns the parameter of a simple binary probability model. These methods were all based on the Bernoulli likelihood. In this section we shall describe the corresponding methods for the rate parameter, λ, for a cohort study. Here the log likelihood takes the Poisson form:

$$D \log(\lambda) - \lambda Y,$$

where D is the number of failures observed and Y is the person-years observation.

The log likelihood ratio test for the null value $\lambda = \lambda_\oslash$ compares the log likelihood at $\lambda_\oslash$ with the log likelihood at $\lambda = D/Y$, the most likely value. The log likelihood ratio is, therefore,

$$[D \log(\lambda_\oslash) - \lambda_\oslash Y] - \left[D \log \left(\frac{D}{Y} \right) - \frac{D}{Y} Y \right]$$

which simplifies to

$$-D \log \left(\frac{D}{E} \right) + (D - E),$$

where $E = \lambda_\oslash Y$ is the 'expected' number of failures obtained by multiplying the null value of the rate parameter by the person-years observation in the study. Minus twice this value can be compared with the chi-squared distribution with one degree of freedom.

The Wald test is based on the best Gaussian approximation to the log likelihood in the region of the most likely value. It is best carried out on the $\log(\lambda)$ scale, where $M = \log(D/Y)$ and $S = \sqrt{1/D}$.

Finally, the score test is based on the best Gaussian approximation to the log likelihood in the region of $\lambda_\oslash$. Some simple calculus shows that the score and score variance (on the $\log(\lambda)$ scale) are given by

$$U = D - E, \qquad V = E,$$

so that the score test is $(D - E)^2/E$.

The null hypothesis most frequently of interest is that the rate in the cohort is no different from the rate in a *reference population*. Typically this reference rate is based on official statistics for a whole country and is estimated from so many events that it can be assumed to be a known constant. In practice the expected number of failures is usually calculated separately for different age bands and summed and E refers to the total expected number added over age bands. In Chapter 15 we show that the theory described above extends without change to this situation.

Exercise 11.8. In the vicinity of a nuclear reprocessing plant, 4 cases of childhood leukaemia were observed over a certain period while, from national registration rates, we would have expected only 0.25. Compare the log likelihood ratio and score tests of the null hypothesis that the incidence rates of leukaemia in the area do not differ from the national rates.[*]

In this case the two methods differ considerably, although both suggest a very small p-value. This reflects the fact that D is very small and the

---

[*]These data are discussed in detail by Gardner, M.J. (1989) *Journal of the Royal statistical Society, Series A*, **152**, 307–326.

Gaussian approximations are unreliable. We shall discuss methods for use in such situations in Chapter 12.

11.8   Misinterpretation of p-values

Reporting of p-values has come into disfavour because they have been widely misinterpreted. Although the same is true of confidence intervals, the nature of the misinterpretation of these is much less serious.

Most scientists interpret the 90% confidence interval as a range within which there is a 90% *probability* that the parameter value lies. We saw in Chapter 10 that, in the frequentist view of statistics, this is not correct — such an interpretation requires probability to be interpreted in terms of subjective degree of belief. In practice, however, it is not a serious error and does not usually lead to serious scientific misjudgement. The corresponding misinterpretation of the p-value, as the probability that the null hypothesis is *true*, is a much more serious error. Small studies which should be quite unconvincing are quoted as strongly negative findings because they have large p-values. The fact that this error is still widespread is the main reason why many authors currently discourage the use of p-values.

11.9   Lod scores and p-values   ⋆

Our example in this chapter concerns genetic linkage and geneticists have taken a rather different approach to measuring the amount of evidence against the null hypothesis. Typically the result of a linkage analysis is presented as a *lod score* defined in terms of the log (base 10) likelihood for a parameter, θ, where this is defined as one minus the probability that two genes are passed from parent to offspring together. This probability is 0.5 when the two loci are unlinked but greater than 0.5 when there is linkage. Thus the null value of θ, which is called the *recombination fraction*, is 0.5 and linkage is represented by $\theta < 0.5$. The lod score for any specified value of θ compares the log likelihood with its value at $\theta = 0.5$. It is conventional to consider linkage to have been demonstrated if the most likely value of θ is less than 0.5 and gives a lod score greater than 3.0.

Using the relationship between the different systems of logarithms explained in Appendix A, a lod score of 3.0 corresponds to

$$-2 \times (\text{log likelihood ratio}) = 13.82$$

and, referring this to the chi-squared distribution on one degree of freedom shows this to be approximately equivalent to a p-value of 0.0002. However, since we are only interested in values of θ less than 0.5, the test is one-sided and this value must be halved to yield $p \approx 0.0001$. This is much smaller than we would require p-values to be in other areas of research, and it would appear that geneticists are much more difficult to dissuade from the null hypothesis than other scientists. This is usually justified on the grounds that the human genome is immense and, *a priori*, it is very unlikely that any one marker locus is linked to a disease susceptibility gene. This argument has considerable force when searching a large number of markers in a 'blind fishing expedition', but would not hold if there were good *a priori* reasons to suspect linkage in a specified region. The interpretation of lod scores, like that of p-values, must take account of the scientific context and rigid criteria should be avoided.

Solutions to the exercises

11.1 At the most likely value, $\Omega = 16/11 = 1.455$, the log likelihood is

$$16 \log(1.455) - 27 \log(2.455) = -18.249$$

while at the null value $\Omega = 0.333$, the log likelihood is

$$16 \log(0.333) - 27 \log(1.333) = -25.354.$$

The log likelihood ratio at the null value is therefore

$$-25.354 - (-18.249) = -7.105.$$

11.2 The value of the log likelihood ratio at $\mu = 100$ is

$$-\frac{1}{2} \left(\frac{116 - 100}{10} \right)^2 = -1.28.$$

11.3 The first four observations of the computer simulation were 104, 115, 82 and 92 and the solution to Exercise 10.1 showed that the corresponding values of the log likelihood ratio at $\mu = 100$ are -0.08, -1.125, -1.62 and -0.32. Only 1 of these is less than the observed log likelihood ratio — a proportion of 0.25.

11.4 The value of minus twice the observed log likelihood ratio is 2.56 and referring this to the table of the chi-squared distribution in Appendix D shows the p-value to be a little over 0.10.

11.5 Minus twice the log likelihood ratio is 14.21. This corresponds to a very small p-value, 0.00016. Such results are usually reported as $p < 0.001$.

11.6 The most likely value of the log odds parameter is

$$M = \log(16/11) = 0.375,$$

and the standard deviation of the Gaussian approximation to the log like-lihood around M is

$$S = \sqrt{\frac{1}{16} + \frac{1}{11}} = 0.392.$$

The null value of the log odds is $\log(0.333) = -1.100$ so that the Wald test is

$$\left(\frac{0.375 - (-1.100)}{0.392}\right)^2 = 14.16.$$

This is very close to minus twice the log likelihood ratio and the approximate p-value is 0.00017.

11.7 The null value for the probability parameter is $\pi_\oslash = 0.25$ so that

$$U = 16 - 27 \times 0.25 = 9.25,$$
$$V = 27 \times 0.25 \times 0.75 = 5.0625.$$

The score test is

$$\frac{(9.25)^2}{5.0625} = 16.90$$

and p-value is less than 0.001.

11.8 The log likelihood ratio chi-squared value is

$$-2 \times \left[-4\log\left(\frac{4}{0.25}\right) + (4 - 0.25)\right] = 14.681.$$

The score test is

$$\frac{(4 - 0.25)^2}{0.25} = 56.250.$$

Both give $p < 0.001$.

12
⭐ Small studies

In small studies the shape of the log likelihood for a parameter can be appreciably different from the quadratic shape of the Gaussian log likelihood and p-values and confidence intervals based on Gaussian approximations can then be misleading. It is conventional in such situations to report *exact* p-values and confidence intervals. In this chapter we will explain how these are conventionally calculated, while drawing attention to some serious difficulties.

12.1 Exact p-values based on the binomial distribution

Consider again the example in Chapter 11 concerning genetic linkage between a gene which renders a subject susceptible to a disease, and a marker gene. The test for linkage was based on the 16 sib pairs with two haplotypes in common and the 3 pairs with no haplotypes in common, so the log likelihood for Ω, the odds of having two haplotypes in common, is

$$16 \log(\Omega) - 19 \log(1 + \Omega).$$

The most likely value of Ω is $16/3 = 5.33$ and the log likelihood takes its maximum value of -8.29 at this value of Ω. The value $\Omega = 1$ corresponds to no linkage and the log likelihood ratio for $\Omega = 1$ is therefore

$$16 \log(1) - 19 \log(1 + 1) - (-8.29) = -4.88.$$

The corresponding p-value is defined as the probability of obtaining a log likelihood ratio, less than -4.88, during many repetitions of the study in which $\Omega = 1$. In the last chapter this probability was obtained approximately from the chi-squared distribution; the problem now is to find its exact value.

Each new repetition of the study will give rise to a log likelihood ratio for $\Omega = 1$. To calculate this it is necessary to go through the same steps as for the split of 16:3. For example, a repetition in which the split was 10:9 gives a log likelihood for Ω of

$$10 \log(\Omega) - 19 \log(1 + \Omega).$$

Table 12.1. A computer simulation and the binomial distribution

	Log likelihood ratio		Simulated	Binomial
Split	Two-sided	One-sided	frequency	probability
0:19	−13.17	0	0	0.000002
1:18	−9.25	0	1	0.000036
2:17	−6.78	0	17	0.000326
3:16	−4.88	0	112	0.001848
4:15	−3.39	0	512	0.007393
5:14	−2.22	0	1777	0.022179
6:13	−1.32	0	4519	0.051750
7:12	−0.67	0	9238	0.096107
8:11	−0.24	0	14523	0.144161
9:10	−0.03	0	18160	0.176197
10:9	−0.03	−0.03	18035	0.176197
11:8	−0.24	−0.24	14857	0.144161
12:7	−0.67	−0.67	9675	0.096107
13:6	−1.32	−1.32	5278	0.051750
14:5	−2.22	−2.22	2306	0.022179
15:4	−3.39	−3.39	750	0.007393
16:3	−4.88	−4.88	194	0.001848
17:2	−6.78	−6.78	38	0.000326
18:1	−9.25	−9.25	7	0.000036
19:0	−13.17	−13.17	1	0.000002

The most likely value for Ω is $10/9 = 1.11$ and the maximum value of the log likelihood is

$$10\log(1.11) - 19\log(1 + 1.11) = -13.14.$$

The log likelihood for $\Omega = 1$ based on this split is therefore

$$10\log(1) - 19\log(1 + 1) - (-13.14) = -0.03.$$

Exercise 12.1. Calculate the log likelihood ratio for $\Omega = 1$ when the split between the two outcomes is 15:4.

For a split such as 4:15, the log likelihood ratio depends on whether we regard the model as allowing values of Ω less than one. If not, then the best supported value of Ω given such a split is 1, and the log likelihood ratio is zero. In this case a one-sided p-value is appropriate.

The way the log likelihood ratio for $\Omega = 1$ depends on the observed split is shown in full in Table 12.1, for both two-sided and one-sided views

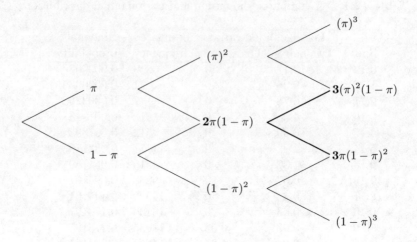

Fig. 12.1.   Generating the binomial distribution.

of the problem.* In the two-sided case, the splits 2:17, 1:18, 0:19 and 17:2, 18:1, 19:0 all produce log likelihood ratios which are less than −4.88, and the splits 3:16 and 16:3 produce log likelihood ratios equal to −4.88. In the one-sided case, the splits 17:2, 18:1, and 19.0 give log likelihood ratios less than −4.88 and the split 16:3 gives a log likelihood ratio equal to −4.88. To find the p-values exactly we need to find the probabilities of the different splits when $\Omega = 1$.

One way of calculating these p-values is to use a Monte Carlo approach similar to that described in Chapter 11. A computer program is written which splits the 19 sib pairs between the two outcomes with odds 1, and repeats the process (say) 100 000 times. The result of doing this is shown in the third column of Table 12.1. Out of 100 000 repetitions of the study, none produced the split 0:19, one produced the split 1:18, 17 produced the split 2:17, and so on. The probabilities of the different splits are therefore estimated by the computer to be 0.00000, 0.00001, 0.00017, and so on.

As in the case of the Gaussian mean, the probabilities can also be worked out theoretically, in this case using the *binomial distribution*. Fig. 12.1 illustrates the derivation of the binomial distribution. The first level of branching represents the possible outcomes of the first observation, the upper branch indicating failure (with probability π) and the lower branch indicating survival (with probability $1 - \pi$). The second level of branching represents the outcome of the second observation. The probability that both subjects fail is $(\pi)^2$ and the probability that both survive is $(1 - \pi)^2$; the remaining two possibilities both have one failure and one sur-

---

*When calculating these log likelihood ratios when the splits are 0:19 or 19:0, note that the expression $0 \log(0)$ takes the value 0.

vivor and, since we do not need to differentiate between these, the branches are allowed to merge, with a total probability of $2\pi(1 - \pi)$. The diagram continues with the inclusion of a third observation. The probability that all three observations are failures is now $(\pi)^3$ and that all three are survivors is $(1 - \pi)^3$. The remaining probabilities correspond to 2:1 and 1:2 splits of failures to survivors and have probabilities $3(\pi)^2(1 - \pi)$ and $3\pi(1 - \pi)^2$ respectively, the multiplier 3 arising because each of these points represents the merging of 3 paths through the tree.

Exercise 12.2. Continue the diagram to generate the probabilities for all possible splits of $N = 4$ observations and also for $N = 5$.

When this process is continued it leads to the general result that the probability that N observations split as D failures and $N - D$ survivors is

$$C(D, N)(\pi)^D(1 - \pi)^{N-D}.$$

where $C(D, N)$, the number of ways of selecting D objects from N, is 1 when $D = 0$ or $D = N$ and

$$\frac{N \times (N - 1) \times \cdots \times (N - D + 1)}{D \times (D - 1) \cdots \times 2 \times 1}$$

otherwise. Binomial probabilities may easily be calculated by computer, and tables are available for values of N and D up to about 20.

The binomial distribution with $N = 19$ and $\pi = 0.5$ is shown in the fourth column of Table 12.1. A comparison between the third and fourth columns of this table shows that the values estimated by the Monte Carlo method are quite close to the correct values, particularly in the centre of the distribution.

One of the areas of dispute when defining an exact p-value is whether to define this as the probability of obtaining a log likelihood ratio less than -4.88 or less than *or equal* to -4.88. This difficulty does not arise with the Gaussian log likelihood because the probability of any one *precise* outcome is zero, but it does arise here; in the two-sided case the splits 3:16 and 16:3 both give rise to the observed log likelihood ratio of -4.88 and have probabilities 0.001848. If these splits are excluded, the two-sided p-value is

$$0.000002 + 0.000036 + 0.000326 + 0.000002 + 0.000036 + 0.000326$$

which adds up to 0.000728. If these splits are included, two further contributions of 0.001848 must be included and the two-sided p-value is 0.004424. Conventionally, splits giving rise to the observed log likelihood ratio are included, but there are arguments in favour of including only one half of the probability for these splits. This course of action gives the *mid-p* value. In our example the mid-p value is 0.002576.

Table 12.2.   Log likelihood ratios and probabilities ($N = 27$, $\pi = 0.25$)

Split	LLR	Probability	Split	LLR	Probability
0:27	-7.767	0.000423	14:13	-4.452	0.001775
1:26	-4.589	0.003810	15:12	-5.699	0.000513
2:25	-2.835	0.016509	16:11	-7.096	0.000128
3:24	-1.645	0.045858	17:10	-8.647	0.000028
4:23	-0.836	0.091716	18:9	-10.357	0.000005
5:22	-0.323	0.140632	19:8	-12.233	0.000001
6:21	-0.057	0.171883	20:7	-14.288	
7:20	-0.006	0.171883	21:6	-16.536	
8:19	-0.149	0.143236	22:5	-18.999	
9:18	-0.469	0.100796	23:4	-21.709	
10:17	-0.956	0.060477	24:3	-24.716	
11:16	-1.603	0.031155	25:2	-28.103	
12:15	-2.403	0.013847	26:1	-32.054	
13:14	-3.353	0.005326	27:0	-37.430	

If these arguments are repeated for one-sided p-values it can be seen that, whichever convention is adopted, the one-sided p-value is half of the two-sided value. This is not generally true and is only the case here because of the symmetry of the binomial distribution in this case. This in turn derives from the fact that the null value of Ω is 1, corresponding to $\pi = 0.5$. For a test of the null value $\pi = 0.25$, the relationship between one- and two-sided p-values is not as simple.

Exercise 12.3. In the genetic linkage example, one of the tests for linkage compares the observed split of the 27 sib pairs into 16 with two haplotypes in common and 11 with one or zero in common with the probabilities 0.25 and 0.75 under the hypothesis of no linkage. The log likelihood ratios and probabilities corresponding to the different possible splits are shown in Table 12.2 (probabilities less than 0.000001 are omitted). Find the exact two-sided p-value for the hypothesis of no linkage.

In this exercise the probability distribution for the different splits is not symmetric and the one-side p-value cannot be obtained by halving the two-sided value. In such situations there is no general agreement about how two-sided p-values should be calculated, because there is no general agreement about how to compare extremeness of splits at opposite ends of the distribution. We have chosen to measure extremeness in terms of the log likelihood ratio, but other criteria are also used and lead to different two-sided p-values.

Table 12.3. Log likelihood ratios and probabilities ($\eta = 0.25$)

Cases	LLR	Probability
0	−0.25	0.778801
1	−0.64	0.194700
2	−2.41	0.024338
3	−4.70	0.002028
4	−7.34	0.000127
5	−10.23	0.000006
6	−13.32	0.000000
etc.		

12.2 The Poisson distribution

When the population at risk, N, is very large and the probability of failure, π, is very small, the binomial distribution takes on a very simple form, called the Poisson distribution:

$$\frac{1}{D!}(\eta)^D \exp(-\eta)$$

where $D!$ denotes D *factorial*

$$D \times (D-1) \cdots \times 2 \times 1$$

and $\eta = N\pi$. The same is approximately true of the number of failures in a cohort subject to rate λ and with Y person-years of observation. Providing we can regard Y, at least approximately, as a fixed constant then the probability of D failures is given by the Poisson distribution with $\eta = \lambda Y$.

The main use of the Poisson distribution is to calculate the p-value corresponding to the null hypothesis which states that the rate in the study cohort is the same as a reference rate, $\lambda_{\rm R}$. The null value of η is $E = \lambda_{\rm R} Y$, the expected number of cases. Given $\eta = E$, the Poisson distribution tells us the probability for any value of D. The idea extends to the case where the expected number of cases is calculated taking account of variation of rates with time.

To illustrate the use of the Poisson distribution, we return to our example of leukaemia surrounding a nuclear reprocessing plant (Exercise 11.8). In that case the expected number of failures was 0.25 and the Poisson probabilities for each possible value of D are shown in Table 12.3. The table also lists the corresponding values of the log likelihood ratio for the null hypothesis, which we showed in Chapter 11 to be given by the expression

$$-D \log \left(\frac{D}{E}\right) + (D - E).$$

Table 12.4.   Definition of the exact confidence interval

	Probability	
Cases	($\eta = 1.3663$)	($\eta = 9.1535$)
0	0.25505	0.00011
1	0.34847	0.00097
2	0.23806	0.00443
3	0.10842	0.01353
4	0.03703	0.03096
5	0.01012	0.05668
6	0.00230	0.08647
7	0.00045	0.11307
8	0.00001	0.12938
etc.		

The observed number of cases of leukaemia was 4 and the corresponding log likelihood ratio -7.34. To find the p-value we add the probabilities of all values of D with log likelihood ratio less than or equal to -7.34 :

$$0.000127 + 0.000006 + 0.000000 = 0.000133.$$

Note that, in this case, there is no difference between the one- and two-sided p-values.

12.3   Exact confidence intervals

An *exact confidence interval* for a parameter is defined in terms of exact p-values. The lower limit of the 90% interval for a parameter θ is found by searching for the null value, $\theta_\oslash$, whose p-value is exactly 0.05. Here, the *one-sided* p-value which assumes that $\theta \geq \theta_\oslash$ is used. The upper limit is defined similarly, save for the fact that the reverse one-sided p-value is used, that is the p-value under the assumption $\theta \leq \theta_\oslash$. The search for these values must be carried out by computer and is laborious, although computational methods have been considerably improved in recent years.

Table 12.4 illustrates the idea of exact confidence intervals using the leukaemia data discussed above. Poisson distributions are shown for two values of $\eta = \theta E$. Both values give one-sided p-values of approximately 0.05 when the observed number of cases is 4, since

$$0.03703 + 0.01012 + 0.00230 + 0.00045 + 0.00001 = 0.04991$$

and

$$0.00011 + 0.00097 + 0.00443 + 0.01353 + 0.03096 = 0.05000.$$

Thus values of θE smaller than 1.3663 and values larger than 9.1535 have one-sided p-values smaller than 0.05. Since $E = 0.25$, the exact confidence interval for θ lies between $1.3663/0.25 = 5.465$ and $9.1535/0.25 = 36.614$.

Exact confidence intervals are only exact in the sense that they are derived from exact p-values. They do *not* necessarily have coverage probabilities exactly equal to 0.90. For the Gaussian mean, μ, when the standard deviation is known, an exact 90% confidence interval does have a coverage probability of exactly 0.90, but for parameters of other models this is often not the case. This is because, in these cases, the coverage probability depends on the unknown true value of the parameter. Thus, exact confidence intervals are not exact in any *scientifically useful* sense.

This observation, taken together with the fact that there are several different ways in which exact p-values may be defined, lead us to doubt the practical usefulness of exact methods. Instead we would argue that, since it is the *log likelihood* which measures the support for different values of the parameter, scientific papers should aim to communicate the log likelihood accurately and concisely. For large studies Gaussian approximations allow us to communicate the log likelihood curve using only M and S, the most likely value and a standard deviation. For small studies it might be necessary to report the log likelihood in greater detail.

12.4   A Bayesian approach

The Bayesian approach goes further and uses the likelihood to update a prior distribution for the parameter into a posterior distribution, using Bayes' rule as described in Chapter 10. No new difficulties are introduced by the fact that a study is small, apart from the inevitable consequence that the information in the likelihood will also be small, so the posterior distribution will not be much different from the prior distribution. This means that conclusions depend more upon our prior beliefs about the parameter in a small study than they would in a large study.

Similar answers to those yielded by the classical exact approach can be obtained using Bayesian arguments if it is assumed *a priori* that we are completely ignorant about the value of the parameter. Such an assumption is called a *vague* prior belief and holds that no value of the parameter is any more probable than any other value, so that the prior distribution is flat. One difficulty is that a flat prior for a parameter θ is not flat with respect to $\log(\theta)$, so a flat prior for θ and a flat prior for $\log(\theta)$ lead to different posterior beliefs.

This may be illustrated by our example of leukaemia in the neighbourhood of a nuclear plant, where the observed number of cases was $D = 4$ while the expected number from national rates was $E = 0.25$. It is conventional to compare rates in the study population with reference rates by the ratio of observed to expected cases, in this case $4/0.25 = 16.0$. This

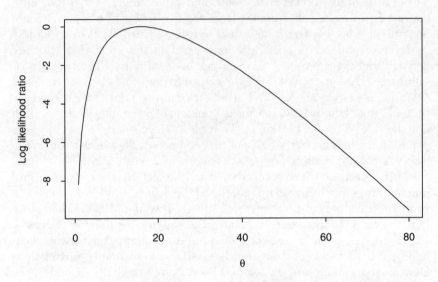

Fig. 12.2.   Log likelihood for the leukaemia data ($D = 4$, $E = 0.25$).

Table 12.5.   Posterior distributions for θ for three vague priors

| Prior (flat with respect to) | Posterior probability distribution for θ | | | |
| | Mean | 90% probability interval | | Probability $\theta < 1.0$ |
		Lower limit	Upper limit	
$\log(\theta)$	16.0	5.5	31.0	0.000133
θ	20.0	7.9	36.6	0.000007
$\sqrt{\theta}$	18.0	6.6	33.8	0.000030

may be regarded as the most likely value of the parameter, θ, of the Poisson probability model with $\eta = \theta E$. The parameter θ may be regarded as an index of mortality in the cohort, relative to national rates.[†] The log likelihood for θ remains Poisson in form and is plotted in Fig. 12.2.

In Bayesian statistics we start with the prior distribution for θ and multiply it by the likelihood to obtain the posterior distribution. The posterior distribution is then used to calculate the (subjective) probability that θ lies in a given range. Table 12.5 summarizes the results of such calculations for the leukaemia data for three different prior belief distributions — each of them vague in some sense.

According to these analyses, it is almost certain that there is an effect

---

[†]A fuller discussion of this model will be encountered in Chapter 15.

Table 12.6. Posterior distributions for θ for three *realistic* priors

Prior belief (90% limits)	Posterior probability distribution for θ			
		90% probability interval		Probability
	Mean	Lower limit	Upper limit	$\theta < 1.0$
0.3–2.0	2.00	0.97	3.33	0.06
0.5–1.6	1.37	0.83	2.02	0.15
0.7–1.3	1.15	0.82	1.52	0.25

of living near Sellafield and the magnitude of this effect, as measured by the mean of the posterior distribution, is very large. Unfortunately, these conclusions are not scientifically credible. Ratios of observed to expected cases of 5 are extremely rare in epidemiology when the numbers of cases are large. This is true even for studies of heavily exposed versus completely unexposed groups, and we would expect much smaller ratios for groups defined only in terms of area of residence. That 5.5 is the *lowest* plausible value for θ does not seem to be a reasonable conclusion.

The problem lies with the choice of prior distributions. Prior to seeing these data, no epidemiologist would seriously have believed that $\theta = 1000$ and $\theta = 2$ are equally probable. Bayesian analyses with more realistic prior distributions give more sensible answers. Table 12.6 shows the results of analysis for three epidemiologists with more realistic prior beliefs. All these prior distributions have mean 1.0, indicating that the epidemiologists have no prior expectation of elevated rather than reduced risk of disease, but they do differ in the *range* of values of θ, around 1.0, which they consider believable.[‡]

Exercise 12.4. With which of the three epidemiologists would you most closely identify yourself?

The conclusions of the three epidemiologists after seeing the data still differ substantially. All tend towards the belief that there is an elevated risk but the extent of the increase is now a lot less than before. The Bayesian approach has therefore shown that such a small study as this cannot lead to identical beliefs within the scientific community. The posterior distribution is too influenced by prior belief and too little by the data.

[‡]For mathematical convenience only, all three distributions have been chosen from the chi-squared family.

Solutions to the exercises

12.1 For a 15:4 split, the log likelihood is

$$15\log(\Omega) - 19\log(1 + \Omega),$$

which takes its maximum value when $\Omega = 15/4 = 3.75$. The values of the log likelihood when Ω takes on values of 3.75 and 1 are, respectively

$$15\log(3.75) - 19\log(4.75) = -9.778,$$
$$15\log(1) - 19\log(2) = -13.170.$$

The log likelihood ratio at $\Omega = 1$ is the difference between these, which is -3.392.

12.2 Fig. 12.3 shows the extension of the diagram from $N = 3$ to $N = 4$ and $N = 5$. The numbers in boldface represent the values of $C(D, N)$.

12.3 Table 12.2 shows that when the observed data are a 16:11 split, the log likelihood ratio for $\pi = 0.25$ is -7.096. The two-sided p-value is the sum of the probabilities for those outcomes leading to log likelihood ratios at least this small, that is

$$\frac{0.000128 + 0.000028 + 0.000005 + 0.000001}{+0.000423} = 0.000585.$$

12.4 There is no solution to this exercise!

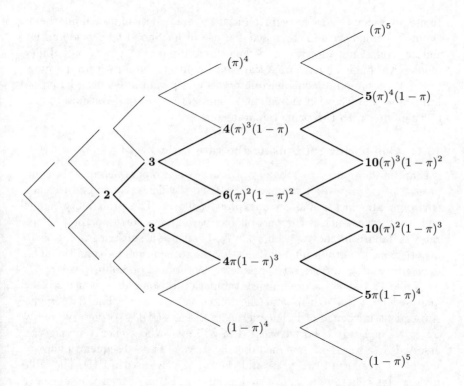

Fig. 12.3. Binomial distributions with $N = 4$ and $N = 5$.

13
Likelihoods for the rate ratio

In previous chapters we have introduced the main ideas of probability models in epidemiology and discussed the use of likelihood to provide an estimate, confidence interval or p-value for the parameter of a probability model. Although we have used the joint log likelihood for several parameters our discussion of confidence intervals and p-values has been based on probability models with only a single parameter. We now consider probability models with two or more parameters.

13.1 Comparing rates using the rate ratio

A simple and important problem which involves two parameters is the comparison of two rates, for example for a cohort which was exposed to some environmental factor and an unexposed cohort. The probability model which underlies such a comparison has parameters corresponding to the rates of failure in the two cohorts. We shall use a subscript notation to denote exposure groups and write λ_1 for the rate parameter conditional on exposure, and λ_0 for the rate parameter conditional on non-exposure.

Table 13.1 shows a preliminary tabulation of some data which will be analysed in detail in this and the following chapter.* The data relate subsequent incidence of ischaemic heart disease (IHD) to dietary energy intake. The study cohort consisted of 337 men whose energy intake was assessed by a seven-day weighed dietary survey. The subsequent follow-up was for an average of 13.7 years and yielded 45 new cases of IHD. The table divides this cohort into an exposed group consisting of men whose energy intake was less than 2750 kcals per day, the remaining men being regarded as unexposed. Although it might seem odd to denote the low energy intake group as exposed, this is because low energy intake is a surrogate measure for physical inactivity. Table 13.1 also introduces some algebraic notation: D_0, D_1 for the number of disease events observed in the unexposed and exposed cohorts respectively, and Y_0, Y_1 for the corresponding person-years observation.

---

*Unpublished data. The study is described by Morris, J.N. *et al.* (1977) *British Medical Journal*, 19 November 1977, **2**, 1307–1314.

Table 13.1.   Incidence of ischaemic heart disease by energy intake

	Energy intake	
	< 2750 kcals (exposed)	≥ 2750 kcals (unexposed)
Person years	1857.5 (Y_1)	2768.9 (Y_0)
New cases	28 (D_1)	17 (D_0)
Estimated rate	15.1	6.1
90% interval	(11.1 → 20.6)	(4.1 → 9.1)

The data from the unexposed group leads to

$$D_0 \log(\lambda_0) - \lambda_0 Y_0 = 17 \log(\lambda_0) - 2\,768.9\lambda_0$$

as the log likelihood for λ_0. The most likely value of λ_0 is the observed incidence rate, $17/2768.9 = 6.1$ per 1000 person-years. The fact that this estimate is based on only 17 observed cases is reflected in the rather wide 90% confidence interval for λ_0 stretching from 4.1 to 9.1 per 1000 person-years. Similarly, the data from the exposed group leads to

$$D_1 \log(\lambda_1) - \lambda_1 Y_1 = 28 \log(\lambda_1) - 1857.5\lambda_1$$

as the log likelihood for λ_1. The most likely value of λ_1 is $28/1857.5 = 15.1$ per 1000 person-years, and the 90% confidence interval stretches from 11.1 to 20.6 per 1000 person-years. The two groups provide independent sets of data, so that the two log likelihoods are added to yield the joint log likelihood

$$17 \log(\lambda_0) - 2\,768.9\lambda_0 + 28 \log(\lambda_1) - 1\,857.5\lambda_1.$$

This is the likelihood for any specified pair of values for the two parameters λ_0 and λ_1. Its maximum value is achieved when these parameters take values equal to the corresponding observed rates — 6.1 and 15.1 per 1000 person-years respectively.

The 90% confidence intervals for the two rates do not overlap and it might seem that the data support the proposition that the two rates are different. In general, however, the degree of overlap of confidence intervals is a poor criterion for comparing rates. If the interval in the high intake group had stretched from, say, 3.0 to 12.0 then it could be argued that, since values of the rate parameter in the range from 11.1 to 12.0 are included in both intervals, the data do not support the idea that the rates are different. The flaw in this argument is that this range is at the extreme of both ranges; the support for the proposition that the rates are similar requires two rather poorly supported propositions to hold simultaneously.

The way to approach such problems is to reparametrize the model in such a way that one of the new parameters makes a comparison. The usual comparison parameter for two rates is the *rate ratio*, which we shall denote by the Greek letter θ. Since $\theta = \lambda_1/\lambda_0$, the rate in the exposed cohort may be written as $\theta\lambda_0$ instead of λ_1 and our model can be written in terms of the parameters (θ, λ_0) instead of (λ_1, λ_0).

The log likelihood for λ_0 and λ_1 in terms of D_0, D_1, Y_0, Y_1 is

$$D_0 \log(\lambda_0) - \lambda_0 Y_0 + D_1 \log(\lambda_1) - \lambda_1 Y_1.$$

To express the log likelihood in terms of the new parameter system, we substitute $\theta\lambda_0$ for λ_1, to get

$$D_0 \log(\lambda_0) - \lambda_0 Y_0 + D_1 \log(\theta\lambda_0) - \theta\lambda_0 Y_1,$$

which reduces to

$$D \log(\lambda_0) + D_1 \log(\theta) - \lambda_0 Y_0 - \theta\lambda_0 Y_1,$$

where $D = D_0 + D_1$ is the total number of observed disease events. For the example in Table 13.1, the log likelihood is

$$45 \log(\lambda_0) + 28 \log(\theta) - 2768.9\lambda_0 - 1857.5\theta\lambda_0$$

The purpose of this choice of new parameters for the model is to concentrate the comparison of the rates into the parameter θ, but unfortunately, the log likelihood for these new parameters cannot be divided into a sum of separate parts, one for each parameter. The appearance of the term $1857.5\theta\lambda_0$ means that the shape of the log likelihood with respect to θ depends on the value of λ_0, and this is unknown. When assessing the support for different values of θ, not knowing λ_0 is somewhat of a problem and in this context λ_0 is called a *nuisance parameter*.

There are two ways of dealing with a nuisance parameter when constructing a likelihood for the parameter of interest. These will be described in the next two sections.

13.2   Profile likelihood

The obvious way to deal with a nuisance parameter is to *estimate* its value. For each value of the rate ratio θ, the value of λ_0 which maximizes the likelihood can be determined and substituted into the joint log likelihood. The resulting maximized log likelihood can then used as a measure of support for this value of θ.

This idea is illustrated in Fig. 13.1. The top graph shows the log likelihood ratio for $\log(\lambda_0)$ and $\log(\theta)$ as a contour map. The contour lines, corresponding to parameter values which have equal log likelihood, are approximately elliptical (this has been aided by the choice of log scales for both parameters, so that they are not bounded). The contours shown correspond to log likelihood ratios of -1, -2, -3, -4, and -5 relative to the maximum value.

The vertical arrows denote specified values of $\log(\theta)$ for which we require to measure the support. For each fixed value of $\log(\theta)$, we find the value of $\log(\lambda_0)$ which maximizes the log likelihood and plot this maximized log likelihood on the lower graph. This is then used to measure the relative support lent by the data to different values of $\log(\theta)$. By analogy with physical maps, this curve is called a *profile* log likelihood. A profile log likelihood is not a true log likelihood since it cannot be directly obtained by taking the log of the probability of the data. However, in most situations it behaves in exactly the same way as a log likelihood. It can be seen from Fig. 13.1 that the value of θ which gives the largest value of the profile log likelihood is also the value corresponding to the maximum of the total log likelihood. The curvature of the profile log likelihood at this maximum point can be used to calculate approximate confidence intervals and Wald tests, and score tests for null values of θ can be carried out using the gradient and curvature of the profile log likelihood at the null value. Similarly, a log likelihood ratio test can be carried out by calculating minus twice the profile log likelihood ratio at the null value of θ.

In the case of the the rate ratio, this process is simplified since the derivation of the profile log likelihood can be carried out algebraically, leading to a mathematical equation for the curve. The value of λ_0 which maximizes the log likelihood for any given value of θ may be shown to be

$$\frac{D}{Y_0 + \theta Y_1}$$

and substituting this for λ_0 in the log likelihood expression gives the profile log likelihood:

$$D_1 \log(\theta) - D \log(Y_0 + \theta Y_1) + D \log(D) - D.$$

Since the last two terms do not depend upon θ, they are irrelevant and may be omitted. We are also at liberty to *add* terms which do not involve θ, and addition of

$$D_1 \log(Y_1) + D_0 \log(Y_0)$$

yields, after some rearrangement, the expression:

$$D_1 \log \left(\frac{\theta Y_1}{Y_0} \right) - D \log \left(1 + \frac{\theta Y_1}{Y_0} \right).$$

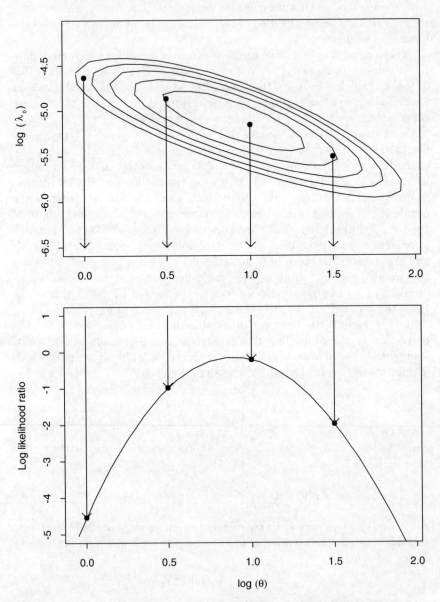

Fig. 13.1. Log likelihood surface for θ and λ (above) and profile log likelihood for θ (below).

This is exactly the same as a Bernoulli likelihood for the odds parameter

$$\Omega = \frac{\theta Y_1}{Y_0}$$

based on a split of D cases as D_1 exposed and $D_0 = D - D_1$ unexposed. It follows that estimation of θ using the profile log likelihood is equivalent to estimating the odds, Ω, in the binary model; the two estimates differ only by the known multiplier, Y_1/Y_0.

From the Bernoulli likelihood, the most likely value of Ω is D_1/D_0 and the standard deviation of $\log(\Omega)$ is

$$\sqrt{\frac{1}{D_0} + \frac{1}{D_1}}.$$

It follows that the most likely value of θ is

$$\frac{D_1/D_0}{Y_1/Y_0} = \frac{D_1/Y_1}{D_0/Y_0}$$

which is the ratio of the most likely values of the two rates and since $\log(\theta)$ differs from $\log(\Omega)$ only by a known constant, the shape of the log likelihoods are identical, and the standard deviation of $\log(\theta)$ is also

$$\sqrt{\frac{1}{D_0} + \frac{1}{D_1}}.$$

Exercise 13.1. Calculate the maximum likelihood estimate of the rate ratio for the data of Table 13.1 and give 90% confidence limits.

For the calculation of p-values, the null hypothesis generally of interest is that the two rates are equal, so that $\theta_\oslash = 1$ and $\Omega_\oslash = Y_1/Y_0$. In terms of the corresponding risk parameter the null hypothesis is that

$$\pi_\oslash = \frac{\Omega_\oslash}{1 + \Omega_\oslash} = \frac{Y_1}{Y_0 + Y_1}.$$

The score is

$$U = D_1 - D\pi_\oslash,$$

which can be written as

$$U = D_1 - E_1$$

where $E_1 = D\pi_\oslash$ is the expected number of exposed cases under the null hypothesis. The score variance is

$$V = D\pi_\oslash(1 - \pi_\oslash).$$

Exercise 13.2. Test the significance of the effect of low energy intake in the data of Table 13.1.

13.3   Conditional likelihood

The approach outlined above starts from the question: what is the probability that, during follow-up, D_0 events occur in the unexposed cohort and D_1 in the exposed cohort? The resulting likelihood involves not only the rate ratio θ (the parameter of interest), but also a nuisance parameter, λ_0. Replacing the unknown nuisance parameter by its most likely value leads to the profile log likelihood for θ. This argument is appealing in that it closely follows the way in which cohort studies are designed and executed — we decide in advance upon the cohort to be followed and the duration of follow-up and wait to see how many disease events occur in different subgroups. However, it is not essential that the likelihood argument should correspond so closely with the study design. In particular, if some aspect of the result contains little or no information about the parameter of interest, then we are free to treat it as if it were fixed by the study design. The aim of such an argument, which is called a *conditional argument*, is to obtain a new probability model for the data which does not involve the nuisance parameter.

In this case the total number of cases tells us nothing about the effect of exposure, which depends on the split among cases between exposed and not exposed. We therefore take the total number of events as fixed, corresponding to a study in which the follow-up continues for just long enough for D events to be observed. The analysis of the study then concentrates on the split of cases between the exposed and unexposed sections of the cohort, and starts from the question: given that D failures occurred, what is the probability that D_0 of them occurred in the unexposed group and D_1 in the exposed group?

The split of the D failures between exposed and unexposed groups may be described using the binary probability model. This is illustrated in Fig. 13.2. The left-hand tree shows the observed split of the failures and the right-hand tree shows the expected split of cases. If Y_1 and Y_0 can be regarded as fixed, the odds that a case was exposed is

$$\Omega = \frac{\lambda_1 Y_1}{\lambda_0 Y_0} = \frac{\theta Y_1}{Y_0},$$

and the log likelihood for θ is

$$D_1 \log\left(\frac{\theta Y_1}{Y_0}\right) - D \log\left(1 + \frac{\theta Y_1}{Y_0}\right).$$

Thus regarding the number of cases as fixed leads directly to a *conditional* log likelihood which depends only upon θ. The log likelihood is conditional

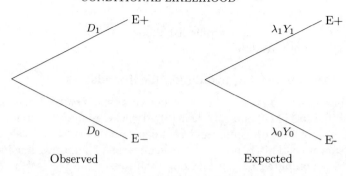

Fig. 13.2. The conditional argument.

in the sense that it takes as fixed an aspect of the data (the total number of events, D) that was, in reality, an unpredictable outcome of the study. In this case the profile and conditional likelihood approaches have led to the same log likelihood and, therefore, to identical estimates and confidence intervals, but in general this will not be the case.

The conditional approach always yields a true log likelihood, being based upon a probability (albeit a *conditional* probability) of observed data. Also, because this probability depends only on the parameter of interest, it can be used to calculate exact p-values and confidence intervals. In our current example, the probabilities for different splits of cases between exposed and unexposed groups, given θ, can be obtained from the binomial distribution. However, the conditional approach is not an automatic method, but relies on our ingenuity in recognizing a suitable conditional argument. Such arguments are not always possible. For example, it has not proved possible to find an argument which leads to a conditional likelihood for the *rate difference*, $\lambda_1 - \lambda_0$.

In contrast, the profile method has the considerable virtue that it can *always* be employed. Even if it is impossible to use an algebraic method to obtain an explicit formula for the profile log likelihood curve, the derivation of the curve numerically by the procedure illustrated in Fig. 13.1 can always be carried out by computer. The difficulty with this approach is that the profile curve is not necessarily a true log likelihood. However, in most situations it does approximately possess the properties of a true log likelihood. These properties can safely be assumed when the number of nuisance parameters is small in comparison with the total quantity of data.

We should note that our current use the conditional approach requires $\lambda_0 Y_0$ and $\lambda_1 Y_1$, the expected numbers of cases in the two groups, to be constants not influenced by the study outcome. Although this is approximately true for the rare events usually studied by epidemiologists (see section 6.3), it may not be an acceptable argument when the probabilities of failure are high. In these cases, the likelihood derived in this chapter can only be regarded as a profile likelihood and exact tests and confidence intervals are not available.

⋆ 13.4 Approximating profile log likelihoods

For the rate ratio it is possible to derive a *mathematical expression* for the profile log likelihood and hence find a Gaussian approximation from which approximate p-values and confidence intervals can be calculated in the usual way. This is not possible in general. The profile likelihood can always be computed by going through the steps indicated in Fig. 13.1, but the resulting curve usually cannot be represented by a simple algebraic expression. Fortunately some simple rules, derived from calculus, allow us to calculate Gaussian approximations to such profile log likelihoods, and hence algebraic expressions for M, S, U, and V, which we can go on to use in the usual way. These rules and their derivation are explained in Appendix C. Here we briefly summarize the most important rules.

An important general problem is the estimation of the difference between two parameters β_0 and β_1 when these are estimated from two independent bodies of data. If the log likelihood for β_0 has a Gaussian approximation defined by the most likely value M_0 and standard deviation S_0 and the approximation to the log likelihood for β_1 is defined by M_1 and S_1, then the Gaussian approximation of the log likelihood for $\beta_1 - \beta_0$ has

$$
\begin{aligned}
M &= M_1 - M_0, \\
S &= \sqrt{(S_1)^2 + (S_0)^2}.
\end{aligned}
$$

The rate ratio is a special case of this more general problem since its logarithm may be written

$$
\log\left(\frac{\lambda_1}{\lambda_0}\right) = \log(\lambda_1) - \log(\lambda_0)
$$

and in Appendix C it is shown that these rules lead to the same Gaussian log likelihood approximation as we obtained earlier. Here we use them to approximate the profile log likelihood for the rate difference. The most likely value is the difference between the most likely values of the rates,

$$
M = \frac{D_1}{Y_1} - \frac{D_0}{Y_0},
$$

and, from Chapter 9, $S_1 = \sqrt{D_1}/Y_1$ and $S_0 = \sqrt{D_0}/Y_0$ so the value of S for the rate difference is

$$
\sqrt{\frac{D_1}{(Y_1)^2} + \frac{D_0}{(Y_0)^2}}.
$$

Exercise 13.3. Calculate an approximate 90% confidence interval for the difference between the rates using the data of Table 13.1.

A still more general problem concerns a weighted sum of parameters, of the form

$$W_1\beta_1 + W_2\beta_2 + W_3\beta_3 + \cdots \qquad ,$$

each β parameter again being estimated from independent bodies of data. The Gaussian approximation to the profile log likelihood for the weighted sum has

$$
\begin{aligned}
M &= W_1M_1 + W_2M_2 + W_3M_3 + \cdots \\
S &= \sqrt{(W_1S_1)^2 + (W_2S_2)^2 + (W_3S_3)^2 + \cdots} \qquad ,
\end{aligned}
$$

where $M_1, S_1, \ldots$ etc. are the most likely values and standard deviations for $\beta_1, \ldots$ etc.. An example is the profile log likelihood for the cumulative failure rate. In Chapter 5 we defined the cumulative rate by

$$\lambda^1 T^1 + \lambda^2 T^2 + \cdots$$

where $\lambda^1, \lambda^2, \ldots$ are probability rates operating for time periods $T^1, T^2, \ldots$. The cumulative rate is, therefore, a weighted sum of the form discussed in this section.

Exercise 13.4. Using the Gaussian approximation given in Chapter 9 for the log likelihoods for rate parameters, derive an expression for the Gaussian approximation to the profile log likelihood for the cumulative rate.

Solutions to the exercises

13.1 The most likely value of θ is

$$\frac{D_1/Y_1}{D_0/Y_0} = \frac{28/1857.5}{17/2768.9} = 2.48.$$

The standard deviation of the estimate of $\log(\theta)$, is

$$S = \sqrt{1/28 + 1/17} = 0.3075,$$

so that the 90% error factor for θ is

$$\exp(1.645 \times 0.3075) = 1.66.$$

The 90% confidence limits for the rate ratio are $2.48/1.66 = 1.49$ (lower limit) and $2.48 \times 1.66 = 4.12$ (upper limit).

13.2   The observed number of events in the low energy intake group is 28. There were 45 events in total and, under the null hypothesis, the probability of having been exposed is $\pi_0 = 1857.5/4626.4 = 0.402$. The score is

$$U = 28 - 45 \times 0.402 = 9.93,$$

and the score variance is

$$V = 45 \times 0.402 \times (1 - 0.402) = 10.81.$$

The score test is $(U)^2/V = 9.12$, giving $p \approx 0.003$.

13.3

$$M = \frac{28}{1857.5} - \frac{17}{2768.9} = 0.00893 \ (8.93 \text{ per } 1000 \text{ person-years}).$$

$$S = \sqrt{\frac{28}{(1857.5)^2} + \frac{17}{(2768.9)^2}} = 0.00321 \ (3.21 \text{ per } 1000 \text{ person-years}).$$

The 90% confidence interval is

$$M \pm 1.645S = 3.65 \text{ to } 14.2 \text{ per } 1000 \text{ person-years}.$$

13.4   The log likelihood for λ^1 is approximated by a Gaussian curve with

$$M^1 = \frac{D^1}{Y^1}, \qquad S^1 = \frac{\sqrt{D^1}}{Y^1}.$$

Similarly for $\lambda^2, \lambda^3, \ldots$ etc. The weights are the durations of observation, $T^1, T^2, \ldots$, so that the profile log likelihood for the cumulative rate has its maximum at

$$M = \frac{D^1}{Y^1}T^1 + \frac{D^2}{Y^2}T^2 + \cdots$$

and the standard deviation of the Gaussian approximation is

$$S = \sqrt{D^1 \left(\frac{T_1}{Y^1}\right)^2 + D^2 \left(\frac{T^2}{Y^2}\right)^2 + \cdots}.$$

Note that, as we narrow the time bands to clicks, the ratio T/Y approaches $1/N$, where N is the number of subjects under observation during the click. In these circumstances, M is the Aalen–Nelson estimate of the cumulative rate and S may be used to calculate an approximate confidence interval.

14
Confounding and standardization

14.1 Confounding

Epidemiological studies generally involve comparing the outcome over a period of time for groups of subjects experiencing different levels of exposure. Such studies are usually not controlled experiments but 'experiments of nature' of which the epidemiologist is a passive observer. In such investigations, there is always the possibility that an important influence on the outcome, which would have been fixed in a controlled experiment, differs systematically between the comparison groups. It is then possible that part of an apparent effect of exposure is due to these differences, and the comparison of the exposure groups is said to be *confounded*. Statistical approaches to dealing with the problem of confounding aim to correct, during analysis, for such deficiencies in the design of experiments of nature.

A particularly important potential confounding variable (or *confounder* in many epidemiological studies is the age of subjects. We shall consider an example in which subjects in a follow-up study are classified according to whether their age at the start of follow-up was less than 55 years or 55 years or more. Suppose that the breakdown between the two age groups is 0.8 : 0.2 and that the conditional probability of failure is 0.1 in the first age group and 0.3 in the second. When age is ignored the overall or *marginal* probability of failure is

$$(0.8 \times 0.1) + (0.2 \times 0.3) = 0.14.$$

Now suppose that the age distribution differs between the two exposure groups, being 0.8 : 0.2 in the not exposed group but 0.4 : 0.6 in the exposed group (see Fig. 14.1). The marginal probability of failure for the unexposed group is still

$$(0.8 \times 0.1) + (0.2 \times 0.3) = 0.14,$$

but for the exposed group it is now

$$(0.4 \times 0.1) + (0.6 \times 0.3) = 0.22.$$

The marginal probabilities of failure now suggest an apparent effect of

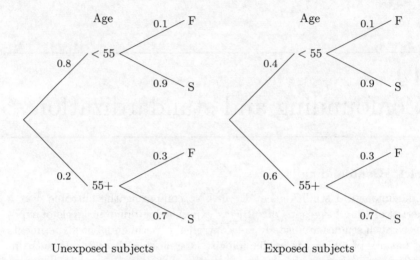

Unexposed subjects   Exposed subjects

Fig. 14.1.   Confounding by age.

exposure, but this is entirely due to the difference in age distributions between the exposed and unexposed subjects.

In this example the apparent effect of exposure is entirely due to age differences but confounding may also be partial, acting either to exaggerate or to dilute a real relationship. As an example of this, suppose the effect of exposure is to raise the probability of failure from 0.1 to 0.2 in the younger age group and from 0.3 to 0.5 for older subjects. When the age distribution is 0.8 : 0.2 in both exposure groups the overall effect of exposure is to increase the marginal probability of failure from

$$(0.8 \times 0.1) + (0.2 \times 0.3) = 0.14$$

in the unexposed group to

$$(0.8 \times 0.2) + (0.2 \times 0.5) = 0.26$$

in the exposed group. When the age distribution is 0.8 : 0.2 in the unexposed group and 0.4 : 0.6 in the exposed group the overall effect of exposure is to increase the marginal failure probability of failure from

$$(0.8 \times 0.1) + (0.2 \times 0.3) = 0.14$$

in the unexposed group to

$$(0.4 \times 0.2) + (0.6 \times 0.5) = 0.38$$

in the exposed group. Thus the overall effect of exposure appears greater when the age distributions differ than when they are the same.

These examples demonstrate that a third variable, such as age, can distort the relationship between an exposure and failure provided it is related to both exposure and failure. This dual relationship is often taken as the definition of a confounder. However, although it is a necessary condition for a variable to be a confounder, it is not sufficient: a confounder must also be a variable which would have been held constant in a controlled experiment. For example, in perinatal epidemiology, we might ask whether birthweight could be regarded as confounding the relationship between the receipt of proper antenatal care and the risk of perinatal death. Although birthweight is related to both antenatal care and perinatal risk, it cannot be regarded as a confounder since one of the *results* of successful antenatal care should be adequate birthweights. Since it would not make sense to envisage an experiment in which we varied the provision of antenatal care while maintaining the distribution of birthweight constant, differences in birthweight distribution cannot be regarded as a deficiency in the design of the experiment of nature. It is not, therefore, a confounder.

14.2   Correction for confounding

The linking of confounding to an imaginary experiment helps to clarify the ideas which lie behind statistical methods for dealing with the problem. There are two rather different approaches, and these closely mimic the ways in which extraneous influences are dealt with in experimental science.

The classical approach to experimentation is to hold constant all influences other than the experimental variable(s) of interest. For example, to avoid confounding by age, we would simply compare failure risks in exposed and unexposed subjects *of a fixed age* or, at least, falling within a narrow range of ages. The statistical comparison would then be of failure probabilities conditional upon age. The same comparison can be made in an non-experimental study by the analytical strategy called *stratification*. By dividing (or stratifying) the data according to age, the single experiment of nature in which age has not been adequately controlled is transformed into a series of smaller experiments within which age is closely controlled. The analysis then compares probabilities of failure between exposure groups within age bands. However, a consequence of this strategy is that individual strata may contain too little data to be informative on their own. The more finely we stratify the data, the more closely we control for confounding, but the sparser our data becomes within strata. This impasse may only be broken by making the further assumption that the comparisons estimate the same quantity within each stratum, and then combining the information from the separate strata. We shall defer further discussion of this approach to Chapter 15.

Holding extraneous variables constant is not the only model for good experimentation, although it is certainly the most familiar. In the twentieth century, experimentation has become a valuable tool in fields of study such as biology, in which such close control of experimental material and conditions is not possible. The idea of *randomization* has been central to this development; if we cannot ensure that experimental groups are identical in all important respects, then by assigning subjects to groups *at random*, we ensure that the probability distributions for extraneous variables do not differ between exposure groups. Comparisons between the groups can then be safely made.

Returning to the comparison of failure probabilities between exposure groups, it is rarely possible, in epidemiology, to use randomization to ensure that extraneous variables have equal distributions in the different exposure groups. However, it is possible to take account of differences in the distribution of a specific variable, such as age, by predicting the outcome for exposure groups which have the same age distribution. This is done by first estimating the age-specific probabilities of failure for each exposure group, and then using these to predict the marginal probabilities of failure for exposure groups which have a standard age distribution. This forms the basis of the second statistical approach to dealing with confounding, known in epidemiology as *direct standardization*.

14.3   Standardized rates

The remainder of this chapter concerns the use of direct standardization to compare *rates*. Since rates are probabilities per unit time they can be compared in the same way as failure probabilities. Age-specific failure rates are estimated for each of the groups being compared, and these are used to predict the marginal rates which would have been observed if the age distributions in the comparison groups had been the same as the standard age distribution. These estimates are called *standardized rates*.

The choice of the age distribution to use for standardization depends on the purpose of the analysis. It is quite common for the overall distribution of age, added over exposure groups, to be used as the standard, thus simulating the results of an experiment in which the total study group was randomly allocated between exposure categories. However, if one of our aims is to facilitate comparisons with other published studies, it is more useful to use an age distribution which is in general use. Several distributions are commonly used for this purpose. One is the age distribution of the world population, another is the age distribution for developed countries. Since there is no 'correct' standard there is much to be said in favour of using a *uniform* age distribution where the percentage falling in each age group is the same. One advantage of using a uniform age distribution is that the standardized rate is then directly proportional to the *cumulative rate* for a subject experiencing the age-specific rates from the study

Table 14.1.   IHD incidence rates per 1000 person-years

Age	Exposed (< 2750 kcal)			Unexposed (≥ 2750 kcal)		
	Cases	P-yrs	Rate	Cases	P-yrs	Rate
40–49	2	311.9	6.41	4	607.9	6.58
50–59	12	878.1	13.67	5	1272.1	3.93
60–69	14	667.5	20.97	8	888.9	9.00
Total	28	1857.5	15.07	17	2768.9	6.14

throughout life.

Direct standardization is most commonly used when comparing quite large groups, such as the populations of different countries or regions. When used with less extensive data it will yield statistically unreliable estimates if some of the age-specific rates, although based on very few cases, receive appreciable weight in the analysis.

To illustrate the technique of direct standardization we shall return to study of ischaemic heart disease and energy intake, discussed in Chapter 13. The incidence of ischaemic heart disease in the exposed group (low energy-intake) is 15.1 per 1000 person-years while the rate in the unexposed group is 6.1 per 1000 person-years. These rates, which take no account of any possible confounding effect of age, are often referred to as *crude* rates to distinguish them from standardized rates.

Table 14.1 shows the data stratified by 10-year age bands. The age distribution is different in the two exposure groups; this may be seen by converting the person-years to a proportion of the total person-years in each group giving 0.168, 0.472, and 0.359 in the three age bands for the exposed (low energy-intake) group and 0.210, 0.459, and 0.321 for the unexposed (high energy-intake) group. These age differences might explain some of the difference in the crude IHD incidence rates.

Using the uniform age distribution as standard, our estimate of the marginal rate for a group of exposed subjects with a uniform age distribution is

$$(0.333 \times 6.41) + (0.333 \times 13.67) + (0.333 \times 20.97) = 13.67$$

per 1000 person years and, for a group of unexposed subjects with a uniform age distribution, it is

$$(0.333 \times 6.58) + (0.333 \times 3.93) + (0.333 \times 9.00) = 6.50$$

per 1000 person-years. The standardized rates for the two groups are therefore 13.7 and 6.5 per 1000 person-years. These do not differ greatly from the crude rates of 15.1 and 6.1 per 1000 person-years, showing that the confounding effect of age is small in this case.

Exercise 14.1. Find the standardized rates for the exposed and not exposed groups using as standard the age distribution with probabilities of 0.2, 0.5, and 0.3 in the three age bands.

★ ## 14.4 Approximating the log likelihood

When there are three age bands, as in the IHD and energy example, the standardized rate parameter takes the form of a weighted sum of the age-specific rate parameters,

$$W^1\lambda^1 + W^2\lambda^2 + W^3\lambda^3,$$

where

$$\lambda^1, \lambda^2, \lambda^3$$

are the rate parameters for the age bands and

$$W^1, W^2, W^3$$

are the probabilities of the standard age distribution. Since λ^1, λ^2 and λ^3 have independent log likelihoods, we can use the ideas introduced in section 13.4 and Appendix C to derive a Gaussian approximation to the profile log likelihood for the standardized rate. The most likely value is

$$W^1M^1 + W^2M^2 + W^3M^3$$

where $M^1 = D^1/Y^1$ is the most likely value of the age-specific rate parameter in band 1, and similarly expressions hold for bands 2 and 3. The standard deviation of the Gaussian approximation is

$$\sqrt{(W^1S^1)^2 + (W^2S^2)^2 + (W^3S^3)^2}$$

where $S^1 = \sqrt{D^1}/Y^1$ is the standard deviation of the Gaussian approximation to the log likelihood for λ^1, again with similar expressions for bands 2 and 3.

For the IHD and energy example the proability weights are

$$W^1 = W^2 = W^3 = 0.333.$$

The age-specific rate for the first age band of the exposed group is 6.41 and the corresponding standard deviation is

$$\sqrt{2}/311.9 = 0.00453,$$

or 4.53 per 1000 person-years. The most likely values for the rates in the other two age bands are 13.67 and 20.97 with standard deviations 3.94 and

5.61 per 1000 person-years. The standard deviation of the standardized rate is therefore

$$\sqrt{(0.333 \times 4.53)^2 + (0.333 \times 3.94)^2 + (0.333 \times 5.61)^2} = 2.74$$

per 1000 person-years.

Exercise 14.2. Show that the standard deviation of the standardized rate for the unexposed group is 1.63 per 1000 person-years.

LOG TRANSFORMATION OF STANDARDIZED RATES

Just as for any other rate, Gaussian approximations to the log likelihood are more accurate when related to the *log* of the standardized rate. The most likely value on the log scale is, of course, just the log of the standardized rate, and the corresponding standard deviation can be calculated by using the rule described in Chapter 9. There we saw that the standard deviation of the Gaussian approximation to the likelihood for $\log(\lambda)$ is obtained from the standard deviation of the Gaussian approximation to the likelihood for λ by multiplying by $1/M$, where M is most likely value of λ. It follows that for the example of energy intake and IHD incidence, the standard deviations of the standardized rates on a log scale are $2.74/13.67 = 0.200$ and $1.63/6.50 = 0.251$.

A simple extension of the same ideas allows us to calculate estimates and confidence intervals for the ratio of two standardized rates. The log of this ratio is equal to the difference between the logarithms of the two standardized rates, and from section 13.4 and Appendix C the standard deviation of the log of the ratio of the standardized rates is

$$\sqrt{(0.200)^2 + (0.251)^2} = 0.321.$$

This can be used to obtain a confidence interval for the ratio of the standardized rates by using the error factor

$$\exp(1.645 \times 0.321) = 1.696.$$

Exercise 14.3. Use this error factor to find an approximate 90% confidence interval for the ratio of the two standardized rate parameters.

Solutions to the exercises

14.1 The estimated standardized rates are

$$(0.2 \times 6.41) + (0.5 \times 13.67) + (0.3 \times 20.97) = 14.41$$

for the exposed group, and

$$(0.2 \times 6.58) + (0.5 \times 3.93) + (0.3 \times 9.00) = 5.98$$

for the unexposed group.

14.2 The standard deviations of the age-specific rates are 3.29, 1.76, and 3.18 respectively. The standard deviation of the standardized rate is

$$\sqrt{(0.333 \times 3.29)^2 + (0.333 \times 1.76)^2 + (0.333 \times 3.18)^2} = 1.63.$$

14.3 The ratio of standardized rates is $13.67/6.50 = 2.10$ and the 90% range for this is from $2.10/1.696 = 1.24$ to $2.10 \times 1.696 = 3.56$.

15
Comparison of rates within strata

15.1 The proportional hazards model

Direct standardization is a very simple way of correcting for confounding but it does have some limitations. This chapter deals with the alternative and more generally useful approach of stratification. We shall again illustrate our argument using the study of the relationship between energy intake and IHD first introduced in Chapter 13 and further analysed in Chapter 14. There, in Table 14.1, we showed the data stratified by 10-year age bands and demonstrated that the low energy intake group is, on average, rather older. This might explain some, or all, of the increase in IHD incidence rate. The method of direct standardization predicts the marginal rates for energy intake groups with the same standard age distribution. This chapter explores the alternative approach which compares age-specific rates within strata. Table 15.1 extends Table 14.1 by calculating rate ratios within each age band. This demonstrates the main problem with this approach to confounding; holding age constant and making comparisons within age strata leads to variable and unreliable estimates, because the age-specific rates are based on so few data.

This problem is resolved is by combining the age-specific comparisons from the separate strata, but any such procedure carries with it a further modelling assumption, because combining the age-specific comparisons can only be legitimate if we believe that they all estimate the same underlying quantity. If we are prepared to believe that the rate ratio between exposure

Table 15.1. Rate ratios within age strata

Age	Exposed (< 2750 kcal)			Unexposed (≥ 2750 kcal)			Rate ratio
	D	Y	Rate	D	Y	Rate	
40–49	2	311.9	6.41	4	607.9	6.58	0.97
50–59	12	878.1	13.67	5	1272.1	3.93	3.48
60–69	14	667.5	20.97	8	888.9	9.00	2.33
Total	28	1857.5	15.07	17	2768.9	6.14	2.45

groups is constant across age-bands, the evidence from the three bands can be brought together to provide a single estimate of the (constant) age-specific rate ratio. Of course the model on which the estimate is based, like all models, is open to question and in later chapters we shall discuss ways in which we can test whether it holds. For the present, we shall be content to believe that the model holds in our example, and that the fluctuation of age-specific rate ratios in Table 15.1 is no more than we would expect given the small numbers of cases in each age band.

Our notation follows naturally from earlier chapters. The age bands are indexed by the superscript t and exposure groups are indexed by subscripts, so that λ_0^t and λ_1^t are the rate parameters in age band t for the unexposed and exposed subjects respectively. We shall write the rate ratio parameter as θ, so that the model of constant rate ratio may be written

$$\frac{\lambda_1^t}{\lambda_0^t} = \theta.$$

This is called the *proportional hazards* model. The parameter θ is called the rate ratio for exposure *controlled for* age, sometimes abbreviated to the *effect* of exposure controlled for age. In this chapter we discuss how θ can be estimated.

15.2   The likelihood for θ

When the rate ratio is constant across age bands, we can replace the rate parameters λ_1^t by $\theta\lambda_0^t$. In our example, this reparametrization replaces the original six rate parameters, which we assume to be constrained to obey the proportional hazards model, with four parameters which are free to take any positive value. One parameter, namely the rate ratio θ, is our prime interest, and the remaining three are regarded as nuisance parameters.

Since each age band serves as an independent study, it is a simple matter to write down the log likelihood for a stratified comparison. Constructing the log likelihood using the prospective argument, each age band contributes a term which depends upon θ and the appropriate λ_0^t. The total likelihood is obtained by adding these terms over age bands. For comparing rates between exposed and unexposed subjects, the parameters λ_0^t are nuisance parameters. As in Chapter 13, replacing these by their most likely value for given θ leads to a profile log likelihood for θ. With the caveat expressed at the end of section 13.3, this log likelihood can also be justified as a conditional likelihood based on the split of cases within each stratum.

The log likelihood ratio curve for $\log(\theta)$ in our illustrative example is shown in Figure 15.1. Using a computer, it is a simple matter to find the most likely value, M, and to use the curvature of the log likelihood ratio to compute a Gaussian approximation. In this case $M = 0.8697$

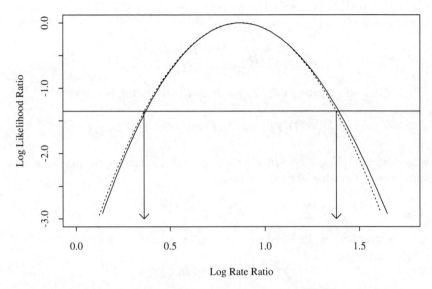

Fig. 15.1. Log likelihood ratio for the common rate ratio.

and $S = 0.3080$, and this approximation is shown as a broken line in the figure. The most likely value of the rate ratio is $\exp(0.8697) = 2.386$ and confidence intervals can be calculated using the error factor:

$$\exp(1.645 \times 0.3080) = 1.660.$$

The fact that the high energy-intake group is, on average, slightly younger than the low energy-intake group is the reason why the estimate of the rate ratio controlled for age is slightly smaller than the crude rate ratio (2.45). However, the difference is extremely small. This is not unusual; rather large differences between exposure groups in important variables are necessary for the effect of confounding to be appreciable.

Unfortunately it is not possible to calculate the values of M and S by hand using simple formulae. The computer programs which are used to carry out such computations are very flexible and allow more complicated models to be fitted. Accordingly discussion of these will be postponed until Part II and the remainder of this chapter will deal with methods which require only a hand calculator.

15.3   A nearly most likely value for θ

We saw in Chapter 13 that, in an unstratified analysis, both profile and conditional arguments led to the Bernoulli likelihood

$$D_1 \log(\Omega) - D \log(1 + \Omega),$$

where Ω, the odds for a case having been exposed, is $\theta Y_1/Y_0$. The gradient of the curve of log likelihood versus $\log(\theta)$ is

$$D_1 - D\frac{\Omega}{1 + \Omega}$$

which, after substituting $\theta Y_1/Y_0$ for Ω and rearranging becomes

$$\frac{1}{Y_0 + \theta Y_1}\left(D_1 Y_0 - \theta D_0 Y_1\right) = W\left(D_1 Y_0 - \theta D_0 Y_1\right),$$

where $W = 1/(Y_0 + \theta Y_1)$. In a stratified analysis, the log likelihood is the sum of contributions of each stratum,

$$\sum \left[D_1^t \log(\Omega^t) - D^t \log(1 + \Omega^t)\right]$$

and the gradient is similarly constructed by adding up gradient contributions:

$$\sum W^t\left(D_1^t Y_0^t - \theta D_0^t Y_1^t\right),$$

where $W^t = 1/(Y_0^t + \theta Y_1^t)$ are stratum *weights*.

The most likely value of θ occurs where the gradient is zero, that is, at

$$\theta = \frac{\sum W^t D_1^t Y_0^t}{\sum W^t D_0^t Y_1^t}.$$

Since calculation of the weights W^t involves θ, and this equation cannot be used directly to find the most likely value. However, it can be used *iteratively* as follows:

1. guess a value for θ, and use this to calculate initial weights;
2. using these, calculate a first estimate of θ;
3. using this new estimate, calculate more accurate weights.

The sequence of calculations may be repeated until there is no change in the estimate. Computer programs for maximum likelihood estimation use similar iterative methods of computation.

In practice, the estimate obtained is not very sensitive to changes in the values of the weights — rather large changes make only a relatively small difference to the estimate. Additionally, it may be argued that it is only really important to achieve the closest approximation to the log likelihood when estimating rate ratios which are fairly close to 1. These considerations suggest using the weights corresponding to the choice $\theta = 1$, and to go no further with the calculations. These weights are the reciprocal of the person-years observations in each age band:

$$W^t = \frac{1}{Y_0^t + Y_1^t} = \frac{1}{Y^t}.$$

Use of these weights leads to the *Mantel–Haenszel* estimate of the rate ratio*,

$$\frac{\sum D_1^t Y_0^t / Y^t}{\sum D_0^t Y_1^t / Y^t}.$$

In this expression, each age band makes contributions of

$$Q^t = \frac{D_1^t Y_0^t}{Y^t}, \qquad\qquad R^t = \frac{D_0^t Y_1^t}{Y^t}$$

to the top (numerator) and bottom (denominator) of the estimate respectively. The estimate of the rate ratio for age band t is Q^t/R^t and the combined estimate of the constant rate ratio is Q/R, where $Q = \sum Q^t$ and $R = \sum R^t$.

Exercise 15.1. Calculate Q^t and R^t for each of the three age bands in Table 15.1, and hence calculate the Mantel–Haenszel estimate of the rate ratio. Compare this with the most likely value.

15.4 Calculating p-values and confidence intervals

Approximate p-values are most easily calculated using the score test. Since the log likelihood for θ for the age-stratified comparison is the sum of contributions from each age band, it follows that its gradient, and hence the *score*, is the sum of scores for each stratum. Similarly, the curvature is the sum of the curvatures of the separate contribution of each stratum so that the overall score variance is the sum of score variances for each stratum. That is,

$$U = \sum U^t, \qquad\qquad V = \sum V^t.$$

Thus to carry out the test we first calculate scores and score variances for each stratum separately and then sum these over strata to obtain the total score and score variance. We then compare $(U)^2/V$ with the chi-squared distribution in the usual way. The contribution of stratum t to the score and score variance are of the same form as given at the end of section 13.2, namely

$$U^t = D_1^t - D^t \pi_{\oslash}^t, \qquad\qquad V^t = D^t \pi_{\oslash}^t (1 - \pi_{\oslash}^t),$$

where $\pi_{\oslash}^t = Y_1^t/Y^t$, the ratio of exposed to total person years.

Exercise 15.2. For our example, what is the p-value for the null hypothesis that, after controlling for age, the rate ratio is 1.

---

*In fact Mantel and Haenszel did not propose *this* method but an extremely similar one for case-control studies. We shall discuss this in Chapter 18.

As before, the value of U may be interpreted as the difference between the number of cases who had been exposed and the number expected under the null hypothesis, taking into account the age structures of exposed and unexposed groups.

The calculation of the score variance, V, also allows us to calculate an approximate confidence interval around the Mantel–Haenszel estimate. A Gaussian approximation on the $\log(\theta)$ scale, with

$$S = \sqrt{\frac{V}{QR}}.$$

can be used to calculate an error factor and the approximate confidence interval in the usual way.[†]

Exercise 15.3. Calculate the standard deviation, S, of the log Mantel-Haenzsel estimate for the energy intake data. Use this to calculate a 90% confidence interval for the rate ratio adjusted for age.

These results are very close to those obtained using a computer program to find the Gaussian approximation to the log likelihood curve. The computer method is better in the sense that, as the quantity of data increases, the approximate interval of support approachs the correct likelihood-based interval, while the Mantel–Haenszel interval remains *slightly* wider no matter how much data we collect. The discrepancy is rarely important.

★ **15.5   The log-rank test**

Our example in this chapter has involved stratification by a time scale, age, into three rather broad bands. In clinical follow-up studies time is measured from diagnosis or start of treatment and the incidence of events may vary rapidly, requiring the choice of narrow bands. This, together with the fact that choice of bands may introduce an arbitrary element into the analysis, has led to the popularity of a version of the test in which time is stratified infinitely finely into clicks, with no click containing any more than one event. This test is called the *log rank*[‡] or *Mantel–Cox* test.

Derivation of this test from that of the previous section is straightforward. The first thing to notice is that clicks which contain no event (i.e. with $D^t = 0$) make no contribution either to the score, U, or the score variance, V. We therefore need only consider those clicks in which we observe the occurrence of an event in one of the groups ($D^t = 1$). These are are

---

[†]This approximation is not widely known, but it would not appropriate to justify it here. It suffices to say that it is adequate for all our purposes.

[‡]This nomenclature may seem rather obscure, since the calculation of the test requires neither logarithms or ranks! It arises from an alternative derivation.

Table 15.2.   Survival times in two groups of patients

Group	Time (days)
Test treatment	$86, 99^*, 119^*, 123^*, 139^*, 161^*, 185^*, 212^*, 231, 253^*,$
($N = 20$)	$262^*, 281^*, 303^*, 355^*, 360^*, 380^*, 392, 467^*, 499^*, 514^*$
Control	$73, 91, 102^*, 120^*, 135, 160^*, 194, 202^*, 209^*, 220^*,$
($N = 20$)	$252, 270^*, 296, 330^*, 347^*, 375^*, 390^*, 414, 475^*, 485^*$

known as *informative* time points.[§] Since each click is very short, we need not consider variation in the time spent by different subjects in the band, and the null probability that a failure was exposed becomes

$$\pi_{\oslash}^t = \frac{N_1^t}{N^t} = \frac{\text{Number of } \textit{exposed} \text{ subjects in study at time } t}{\textit{Total} \text{ number of subjects in study at time } t}.$$

Each failure makes a contribution to the score of the difference between the observed number of events in the exposed group, which is either 0 or 1, and the expected number, which is simply $\pi_{\oslash}^t$. The score variance is obtained by adding the contributions

$$V^t = \pi_{\oslash}^t(1 - \pi_{\oslash}^t).$$

Exercise 15.4. Table 15.2 shows times between entry to a clinical trial and relapse for patients receiving two methods of therapy. (The data are only illustrative — a real trial with so much censoring would need to be much larger than this!) The times marked with an asterisk represent times at which observation ceased without occurrence of relapse. Construct a table showing the times of occurrence of relapses, the number of patients in each group under study at each of these times, and the corresponding observed and expected relapses in the test group. Use this table to carry out the score test.

15.6   Comparison with reference rates: the SMR

An important special case concerns the comparison of age-specific rates in a study cohort, λ^t, with those in a *reference population*, which we shall denote by λ_R^t. We have discussed this informally in Chapter 6. A more formal treatment follows as a simple case of the methods discussed above.

The proportional hazards model holds that the ratio of age-specific rates in the study cohort to the reference rates is constant across age bands,

$$\frac{\lambda^t}{\lambda_R^t} = \theta.$$

[§]Since clicks have no duration, we assume that no more than one event occurs at any time point.

If we observe D^t failures in Y^t person years of observation in each age band of the cohort, the log likelihood contribution is

$$D^t \log(\lambda^t) - \lambda^t Y^t$$

and making the substitution $\lambda^t = \theta \lambda_{\mathrm{R}}^t$ this becomes

$$D^t \log(\theta) + D^t \log(\lambda_{\mathrm{R}}^t) - \theta \lambda_{\mathrm{R}}^t Y^t.$$

Since the reference rates λ_{R}^t are calculated from very large populations, they are effectively known constants, and the above log likelihood depends only on one unknown parameter, θ. The second term in the log likelihood does not depend on θ and can be ignored, and the third term may be simplified after noting that $\lambda_{\mathrm{R}}^t Y^t$ is the expected number of failures obtained by multiplying the age-specific reference rate by the corresponding person-years of observation of the study cohort (see Chapter 6). Denoting this by E^t, the log likelihood contribution of one age band becomes

$$D^t \log(\theta) - \theta E^t$$

and summation over age bands leads to the total log likelihood

$$D \log(\theta) - \theta E,$$

where D, E are the total observed and expected numbers of failures. This is a Poisson log likelihood, but the rate ratio parameter θ replaces the rate parameter λ, and the expected number of failures E replaces the person-years Y. Thus estimating θ in this case is just the same as estimating a rate. The most likely value is the ratio of observed to expected cases, D/E, and in epidemiology this is called the standardized mortality ratio, or *SMR*. A 90% confidence interval can be calculated using the error factor

$$\exp\left(1.645\sqrt{\frac{1}{D}}\right).$$

An approximate p-value for the null hypothesis $\theta = 1$ can be carried out using the score and score variance

$$U = D - E, \qquad V = E.$$

Comparison of rates with reference rates in this way is known in epidemiology as *indirect standardization*.

Exercise 15.5. In the follow-up study of ankylosing spondylitis patients discussed in Chapter 6, the observed number of deaths from leukaemia was 31 while the expected number calculated from reference rates was 6.47. Calculate the 90% confidence interval for the common ratio of cohort age-specific rates to reference rates. Also calculate an approximate p-value for the null hypothesis $\theta = 1$.

Exercise 15.6. The calculation of the expected number of deaths in the ankylosing spondilitis study was based on person-years classified by both age and calendar period (see Chapter 6). What further modelling assumption is formally necessary to justify the analysis carried out in the previous exercise?

15.7 Comparing standardized rates

We showed in Chapter 14 that standardized rates estimate the marginal rates when the age distributions are corrected to a common standard. These are weighted sums of age-specific rates. In the case of three age bands, the marginal rate is

$$W^1\lambda^1 + W^2\lambda^2 + W^3\lambda^3$$

where (W^1, W^2, W^3) are the relative frequencies of the three age bands in the standard distribution, and the ratio of two marginal rates, corrected to the same age distribution, is

$$\frac{W^1\lambda_1^1 + W^2\lambda_1^2 + W^3\lambda_1^3}{W^1\lambda_0^1 + W^2\lambda_0^2 + W^3\lambda_0^3}.$$

When the proportional hazards model holds, every term in the numerator of this expression is θ times the corresponding term in the denominator, and it follows that the ratio of marginal rates will also be θ — the relationship between marginal rates is the same as that between the conditional (age-specific) rates. Thus, the ratio of standardized rates can be used as an estimate of θ. However it may not be a very good estimate if the standard age distribution gives high weight to age bands with few failures.

Note that the equivalence demonstrated above between the conditional and marginal comparisons does not hold for *all* stratification models. For example, if the ratio of the age-specific *odds* of failure for exposed and unexposed subjects is a constant, θ, for all ages then the ratio of marginal odds is not equal to θ, even when there is no confounding and the age distributions are identical. Thus we cannot always rely on the method of direct standardization if we are interested in comparisons within strata. In Chapter 18 we shall encounter an important example of this.

15.8 Comparison of SMRs

Although the ratio of standardized rates can be used as an alternative estimate of θ, there has been some controversy as to whether the ratio of two SMRs can also be used in this way.

An understanding of the formal model which lies behind indirect standardization clarifies this argument. Calculation of an SMR for an exposed cohort, using reference rates λ_R^t implies the model

$$\lambda_1^t = \theta_1 \lambda_R^t,$$

where θ_1 is the constant ratio of rates in this cohort to reference rates. Similarly, calculation of an SMR for an unexposed cohort implies the model

$$\lambda_0^t = \theta_0 \lambda_R^t.$$

A direct consequence of these two models is that the ratio of rates for the two cohorts is also constant across age. This can be demonstrated by simply dividing the two equations, when λ_R^t cancels leaving

$$\frac{\lambda_1^t}{\lambda_0^t} = \frac{\theta_1}{\theta_0} = \theta.$$

Thus if the age-specific rates for both exposed and unexposed cohorts are proportional to the reference rates, the comparison of SMRs is legitimate. Since the likelihoods for θ_1 and θ_0 are Poisson in form, with expected numbers of failures E_1 and E_0 replacing person-years observation Y_1 and Y_0, the likelihood for their ratio, θ, is the same as for the rate ratio in Chapter 13.

This method, however, relies on the assumption that both sets of age-specific rates are proportional to the reference rates. If they are proportional to each other, but not to the reference rates, then the ratio of SMRs will not correctly estimate the rate ratio θ. Because of this additional assumption concerning reference rates, estimation of θ by the ratio of SMRs is not usually to be recommended.

Solutions to the exercises

15.1 The calculations are as follows:

Age	Q^t	R^t
40–49	$2 \times 607.9/919.8 = 1.32$	$4 \times 311.9/919.8 = 1.36$
50–59	$12 \times 1272.1/2150.2 = 7.10$	$5 \times 878.1/2150.2 = 2.04$
60–69	$14 \times 888.9/1556.4 = 8.00$	$8 \times 667.5/1556.4 = 3.43$
Total	16.42	6.83

The Mantel–Haenszel estimate is $16.42/6.83 = 2.40$ while the most likely value is 2.39.

15.2 The score is:

$$U = \left(2 - 6\frac{311.9}{919.8}\right) + \left(12 - 17\frac{878.1}{2150.2}\right) + \left(14 - 22\frac{667.5}{1556.4}\right)$$

$$= \quad 28 - 18.41$$
$$= \quad 9.59$$

and the score variance is

$$V = 6 \times \frac{311.9 \times 607.9}{(919.8)^2} + 17 \times \frac{878.1 \times 1\,272.1}{(2\,150.2)^2} + 22 \times \frac{667.5 \times 888.9}{(1\,556.4)^2}$$
$$= 1.34 + 4.11 + 5.39$$
$$= 10.84.$$

The chi-squared value (1 degree of freedom) is $(9.59)^2/10.84 = 8.48$ and $p < 0.005$.

15.3 The standard deviation for the approximation is

$$S = \sqrt{\frac{V}{QR}} = \sqrt{\frac{10.84}{16.42 \times 6.83}} = 0.311.$$

The error factor for the 90% confidence interval is $\exp(1.645 \times 0.311) = 1.67$, and recalling that the Mantel–Haenszel estimate was 2.40, the confidence limits are $2.40/1.67 = 1.44$ (lower limit) and $2.40 \times 1.67 = 4.01$ (upper limit).

15.4 The times at which events occurred, the numbers of patients under observation, and the observed and expected relapses in the test group are shown below.

t	N_1^t	N_0^t	N^t	D_1^t	E_1^t
73	20	20	40	0	$20/40 = 0.50$
86	20	19	39	1	$20/39 = 0.51$
91	19	19	38	0	$19/38 = 0.50$
135	16	16	32	0	$16/32 = 0.50$
194	13	14	27	0	$13/27 = 0.48$
231	12	10	22	1	$12/22 = 0.55$
252	11	10	21	0	$11/21 = 0.52$
296	8	8	16	0	$8/16 = 0.50$
392	4	3	7	1	$4/7 = 0.57$
414	3	3	6	0	$3/6 = 0.50$

The overall score is

$$U = 3 - (.50 + .51 + .50 + \cdots + .57 + .50) = -2.13$$

and the score variance is

$$V = (.50 \times .50) + (.51 \times .49) + \cdots + (.50 \times .50) = 2.49.$$

The score test is $(U)^2/V = 1.82$ and $p > 0.10$. This test is the score test for $\theta = 1$ in the proportional hazards model which holds that the ratio of the relapse rates of the two treatments is constant (at θ) regardless of time since entry into the trial.

15.5   The most likely value of θ is the SMR,

$$\frac{31}{6.47} = 4.791.$$

The error factor is

$$\exp\left(1.645\sqrt{\frac{1}{31}}\right) = 1.344,$$

so that the 90% confidence interval is from $4.791/1.344 = 3.56$ to $4.791 \times 1.344 = 6.44$.

The score test is

$$\frac{(31 - 6.47)^2}{6.47} = 93.00$$

and $p < 0.001$.

15.6   Follow-up was stratified by both age and calendar period when calculating the expected number of deaths. The model which underlies the above analysis therefore assumes that the ratio of rates in the ankylosing spondilitis cohort to those in the reference population is constant for all ages and for all calendar periods.

16
Case-control studies

In a cohort study, the relationship between exposure and disease incidence is investigated by following the entire cohort and measuring the rate of occurrence of new cases in the different exposure groups. The follow-up allows the investigator to register those subjects who develop the disease during the study period and to identify those who remain free of the disease. In a *case-control* study the subjects who develop the disease (the cases) are registered by some other mechanism than follow-up, and a group of healthy subjects (the controls) is used to represent the subjects who do not develop the disease. In this way the need for follow-up is eliminated. If there is no relationship between exposure and disease incidence the distribution of exposure among the cases should be the same as the distribution among the controls.

Historically the aim of case-control studies was limited to testing for association between exposure and disease. Often little thought went into the selection of control groups, or even of cases to be studied. Frequently, studies were carried out using whatever cases could be traced from medical records at a given centre. In this rather careless climate, case-control studies fell into disrepute. However, it is now understood that properly conducted case-control studies allow *quantitative* estimates of exposure effects and this discovery has clarified the fundamental assumptions of the method. It has also contributed to a clearer understanding of the design of case-control studies issues and to a considerable improvement in the quality of studies.

We shall look first at estimating exposure effects and then consider how best to select controls. In the last section of the chapter there is a brief account of some of the difficulties which arise when case-control studies are based on prevalent rather than incident cases.

16.1 The probability model in the study base

Every case-control study of incidence can be seen within the context of an underlying cohort which supplies the cases on which the case-control study depends. A useful terminology refers to this underlying cohort, observed for the duration of the study, as the study *base*.

To estimate the quantitative relationship between exposure and disease incidence we need to look more closely at what is happening in the study base. Consider the simple situation where the study base is divided into two groups, unexposed and exposed, and let π_0, π_1 be the probabilities that a member of the unexposed or the exposed group will fail over the period of the study and become a case.

The branches in the probability tree shown in Fig. 16.1 refer to the different possibilities for a randomly chosen member of the study base, and the events are taken in order of occurrence. The first branching of the tree refers to exposure. The subject may have been exposed (E+), or not (E−); we have taken the probability that a subject was exposed as 0.1, for illustration. The next branching refers to failure. The subject may fail (F), or survive (S); these are the probabilities already referred to as π_1 for the exposed group and π_0 for the unexposed group. The final branching refers to whether the subject is selected into the study or not; for illustration we have chosen a probability of 0.97 that a failure is registered and therefore included as a case, and a probability of 0.01 that a surviving subject is selected as one of the sample of controls. Note that the probability that a failure is registered is assumed to be the same for both exposure groups, and the probability that a healthy subject is chosen as a control is assumed to be the same for both exposure groups.

There are 8 possible outcomes for a member of the study base, corresponding to the 8 tips of the tree, but only 4 of these appear in the study. The four outcomes corresponding to the case-control study are: exposed cases, exposed controls, unexposed cases and unexposed controls. The numbers of subjects in these categories are referred to as D_1, H_1, D_0, H_0, respectively, where D refers to cases, H to healthy controls, and the suffices 1 and 0 refer to exposed and unexposed. The probabilities of the four outcomes appearing in the case-control study are calculated by multiplying conditional probabilities along the branches, and are shown to the right of the figure.

The estimation of the disease exposure relationship in the study base from the results of the case-control study may be approached using either a *retrospective* conditional argument or a *prospective* conditional argument. These correspond to two different ways of reorganizing the probability tree.

16.2   The retrospective probability model

In this argument we re-express our model as a model for the conditional probabilities of exposure given that the subject was a case (F) or a control (S). The reordering of the probability tree to reflect this argument is shown in Fig. 16.2. We define the parameter Ω_1 as the odds of having been exposed for a case. From Fig. 16.2, Ω_1 is related to the odds of failure in the study

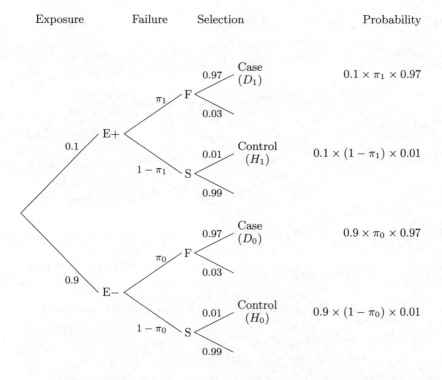

Fig. 16.1.   The probability model in the study base.

base by the equations

$$\Omega_1 = \frac{0.1 \times \pi_1 \times 0.97}{0.9 \times \pi_0 \times 0.97} = \frac{0.1}{0.9} \times \frac{\pi_1}{\pi_0}.$$

The value of Ω_1 can be estimated by D_1/D_0, the ratio of exposed to unexposed cases. Similarly, we define Ω_0 as the odds of a having been exposed for a control. From Fig. 16.2,

$$\Omega_0 = \frac{0.1 \times (1 - \pi_1) \times 0.01}{0.9 \times (1 - \pi_0) \times 0.01} = \frac{0.1}{0.9} \times \frac{1 - \pi_1}{1 - \pi_0},$$

and the value of Ω_0 can be estimated by H_1/H_0, the ratio of exposed to unexposed controls. Finally the *odds ratio*

$$\frac{\Omega_1}{\Omega_0} = \frac{\pi_1/(1 - \pi_1)}{\pi_0/(1 - \pi_0)}$$

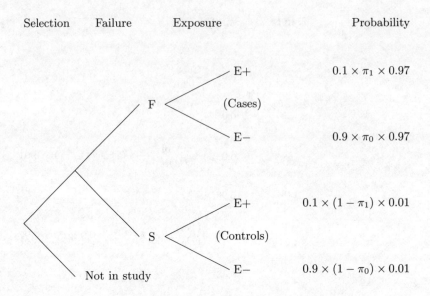

Fig. 16.2.   The probability tree for the retrospective argument.

can be estimated by

$$\frac{D_1/D_0}{H_1/H_0}.$$

Thus although it is not possible to estimate π_0 and π_1 separately from a case-control study it *is* possible to estimate the odds ratio.

EXAMPLE: BCG VACCINATION AND LEPROSY

The data in Table 16.1 are from a rather unusual example of a case-control study in which the controls were obtained from a 100% cross-sectional survey of the study base.* The aim of the study was to investigate whether BCG vaccination in early childhood, whose purpose is to protect against tuberculosis, confers any protection against leprosy, which is caused by a closely related bacillus. New cases of leprosy reported during a given period in a defined geographical area were examined for presence or absence of the characteristic scar left by BCG vaccination. During approximately the same period, a 100% survey of the population of this area had been carried out, and this survey included examination for BCG scar. The tabulated data refer only to subjects under 35, because persons over the age of 35 at the time of the study would have been children at a time when vaccination was not widely available.

---

*From Fine, P.E.M. *et al.* (1986) *The Lancet*, August 30 1986, 499–502.

Table 16.1.   BCG scar status in new leprosy cases and in a healthy population survey

BCG scar	Leprosy cases	Population survey
Present	101	46 028
Absent	159	34 594

Table 16.2.   A simulated study with 1000 controls

BCG scar	Leprosy cases	Population survey
Present	101	554
Absent	159	446

Exercise 16.1. Estimate the odds of BCG vaccination for leprosy cases and for the controls. Estimate the odds ratio and hence the extent of protection against leprosy afforded by vaccination.

This example provides a good illustration of the potential economy of the case-control approach. Here a population survey was available for control but had it not been there would have been no need to carry out such a large-scale exercise. The precision of the odds ratio estimate is dominated by the precision of the odds for BCG scar among the 260 leprosy cases. Perhaps 1000 suitably chosen controls would be enough to estimate the corresponding odds among healthy subjects— there is little gain in precision to be obtained by using 80 000!

Exercise 16.2. Table 16.2 shows the results of a computer-simulated study which picked 1000 controls at random. What is the odds ratio estimate in this study?

16.3   The prospective probability model

In this argument we re-express our model in terms of the conditional probabilities of failure given selection into the study and given exposure status. The re-ordering of the conditional probability tree to reflect this argument is shown in Fig. 16.3. Define the parameter ω_1 as the *odds of being a case* for exposed subjects. By the odds of being a case we mean

$$\frac{\text{Probability of failure given that the subject is in the study}}{\text{Probability of survival given that the subject is in the study}}$$

From Fig. 16.3

$$\omega_1 = \frac{0.1 \times \pi_1 \times 0.97}{0.1 \times (1 - \pi_1) \times 0.01} = \frac{0.97}{0.01} \times \frac{\pi_1}{1 - \pi_1},$$

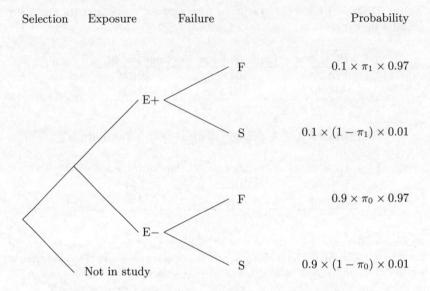

Fig. 16.3. The prospective probability model.

and this can be estimated by the case/control ratio among exposed subjects, D_1/H_1. Similarly the odds of being a case for unexposed subjects is

$$\omega_0 = \frac{0.9 \times \pi_0 \times 0.97}{0.9 \times (1 - \pi_0) \times 0.01} = \frac{0.97}{0.01} \times \frac{\pi_0}{1 - \pi_0},$$

which can be estimated by the case/control ratio among unexposed subjects, D_0/H_0. Finally, the odds ratio

$$\frac{\omega_1}{\omega_0} = \frac{\pi_1/(1 - \pi_1)}{\pi_0/(1 - \pi_0)},$$

can be estimated by

$$\frac{D_1/H_1}{D_0/H_0}.$$

This is the same estimate as that obtained from the retrospective approach since

$$\frac{D_1/D_0}{H_1/H_0} = \frac{D_1/H_1}{D_0/H_0} = \frac{D_1 H_0}{D_0 H_1}.$$

16.4 Many levels of exposure

In the retrospective argument it is the exposure status which is the response (outcome variable); in the prospective argument it is the disease status which is the response. The retrospective argument is more natural,

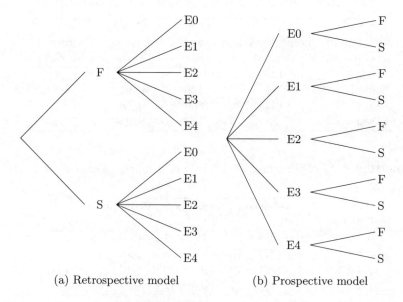

(a) Retrospective model   (b) Prospective model

Fig. 16.4.   Five exposure categories.

but the prospective argument leads to the same answers and is more convenient when studying exposures with many levels. This is illustrated by
Fig. 16.4, which shows probability trees for both arguments when there are
5 exposure categories. Disease status is indicated by F (for cases) or S (for
controls) and the 5 exposure categories are labelled E0 to E4. To construct
a likelihood using the retrospective likelihood we must use a probability
model for a response with 5 possible outcomes, but the prospective argument only requires the binary probability model. The odds of being a
case for subjects in exposure category i is a constant multiple of the corresponding odds of failure in the study base; with the selection probabilities
assumed in Fig. 16.1,

$$\omega_i = \frac{\pi_i}{1 - \pi_i} \times \frac{0.97}{0.01}.$$

As the complexity of the exposure grouping increases, the retrospective
probability model must become ever more complex, while the prospective
model remains binary.

As an example of an exposure with more than two levels we shall look
at a famous study carried out in the middle of the nineteenth century by
William Guy.[†] This was possibly the first case-control study. The level of
physical activity of the occupations of pulmonary tuberculosis outpatients
(cases) was compared with that of other outpatients (controls). The data

[†]From Guy, W.A. (1843) *Journal of the Royal Statistical Society*, **6**, 197–211.

Table 16.3.   Physical exertion at work of 1659 outpatients

Level of exertion in occupation	Pulmonary consumption (Cases)	Other diseases (Controls)	Case/ control ratio	Estimated odds ratio
Little	125	385	0.325	1.64
Varied	41	136	0.301	1.52
More	142	630	0.225	1.14
Great	33	167	0.198	1.00

Table 16.4.   Alcohol and tobacco use by oral cancer cases and (controls)

Alcohol (oz/day)	Tobacco (cigarette equivalents per day)							
	0		1–19		20–39		40+	
0	10	(38)	11	(26)	13	(36)	9	(8)
0.1 – 0.3	7	(27)	16	(35)	50	(60)	16	(19)
0.4 – 1.5	4	(12)	18	(16)	60	(49)	27	(14)
1.6 +	5	(8)	21	(20)	125	(52)	91	(27)

are shown in Table 16.3. There are four levels of exposure corresponding to different levels of activity and the table shows the ratio of cases to controls. Each of these case-control ratios estimates some constant times the odds of failure conditional on exposure level. Since the constant depends on the probability of registration for cases and selection for controls it will be the same for all exposure levels and the case/control ratios can be compared as though they were the odds of failure.

Looking at the case/control ratios in this way, they suggest that there is a steady increase in the odds of failure (and hence the incidence rate) with decreasing level of physical activity. The table also shows odds ratio estimates with the 'great' activity category taken as reference. By definition, the odds ratio for this reference category is 1. The natural choice of reference category is the one with lowest exposure to adverse factor. In some cases, however, the natural reference category might contain very few cases and controls, leading to poor estimation of all the odds ratios; another reference category should then be chosen.

Exercise 16.3. Table 16.4 shows the distribution of 483 cases of oral cancer by level of alcohol consumption and level of tobacco consumption, together with the corresponding distribution for 447 controls.[‡] Calculate the case/control ratios, and describe the joint action of the two exposures.

---

‡From Rothman, K.J. and Keller, A.Z. (1972) *Journal of Chronic Diseases*, **23**, 711–716.

16.5   Incidence density sampling

We saw in Chapter 1 that, when the probabilities of failure are small, the risk and odds parameters are approximately equal. In these conditions, we showed in Chapter 5 that the risk parameter is also approximately equal to the cumulative rate, λt. It follows that

$$\frac{\pi_1/(1-\pi_1)}{\pi_0/(1-\pi_0)} \approx \frac{\pi_1}{\pi_0} \approx \frac{\lambda_1}{\lambda_0}$$

for rare events. These ratios are known as the *odds ratio*, the *risk ratio*, and the *rate ratio*, and the condition for these to be approximately the same is usually described as the *rare disease assumption*. Taken together with the arguments developed in this chapter, we see that the odds ratio in a case-control study may be used to estimate the rate ratio in the underlying study base. There are two additional assumptions in this argument:

1. all subjects in the base are observed from the beginning of the study period, that is, there are no *late entries*;

2. all subjects who do not fail from the cause of interest will remain under observation until the end of the study period, that is, there is no *censoring*.

In practice, these assumptions are more likely to be violated than the rare disease assumption.

All of these assumptions can be guaranteed by the simple device of selecting a short enough study period. If insufficient cases would be obtained from such a study then the remedy is simple – carry out several *consecutive* short studies. The subjects remaining in the base at the end of one study immediately enter the next study. Each study then provides a separate estimate of the rate ratio, and provided this ratio remains constant over the whole study period, the information can be aggregated using methods very similar to those discussed in Chapter 15.

Taken to the limit, the total time available for the study may be divided into clicks which contain at most one case. Those clicks in which no case occurs are not informative so there is no purpose in drawing controls, but controls are drawn for all clicks in which a case occurs. Thus one or more controls are drawn from the study base immediately after the occurrence of each case. This design is termed *incidence density sampling*.

A study carried out in this way involves matching of controls to cases with respect to time. Methods for stratified case-control studies will be discussed in Chapter 18, but in the special case where the ratio of exposed to unexposed persons in the study base does not vary appreciably over the study period, it is legitimate to ignore the matching by time during the analysis.

One practical problem with this sampling method is that it is possible for the same individual to be included in the study more than once. For example, a control drawn at one point in time may later become a case or may be selected as a control a second time. Is it legitimate to carry out analyses which count the same person more than once? In Chapter 4 we saw that a single subject observed through several consecutive time bands can be treated as a series of different subjects, one for each band. In exactly the same way, in a case-control study it turns out to be correct to allow subjects to be sampled again in later time bands and treated as independent controls.

16.6   Nested case-control studies and case-cohort studies

An important use of incidence density sampling is in *nested* case-control studies, where case-control analysis is used in cohort studies. This is an attractive option whenever the assessment of exposure of any subject is, for some reason or other, expensive. For example, in dietary studies, individual diet may have been assessed by very detailed diary records of food intake, perhaps referring to several periods of time. The coding and transcription of such records for computer analysis is laborious and expensive. Much of this work is avoided in a nested case-control study by coding these records only for cases, as they occur, and for groups of controls drawn for each case. Since there is (usually) little to be gained by drawing more than five controls for each case, there are considerable savings to be made by such a strategy. We shall discuss the design and analysis of nested case-control studies in Chapter 33.

In recent years some authors have suggested that there are sometimes practical advantages in selecting controls by taking a single random sample of the cohort at the *beginning* of the study. This type of study has been termed a *case-cohort* or *case-base* study. If the disease is rare and there is little loss to follow-up, then the analysis may be carried out as usual, after first removing from the control sample any individuals who later became cases. However, if stratification by time becomes necessary the analysis is more difficult.

16.7   Selection bias

One important reason for obtaining wrong answers from case-control studies is incorrect sampling of controls (or cases) from the study base. This is called *selection bias*. It should be clear from this chapter that case-control studies will only yield unbiased estimates of

$$\frac{\pi_1/(1 - \pi_1)}{\pi_0/(1 - \pi_0)}$$

if the selection probabilities for both cases and controls do not vary between exposure groups. Selection bias occurs when this is not true.

A study can only be truly convincing in this respect if its base is closely defined. The type of study with the best defined base is a nested case-control study, in which the study base consists of a documented and closely traced cohort. This method has proved particularly useful in occupational studies, where employment records identify an underlying cohort and pension schemes provide a mechanism for long term follow-up.

In a *geographically* based case-control study the base is defined by residence in a particular geographical area during the period of study. Although all such individuals are not specifically identified, it may nevertheless be possible to carry out a study in such a way that all cases are registered and controls drawn in a manner unrelated to exposure. Such studies require complete registration of disease in the study area, including capture of resident cases diagnosed and treated elsewhere. Control selection may also be difficult, since few countries have accurate and accessible population registers.

Another important base for case-control studies is the patient list of the family doctor. These lists offer good possibilities for representative control selection and for complete registration of cases particularly when, as in the United Kingdom, access to all medical services is channelled through the family practitioner.

For reasons of economy and convenience, a common choice is the *hospital-based* case-control study in which the case series is made up of all new cases presenting at one or more hospitals during the period of the study. Here the study base consists of the *catchment population* comprising all those persons who would have attended these hospitals if they had developed disease during this period. This is ill defined and it is difficult to demonstrate convincingly that the probability of control selection from the study base is independent of exposure. The device of using other patients, attending for unrelated conditions, has two clear difficulties:

1. catchment populations for different specialities in the same hospital do not necessarily coincide, and

2. patients who are sick with other diseases are not necessarily representative of the population of persons free of the disease of interest. In particular, factors associated with increased risk of these diseases may appear to be *protective* against the disease of interest simply because they are over represented in controls.

Against these difficulties must be set the claim that recall bias and other forms of differential exposure misclassification may be reduced when both case and control groups are hospital patients.

Two further points should be made briefly before concluding this section. First, matching is extremely useful in avoiding selection bias although its use is more frequently advocated on the grounds of efficiency. We shall return to this discussion in Chapter 18. Second, it is important to draw attention to the fact that the best sampling scheme can be invalidated by poor subject compliance. If a substantial number of potential cases and controls refuse to participate there is considerable potential for bias as a result of differential compliance in different exposure groups. All too often case-control studies do not report compliance, and the potential for such bias is hard to assess.

16.8   Prevalent cases

If a case-control study is carried out using prevalent cases it is no longer a study of disease incidence and the odds ratio estimate cannot be interpreted as an estimate of a ratio of incidence rates. However, such studies can be used to study relationships of exposures to the prevalence of disease.

If the cases can be considered a random sample of those with disease in the population, and controls can be considered a random sample of the healthy section of the population, then the odds that a case was exposed divided by the odds that a control was exposed is an estimate of

$$\frac{\text{Prevalence odds in exposed population}}{\text{Prevalence odds in unexposed population}}.$$

When the prevalence in both groups is low this ratio is approximately equal to the prevalence in the exposed population divided by the prevalence in the unexposed population.

The remarks concerning sources of bias in incident case-control studies apply equally here. In particular, recall bias is a serious problem when interviewing prevalent cases who have been sick and in contact with medical professionals for some time. However, the main problems of interpretation are those of interpreting prevalence itself; the odds ratio is affected by factors which influence the *duration* for which a case, once diagnosed, remains in the sampling frame. These include not only factors related to survival, but factors relating to migration which may be complex and difficult to quantify.

Solutions to the exercises

16.1 The estimate of the odds *for* vaccination in leprosy cases is $101/159 = 0.635$ as compared with $46\,028/34\,594 = 1.331$ in the healthy subjects. The odds ratio estimate is $0.635/1.331 = 0.48$.

16.2 The odds ratio is
$$\frac{101/159}{554/446} = 0.51.$$

16.3 The case/control ratios are as follows:

Alcohol	Tobacco (cigs. per day)			
(oz/day)	0	1–19	20–39	40+
0	0.26	0.42	0.36	1.12
0.1–0.3	0.26	0.46	0.83	0.84
0.4–1.5	0.33	1.13	1.22	1.93
1.6 +	0.63	1.05	2.40	3.37

Because the frequencies in the table are small, there is much random variation, but there is an overall tendency for the ratios to increase both from left to right along rows, and from top to bottom down columns. This indicates that *both* variables have an effect on cancer incidence; there is an effect of tobacco when alcohol intake is held constant, and vice versa.

17
Likelihoods for the odds ratio

The data from a simple case-control study (exposed and unexposed) can be arranged as a 2×2 table such as that set out in Table 17.1. We saw in Chapter 16 that there are two ways in which the probability model for a case-control study can be set up but that, for both models, the ratio of odds parameters are equal to the ratio of odds of failure in the study base.

17.1 The retrospective log likelihood

As in Chapter 16, we write Ω_0 for the odds of exposure among controls, and Ω_1 for the odds of exposure among cases. Our interest is in the odds ratio parameter $\theta = \Omega_1/\Omega_0$, so we change from the parameters Ω_0 and Ω_1 to the parameters Ω_0 and θ, and regard Ω_0 as a nuisance parameter. The total log likelihood is the sum of the log likelihood for Ω_0 based on the split of the H controls between exposed and unexposed, and the log likelihood for Ω_1 $(= \theta\Omega_0)$ based on the split of D cases,

$$H_1 \log(\Omega_0) - H \log(1 + \Omega_0) \quad + \quad D_1 \log(\theta\Omega_0) - D \log(1 + \theta\Omega_0).$$

To use this log likelihood for estimating of the odds ratio θ, we form a profile log likelihood by replacing Ω_0 by its most likely value for each value of θ. Unlike the profile log likelihood for the rate ratio in cohort studies, this curve cannot be expressed as a simple algebraic expression, but the results of section 13.4 and Appendix C can be used to derive a Gaussian approximation.

This derivation follows from the fact that the *log* odds ratio is the difference between two log odds parameters,

$$\log(\theta) = \log(\Omega_1) - \log(\Omega_0).$$

Table 17.1. Notation for the 2×2 table

Exposure	Cases	Controls	Total subjects
Exposed	D_1	H_1	$N_1 = D_1 + H_1$
Unexposed	D_0	H_0	$N_0 = D_0 + H_0$
Total	D	H	$N = D + H$

These are estimated from two independent bodies of data and have most
likely values

$$M_1 = \log\left(\frac{D_1}{D_0}\right), \qquad M_0 = \log\left(\frac{H_1}{H_0}\right),$$

and standard deviations

$$S_1 = \sqrt{\frac{1}{D_1} + \frac{1}{D_0}}, \qquad S_0 = \sqrt{\frac{1}{H_1} + \frac{1}{H_0}}.$$

It follows from general results given in section 13.4 and Appendix C that
the most likely value of the log odds ratio is

$$\begin{aligned} M &= M_1 - M_0 \\ &= \log\left(\frac{D_1/D_0}{H_1/H_0}\right) \end{aligned}$$

and the standard deviation of the Gaussian approximation to the log likelihood is

$$\begin{aligned} S &= \sqrt{(S_1)^2 + (S_0)^2} \\ &= \sqrt{\frac{1}{D_1} + \frac{1}{D_0} + \frac{1}{H_1} + \frac{1}{H_0}}. \end{aligned}$$

This can be used to calculate an error factor for the odds ratio and hence
an approximate 90% confidence interval.

The expression for S only differs from that for the rate ratio in a cohort
study by the addition of the two last terms. These are reciprocals of the
counts of controls and represent the loss of precision incurred by carrying
out a case-control study rather than a cohort study. Once the number
of controls is substantially larger than the number of cases, this loss of
precision becomes negligible. Hence the common assertion that there is
little to be gained by drawing more than four or five times as many controls
as cases.

Exercise 17.1. For the study of BCG vaccination and leprosy discussed in
Chapter 16, calculate the expected result of the study using
(a) the same number of controls as cases;
(b) twice as many controls as cases; and
(c) five times as many control as cases.
Compare the corresponding values of S with that achieved by using the entire
population as controls.

Carried out algebraically, these calculations lead to the general result that
the ratio of the standard deviation of an estimate from a case-control study
to the standard deviation from a cohort study yielding the same number

of cases is

$$\sqrt{1 + (1/m)}$$

where m is the number of controls expressed as a multiple of the number of cases. When $m = 1$ this expression shows that the standard deviation is 1.41 times higher in a case-control study than in a cohort study. When $m = 5$ the factor reduces to 1.10 and when $m = 10$ this reduces only a little more to 1.05. The behaviour of this expression as m increases confirms the impression of the last exercise — that there is little gain in efficiency to be obtained by selecting more than five times as many controls as cases.

THE NULL HYPOTHESIS $\theta = 1$

We can calculate an approximate p-value for the null hypothesis using using any one of the three methods we have encountered earlier. The log likelihood ratio test is now based on the profile log likelihood. The Wald test is calculated by comparing the most likely value of the odds ratio with the null value, $\log(\theta) = 0$, by calculating

$$\left(\frac{M - 0}{S}\right)^2.$$

Finally, the score test can be derived using the general relationships set out in Appendix C. At the null hypothesis the two odds parameters are equal and their most likely common value is N_1/N_0. The score, U, is found from the gradient of the profile log likelihood with respect to $\log(\Omega_1)$ at this point, which turns out to be

$$
\begin{aligned}
U &= D_1 - E_1 \\
&= -(D_0 - E_0),
\end{aligned}
$$

where

$$E_1 = D\frac{N_1}{N}, \qquad E_0 = D\frac{N_0}{N}$$

can be thought of as the expected numbers of exposed and unexposed cases under the null hypothesis. The score variance is obtained from the curvature of the profile log likelihood at the null value $\theta = 1$, which yields

$$V = \frac{DHN_0N_1}{(N)^3}.$$

As usual, an approximate p-value can be obtained by referring $(U)^2/V$ to the chi-squared distribution on one degree of freedom.

Table 17.2. Tonsillectomy and Hodgkins disease

Tonsillectomy	Cases		Controls		Total subjects	
Positive	90	(D_1)	165	(H_1)	255	(N_1)
Negative	84	(D_0)	307	(H_0)	391	(N_0)
Total	174	(D)	472	(H)	646	(N)

Exercise 17.2. Table 17.2 shows data from a study of the relationship between tonsillectomy and the incidence of Hodgkin's disease.[*] Calculate the maximum likelihood estimate of θ with a 90% confidence interval, and calculate a p-value for $\theta = 1$.

17.2 The prospective log likelihood

We now turn to the log likelihood we obtain using the prospective probability model. As in Chapter 16, we write ω_1 for the odds that an exposed subject is a case, ω_0 for the corresponding odds for an unexposed subject, and change to (ω_0, θ) where $\theta = \omega_1/\omega_2$. The log likelihood is again the sum of two Bernoulli log likelihood terms,

$$D_0 \log(\omega_0) - N_0 \log(1 + \omega_0) \quad + \quad D_1 \log(\theta \omega_0) - N_1 \log(1 + \theta \omega_0),$$

and the profile log likelihood is obtained by replacing ω_0 by its most likely value at each value of θ. As with the retrospective model, this does not lead to a simple algebraic expression, but the Gaussian approximation can easily be derived, since

$$\log(\theta) = \log(\omega_1) - \log(\omega_0)$$

and the log likelihoods for $\log(\omega_1)$ and $\log(\omega_0)$ are based on independent sets of data. The most likely values of ω_1 and ω_0 are

$$M_1 = \log\left(\frac{D_1}{H_1}\right), \qquad M_0 = \log\left(\frac{D_0}{H_0}\right),$$

and the corresponding standard deviations are

$$S_1 = \sqrt{\frac{1}{D_1} + \frac{1}{H_1}}, \qquad S_0 = \sqrt{\frac{1}{D_0} + \frac{1}{H_0}}.$$

As before, the most likely value of $\log(\theta)$ is

$$M \quad = \quad M_1 - M_0$$

[*]From Johnson, S.K. and Johnson, R.E. (1972) *New England Journal of Medicine*, **287**, 1122–1125.

$$= \log\left(\frac{D_1/H_1}{D_0/H_0}\right)$$

and the standard deviation of the Gaussian approximation to the log likelihood is

$$S = \sqrt{(S_1)^2 + (S_0)^2}$$

$$= \sqrt{\frac{1}{D_1} + \frac{1}{H_1} + \frac{1}{D_0} + \frac{1}{H_0}}.$$

These results are exactly the same as we obtained using the retrospective argument. In the same way we can show that the log likelihood ratio and score tests are identical for the two approaches. Indeed, some further mathematics shows that the profile log likelihoods for the two arguments are identical. This continues to be the case for more complex patterns of exposure and, since the prospective approach is more convenient in these situations, it is to be preferred.

17.3 The hypergeometric likelihood

Both the probability models discussed above contain a nuisance parameter in addition to the parameter of interest, θ. Both lead to profile log likelihood for θ and depend on profile likelihood behaving in the same way as a true likelihood.

When there is sufficient data, the profile log likelihood does indeed behave in this way. However, profile likelihoods are obtained by estimating the nuisance parameters, and it is only safe to assume that they have the same properties as true likelihoods if the accuracy of that estimation increases as the total number of subjects increases. If the number of nuisance parameters increases with the number of subjects, this improved estimation is not achieved and profile likelihoods can be misleading. This happens in case-control studies if, as the total number of subjects increases, the study is divided into an increasing number of small strata in an attempt to deal with confounding. For either the prospective or the retrospective likelihood it is necessary to introduce a separate nuisance parameter for each stratum, so the number of parameters will increase with the number of subjects. The worst case is the individually matched case-control study in which the number of strata (and nuisance parameters) is equal to the number of case-control pairs. It turns out that the use of profile likelihood methods in this situation leads to wrong answers.

An alternative way of eliminating the nuisance parameter is a *conditional* approach based on a probability model in which *both* margins of the 2×2 table (Table 17.1) are fixed. The set of probabilities for all splits of subjects which maintain the same marginal totals is known as the *hypergeometric* distribution. For the table shown in Table 17.1, the probability is

$$\frac{1}{K(\theta)} \times \frac{(\theta)^{D_1}}{D_1!D_0!H_1!H_0!}$$

where $K(\theta)$ is chosen so that the probabilities for all possible tables with the same margins add up to one:

$$K(\theta) = \sum_{\text{Possible tables}} \frac{(\theta)^{D_1}}{D_1!D_0!H_1!H_0!}.$$

This distribution depends only on the parameter θ and can be used to calculate exact p-values and confidence intervals for the odds ratio as outlined in Chapter 12. The use of these methods is illustrated in section 17.4.

The likelihood based on this distribution is called the *hypergeometric likelihood*. Because of the function $K(\theta)$, it is difficult to calculate except when the number of possible tables consistent with the margins is small. We shall consider an important special case in Chapter 19 and give a more general treatment of this likelihood in Chapter 29. For the present we note that the hypergeometric likelihood does lead to a simple score test for $\theta = 1$. The score is exactly the same as for the profile log likelihoods, that is

$$U = D_1 - E_1,$$

but the score variance can be shown to be

$$V = \frac{DHN_0N_1}{(N)^2(N-1)}.$$

This differs from the expression derived from the curvature of the *profile* log likelihood by the term $(N-1)$ in place of N in the denominator. The difference this makes to the value of the variance is usually negligible. The one situation where it does make a difference is in matched studies where the number of subjects in each stratum is very small. In the worst case of the 1:1 individually matched study, $N = 2$ in every stratum and the profile likelihood argument wrongly estimates the score variance by a factor of two. We shall, therefore, return to the hypergeometric likelihood when discussing the analysis of individually matched case-control studies in Chapter 19.

17.4   Exact methods

The use of the hypergeometric distribution for exact tests and confidence intervals follows exactly the same principles as set out in Chapter 12. This is illustrated in this section using some data drawn from a case-control study set up to investigate an excess of childhood leukaemia cases in the

Table 17.3. Paternal radiation exposure in leukaemia cases and controls

Paternal exposure	Leukaemia cases	Local controls	Total
≥ 100 mSv (Exposed)	3	1	4
< 100 mSv (Unexposed)	1	19	20
Total	4	20	24

Table 17.4. Hypergeometric log likelihood ratios and probabilities

D_1	LLR $(\theta = 1)$	Hypergeometric probability		
		$(\theta = 1)$	$(\theta = 2.440)$	$(\theta = 1534.1)$
0	-0.785	0.455957	0.202245	
1	-0.105	0.429136	0.464450	0.000001
2	-1.451	0.107284	0.283314	0.000460
3	-4.252	0.007529	0.048511	0.049540
4	-9.271	0.000094	0.001480	0.949998
Total		1.0	1.0	1.0

vicinity of a nuclear reprocessing plant (see Exercise 11.8). The data set out in Table 17.3 concern occupational radiation exposure in fathers of 4 cases and fathers of 20 local controls.[†]

There are five possible tables with the same margins as Table 17.3, with values of D_1 (the number of exposed cases) ranging from zero to four. The hypergeometric distribution gives the conditional probability for each table as a function of the odds ratio parameter, θ, and the log likelihood for any value of θ is calculated by taking the log of the probability of the *observed* outcome $D_1 = 3$. The most likely value of θ is 37.345[‡] and the log likelihood ratio which compares this with the null value ($\theta = 1$) is −4.252. Table 17.4 shows, in the column headed LLR, similar log likelihood ratio comparisons for each of the five possible tables and, in the next column, the conditional probabilities of these tables when the null hypothesis is true. The p-value is the sum of probabilities of the observed table and of all tables which are in greater conflict with the null value. In this case $p = 0.007529 + 0.000094 = 0.007623$. The one-sided and two-sided p-values are identical in this case. This way of calculating the p-value for a 2×2 table is called *Fisher's exact test*.

Similar ideas are used to calculate 'exact' confidence intervals. To find

---

[†]From Gardner, M.J. *et al.* (1990) *British Medical Journal*, **300**, 423–429.

[‡]Note that this is not the same value as that obtained with the profile likelihood which is $(3 \times 19)/(1 \times 1) = 57$.

the limits of the 90% interval we search for values of θ which give one-sided p-values of 0.05. These values are 2.440 (lower limit) and 1534.1 (upper limit) and the corresponding hypergeometric distributions are shown in the last two columns of Table 17.4. At $\theta = 2.440$ the one-sided p-value is $0.048511 + 0.001480 = 0.04991$ and at $\theta = 1534.1$ the one-sided p-value is $0.000001 + 0.000460 + 0.049540 = 0.050001$. Values of θ outside the range from 2.440 to 1534.1 would have smaller p-values than 0.05 and the frequentist theory would therefore suggest that we should pronounce ourselves 90% confident that θ lies within this range. As we have seen in Chapter 12, this is a very technical use of the word confident and no epidemiologist would really believe that θ could really take such large values. The extreme finding is obtained, at least to some extent, because the radiation level chosen here to divide exposed and unexposed groups was chosen *after* seeing the data.

Solutions to the exercises

17.1   The following shows the expected results of the three studies. These have been calculated by splitting the controls between scar present and scar absent categories in the proportions $46\,028/80\,622$ and $34\,594/80\,622$ respectively.

			Expected controls		
BCG scar	Cases	Population	(a)	(b)	(c)
Present	101	46 028	148	296	740
Absent	159	34 594	112	224	560
Total	260	80 622	260	520	1300

The standard deviations for the log odds ratio estimate are worked out using the formula $S = \sqrt{1/D_0 + 1/D_1 + 1/H_0 + 1/H_1}$ and are 0.179, 0.155, and 0.139 respectively. The standard deviation using the full data is 0.127. The gain in precision with increasing numbers of controls clearly follows a law of diminishing returns.

17.2   The maximum likelihood estimate of θ is the observed odds ratio:

$$\frac{90/84}{165/307} = 1.99.$$

and

$$S = \sqrt{\frac{1}{84} + \frac{1}{90} + \frac{1}{307} + \frac{1}{165}} = 0.180.$$

For calculating 90% confidence limits, the error factor is $\exp(1.645\times0.180) = 1.34$. The limits are therefore $1.99/1.34 = 1.48$ (lower limit) and $1.99 \times 1.34 = 2.67$ (upper limit).

The expected number of exposed cases is given by

$$E_1 = 174 \times \frac{255}{646} = 68.68$$

so that the score, U, is $(90 - 68.68) = 21.32$. The score variance is

$$\frac{174 \times 472 \times 255 \times 391}{(646)^3} = 30.37.$$

The score test is $(21.32)^2/30.37 = 14.97$, $(p < 0.001)$.

18
Comparison of odds within strata

This chapter deals with methods for analysing stratified case-control studies which closely parallel the methods for cohort studies discussed in Chapter 15.

18.1 The constant odds ratio model

As an example we return to the study of the effect of BCG vaccination upon the incidence of leprosy. Since leprosy incidence increases with age among young people, age is certainly a variable which would have been controlled in an experiment. In Chapter 16 it was shown that BCG-vaccinated individuals had just under one half of the incidence of leprosy as compared with unvaccinated persons, but age was ignored in the analysis. This could have biased the estimated effect of BCG vaccination because BCG vaccination in the area (Northern Malawi) was introduced gradually in infants and young children, so that people who were older during the study period, having been born at earlier dates, were less likely to have been vaccinated. As a result, on average the vaccinated group will be younger than the unvaccinated group. This means that, even if BCG vaccination were totally ineffective, one would expect to observe lower rates in vaccinated members of the base cohort, simply as a result of their relative youth.

Table 18.1 subdivides these data by strata corresponding to 5-year age

Table 18.1. BCG vaccination and leprosy by age

| | BCG scar | | | | Odds |
| | Leprosy cases | | Healthy population | | ratio |
Age	Absent	Present	Absent	Present	estimate
0–4	1	1	7593	11719	0.65
5–9	11	14	7143	10184	0.89
10–14	28	22	5611	7561	0.58
15–19	16	28	2208	8117	0.48
20–24	20	19	2438	5588	0.41
25–29	36	11	4356	1625	0.82
30–34	47	6	5245	1234	0.54

bands. The table also shows age-specific odds ratios. Although there is random variation, there is no systematic trend of the odds ratio with age, and it seems reasonable to make the assumption that the odds ratio parameter is the same in all age bands. In the next section we show how an estimate of this common odds ratio can be calculated.

18.2   An estimate of the common odds ratio

In the prospective approach to the analysis, the assumption of a common odds ratio implies that ω_1^t/ω_0^t is constant, so that the model can be expressed in terms of the odds ratio parameter θ and the ω_0^t parameters. Alternatively, in the retrospective approach the model is expressed in terms of θ and the parameters Ω_0^t. In both approaches, replacing the nuisance parameters by their estimates leads to the profile likelihood for θ. If there are not too many strata, and the data are not too sparse in each stratum, then the profile likelihood for θ can be used to find the most likely value and the supported range. For coarsely stratified data sets such as Table 18.1, these conditions are met. Such an analysis is not feasible by hand, but would usually be carried out on a computer using *logistic regression* (see Chapter 23).

When the data are very finely stratified so that each stratum contains very few cases and controls, the profile likelihood approach can be unreliable, and the hypergeometric likelihood should be used. The total log likelihood is then obtained by adding together the hypergeometric log likelihoods for the different strata. Again, the most likely value M and the standard deviation S cannot usually be computed by hand, but would be carried out using a *conditional* logistic regression program (see Chapter 29). However, the calculations for the score test for $\theta = 1$ are straightforward. For a single stratum the score under the hypergeometric likelihood is

$$U = D_1 - E_1$$

where D_1 is the observed number of exposed cases and $E_1 = DN_1/N$ is the expected number under the null hypothesis. The score variance is

$$V = \frac{DHN_0N_1}{(N)^2(N-1)}.$$

Since every stratum contributes additively to the overall log likelihood, the overall score is a sum of contributions from each stratum of exactly the same form as above. Thus, the score is

$$U = \sum(D_1^t - E_1^t)$$

where

$$E_1^t = D^t \frac{N_1^t}{N^t}.$$

and the overall score variance is

$$V = \sum \frac{D^t H^t N_0^t N_1^t}{(N^t)^2(N^t - 1)}.$$

Exercise 18.1. Show that the first age band in Table 18.1 makes a contribution of -0.21 to U and 0.48 to V.

The overall test statistic is obtained by repeating these calculations for each stratum and yields

$$U = -0.21 - 0.69 - 6.68 - 6.56 - 8.11 - 1.76 - 4.06 = -28.07$$

and

$$V = 0.48 + 6.05 + 12.18 + 7.38 + 8.22 + 9.22 + 8.09 = 51.62.$$

The approximate chi-squared value on one degree of freedom is

$$(U)^2/V = 787.92/51.62 = 15.26.$$

The statistic U has a negative sign because the exposure is protective — the observed number of vaccinated cases is less than would have been expected had vaccination been ineffective.

Exercise 18.2. Verify that, when there is only one case per stratum, the test becomes identical to the log rank test discussed in section 15.5.

This test was proposed by Mantel and Haenszel. They also proposed a way of calculating a nearly most likely value for θ. This is suggested by an algebraic rearrangement of the equation for the score:

$$\begin{aligned} U &= \sum(D_1^t - E_1^t) \\ &= \sum \frac{D_1^t H_0^t - D_0^t H_1^t}{N^t} \\ &= \sum Q^t - \sum R^t, \end{aligned}$$

where $Q^t = D_1^t H_0^t / N^t$ and $R^t = D_0^t H_1^t / N^t$. The usual estimate of the odds ratio in stratum t is Q^t/R^t, and this suggests estimating the common odds ratio, θ, by

$$\frac{Q^1 + Q^2 + \dots}{R^1 + R^2 + \dots} = \frac{Q}{R}.$$

When the true value of θ is close to 1, this *Mantel–Haenszel estimate* is almost as precise as the the most likely value of θ according to the hypergeometric likelihood. It can only be improved upon for odds ratios which differ substantially from one.

Exercise 18.3. Show that the Mantel–Haenszel estimate of the odds ratio for the data of Table 18.1 is 0.587.

Note that allowing for confounding by age has weakened the estimated protective effect of vaccination. This is now about 41% rather than 52% — a modest adjustment. This is in accord with the general experience that confounding only causes substantial modification of rate ratios in quite extreme circumstances.

The usefulness of the Mantel–Haenszel estimate in practice was limited by the fact that, rather surprisingly, no expression was available for its standard deviation until relatively recently. Several estimates have now been proposed, most of them rather awkward to calculate. For most practical purposes, a good estimate is provided by the same expression as for the cohort study version (Chapter 15):

$$ S = \sqrt{\frac{V}{QR}}. $$

Exercise 18.4. For the data of Table 18.1, calculate the 90% confidence interval for the age-adjusted vaccine effect.

18.3   Improving efficiency by matching

In Exercise 16.2 we repeated the analysis of the leprosy study using a sample of 1000 controls drawn randomly from the healthy population, with only a modest loss in the precision of our estimate of the odds ratio. The position changes, however, when we stratify by age in the analysis.

Table 18.2 shows the way the simulated data lie. It is clear that the precision of the age-controlled odds ratio estimate will not be as good as we would have expected with more than 3 times as many controls as cases. The study has 238 controls for the 2 cases in the 0–4 year age group yet only 80 controls for the 53 cases in the 30–34 year age group.

With such a design, many controls are wasted and the efficiency of the study will be lower than it would be if the ratio of controls to cases were held constant within strata. This is called *matching*. If the study is carried out so as to achieve a constant ratio of cases to controls in broad groups it is called a *group* or *frequency* matching. If a set of matched controls are selected specifically for each case, it is called *individual matching*. Table 18.3 shows a simulated study in which the number of controls has been maintained at 4 times the number of cases in all age groups.

Exercise 18.5. For the data set out in Table 18.2, the values of Q, R, U, V are

Table 18.2. The simulated study stratified by age

| | BCG scar | | | |
| | Cases | | Controls | |
Age	Absent	Present	Absent	Present
0–4	1	1	101	137
5–9	11	14	91	115
10–14	28	22	82	101
15–19	16	28	28	87
20–24	20	19	25	69
25–29	36	11	63	21
30–34	47	6	56	24

Table 18.3. A simulated group-matched study

| | BCG scar | | | |
| | Cases | | Controls | |
Age	Absent	Present	Absent	Present
0–4	1	1	3	5
5–9	11	14	48	52
10–14	28	22	67	133
15–19	16	28	46	130
20–24	20	19	50	106
25–29	36	11	126	62
30–34	47	6	174	38

30.00, 51.57, 21.57, and 39.68. For Table 18.3 the corresponding values are 32.14, 56.54, 24.40, and 43.27. Compare the estimates, confidence intervals, and score tests for the two sets of data.

In practice, age is usually a very strong confounder and almost all case-control studies are matched for age. At one stage, simultaneously matching for as many other confounders as possible was frequently advocated. It is now clear that this is not a good idea, but matching is such an intuitively appealing idea to many epidemiologists that some discussion of the points for and against matching is of interest.

First it should be noted that an appreciable gain in precision is achieved only for a confounding variable which is very strongly related to the exposure of interest. For less strongly related confounders matching leads to only modest gains in precision while complicating the study design. More seriously, if a variable is matched in the design, the ability to examine the effect of that variable is lost since its distribution in the controls will match that in the cases rather than that in the study base. One must be confident

Table 18.4.   Bias due to ignoring matching

	Cases		Controls		Odds
Stratum	Exposed	Unexposed	Exposed	Unexposed	ratio
1	89	11	80	20	2.0
2	67	33	50	50	2.0
3	33	67	20	80	2.0
Total	189	111	150	150	1.7

of the role and status of the variable before accepting such a limitation.

Secondly, much of the early popularity of matching stemmed from a misconception that variables matched in the design can be ignored in analysis, since differences between cases and controls could then not be attributable to these variables. It is now understood that this practice leads, in general, to incorrect estimates of odds ratios. This is demonstrated by Table 18.4. There are 100 cases and 100 controls in each stratum so that, overall, the cases and controls are matched with respect to stratum. However, despite the matching, the marginal odds ratio is 1.7 rather than 2.0, the value within strata. We have already warned of this behaviour of the odds ratio in section 15.7; even when confounding by age is removed by matching, the marginal odds ratio is not equal to the conditional (age-specific) odds ratios.

The bias that arises by ignoring matching in the analysis is always towards $\theta = 1$. The only circumstances under which it does not occur is when the matching variable is unrelated to exposures of interest. Only then may the matching be ignored, but in that case the variable is not a confounder and there would seem to be no purpose in matching for it in the first place. However, we shall see in the next section that there are reasons for matching other than for the efficient control of confounding. Some of these can lead to circumstances in which the matching can be ignored in analysis, but usually this is not the case.

Taken together, these two points lead us to a position where a matching variable *must* be regarded as a confounder and *must* be used in the analysis. From this it follows that estimates of the effects of all other exposures will be controlled for the matching variable. But this may not be what we want to do. For example, in perinatal epidemiology it may be appropriate in some analyses to consider birthweight as a confounder while for other analyses this may not be sensible. If the study is matched for birthweight at the design stage, analyses which seek to hold birthweight constant are easily carried out using stratified comparisons, but analyses which do not hold birthweight constant are much more difficult. Indeed they would be impossible without knowledge of the sampling fractions for drawing controls from the base within strata. These complexities are best avoided and

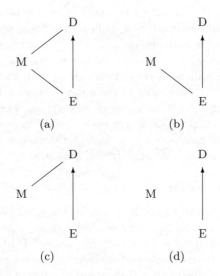

Fig. 18.1.   To match or not to match?

matching for variables which may not be regarded as confounders for some questions is in general a mistake.

Finally, matching may actually *reduce* the efficiency of a study. This occurs when the matching variable is strongly related to the exposure, but not to disease risk (so that, again, it is not a confounder). This is called *overmatching*. It leads to a loss in efficiency because the effect of the matching is only to narrow the range of exposure studied. A good example would be a study of diet and some childhood illness using siblings of cases as controls. While such a study would be expected to yield the correct answer if properly analysed, it would be very inefficient — since siblings usually eat at the same table of the same prepared meals, the only information available for estimating the effects of interest will be from sibling pairs with discordant diets.

This discussion is summarized in Fig. 18.1. The letters D, E, and M refer to disease, exposures of interest, and matching variable respectively. Connecting lines indicate statistical relationship. Case (a) is the only one in which matching leads to a more precise estimate of the odds ratio. Case (b) is overmatching and leads to a *loss* of precision. In cases (a) and (b), the matching must be preserved in the analysis, whereas in cases (c) and (d) it may be ignored.

The above discussion tacitly assumes that controls are matched to cases in rather broad strata, such as 5- or 10-year age bands. It applies equally to individually matched studies; in principle there is no difference between these options, although in practice the latter present rather more difficult analysis problems as a result of the very large number of nuisance parameters introduced by such fine stratification. These will be discussed in Chapter 19. Although matching must usually be preserved during analysis, it is not always necessary to preserve *individual* matching. If matching of controls to cases is only with respect to well defined, accurately measured variables then a coarser grouping at the analysis stage is both possible and acceptable. For example, if matching is only by age, analysis by 5- or 10-year bands will be quite satisfactory even if specific controls were drawn for each case. However, matching by characteristics such as neighbourhood or family does not allow later aggregation of strata.

18.4   Other reasons for matching

Matching is usually justified on the grounds of statistically efficient control for confounding. Close examination of this suggests that matching should be used as little as possible and only for variables, like age, which are strongly related to both disease and exposure and whose status is unequivocally that of confounder. However, a cursory review of the epidemiological literature shows that matching is used much more widely than this argument would support. This is because controls are often matched to cases for reasons which have nothing to do with control for confounding.

INCIDENCE DENSITY SAMPLING

One example is incidence density sampling, which is simply matching controls to cases with respect to *time* (date of occurrence). Although time may be a confounder (when both disease rate and exposure distribution in the study base vary during the study period), incidence density sampling is more usually employed for simple practical reasons. It will often be possible to ignore this matching in the analysis or, at most, to group coarsely on time.

DEFINING THE EXPOSURE WINDOW

Until this point we have assumed that each individual can be classified as exposed or unexposed and that this assignment holds for all time. However, many exposures in epidemiology vary over time, perhaps quite rapidly. When this is the case, it is necessary to specify the time period for assessing relevant exposure. This *exposure window* is usually clearly definable for cases, by working backwards from the point at which disease was first recognized, but comparable rules for controls can be difficult to specify. Things are much easier when one or more controls are matched to each single case with respect to time of diagnosis of the case; the time window used for assessing the relevant exposure of each case is carried over to the

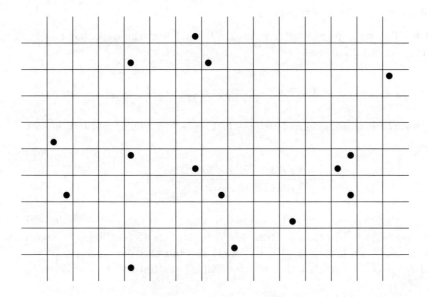

Fig. 18.2. Neighbourhood matching.

matched controls, thus ensuring comparability. We shall encounter a good example of this in Chapter 19.

AVOIDING SELECTION BIAS

Another example is where controls are matched to cases in order to minimize selection bias. This is usually done either because the study base has not been precisely defined or because there is no accurate way of sampling it. For example, in a geographically based study selection bias may be caused by the lack of an accurate population register of the study area. Unfortunately, construction and maintenance of such registers is enormously costly and will rarely be feasible for a single case-control study. However, if the study is closely matched, better sampling may be possible. Fig. 18.2 illustrates this for a geographically based study, divided by the grid into small *neighbourhoods*. The dots represent cases occurring during the study period. A study which matched for neighbourhood would sample controls only from those neighbourhoods in which a case occurred and it would only be necessary to construct lists of eligible controls for these. If neighbourhoods are sufficiently small this involves little work. Of course, the definition of neighbourhood does not have to be in terms of a regular grid for this argument to apply. A similar argument justifies drawing controls from the list of patients of the family doctor of each case.

Solutions to the exercises

18.1   The number of exposed cases, D_1^1, is 1 and the expected number under the null hypothesis is

$$E_1^1 = 2 \times \frac{11720}{11720 + 7594} = 1.21$$

so that the contribution to U is $(1 - 1.21) = -0.21$. The contribution to V is

$$\frac{2 \times 19312 \times 7594 \times 11720}{(19314)^2 \times 19313} = 0.48.$$

18.2   The expression for the 'expected' number of exposed cases in each stratum, E_1^t, is identical to that given in section 15.5. Thus, the score statistics, U, are identical. When there is only one case per stratum, $D^t = 1$ and $H^t = N^t - 1$ so that the contribution of stratum t to V is

$$V^t = \frac{(N^t - 1)N_0^t N_1^t}{(N^t)^2 (N^t - 1)} = \frac{N_0^t N_1^t}{(N^t)^2},$$

which is identical to our previous expression. When using the log rank test with tied event occurrence times (so that $D^t > 1$), the variance formula given in this chapter should be used.

18.3   The first contribution to the numerator (top) and denominator (bottom) of the Mantel–Haenszel estimate are as follows:

$$Q^1 = \frac{1 \times 7593}{1 + 1 + 7593 + 11719}, \qquad R^1 = \frac{1 \times 11719}{1 + 1 + 7593 + 11719}.$$

Continuing the calculation, we get:

Age	Q^t	R^t
0–4	0.39	0.61
5–9	5.76	6.46
10–14	9.34	16.01
15–19	5.96	12.53
20–24	5.74	13.86
25–29	7.95	9.70
30–34	4.82	8.88
Total	39.96	68.05

Note that the ratio Q/R for each row gives the odds ratios calculated in the previous exercise. The Mantel–Haenszel estimate is $39.96/68.05 = 0.587$.

18.4 V is given in the text following the first exercise as 51.62 and Q and R were calculated in the second exercise to be 39.96 and 68.05 respectively. Using the formula $S = \sqrt{V/(QR)}$,

$$S = \sqrt{\frac{51.62}{39.96 \times 68.05}} = 0.138$$

The error factor for 90% confidence limits is $\exp(1.645 \times 0.138) = 1.255$ so that the confidence limits for the odds ratio controlled for age are $0.587/1.255 = 0.47$ (lower limit) and $0.587 \times 1.255 = 0.74$ (upper limit).

18.5 The analysis of the two sets of data yields the following results:

	Table 18.2	Table 18.3
Estimate (θ)	0.582	0.568
S ($\log(\theta)$)	0.160	0.154
Error factor	1.301	1.289
Lower 90% limit	0.447	0.441
Upper 90% limit	0.757	0.732
$(U)^2/V$	11.73	13.76

In this case the increase in precision achieved by matching is not great.

19
Individually matched case-control studies

Analyses which preserve the matching of individual cases to their controls follow similar principles to those of Chapter 18. The strata are now the sets made up of each case and its matched controls. Studies designed to have a fixed number of controls, m say, drawn for each case, will be referred to as $1:m$ matched studies.

19.1 Mantel–Haenszel analysis of the 1:1 matched study

For reasons discussed in Chapter 18, the use of profile likelihood gives misleading estimates of odds ratios when there are a large number of strata with little data in each stratum. However, the Mantel–Haenszel method works perfectly well in these circumstances. The calculations are particularly easy in the 1:1 case, and illustrate ideas which are important for our later discussion of the likelihood approach.

The results of 1:1 matched studies are usually presented in 2×2 tables such as Table 19.1.* These data were drawn from the same study as reported in Chapter 17, and concern the relationship between tonsillectomy history and the incidence of Hodgkin's disease. The total study included 174 cases and 472 controls, but the controls were siblings of the cases, and the authors felt that the matching of cases and sibling controls should be preserved. They also wished to control for age and sex and therefore restricted their analysis to 85 matched case-control pairs in which the case and sibling control were of the same sex and matched for age within a specified margin. Note that, in the construction of matched sets, the original 174 cases and 472 controls have been reduced to only 85 cases and 85 controls.

Tables such as Table 19.1 can be confusing because we are used to seeing tables that count subjects, while this table counts case-control sets. The four cells of the table correspond to the four possible exposure configurations of a case-control set. These are illustrated in terms of a tree in Fig. 19.1. The first branching point is according to whether or not the control was exposed (denoted E+ and E- respectively), while the second

---

*From Cole, P. *et al.* (1973) *New England Journal of Medicine*, **288**, 634.

Table 19.1. Tonsillectomy history in 85 matched pairs

History	History of control	
of case	Positive	Negative
Positive	26	15
Negative	7	37

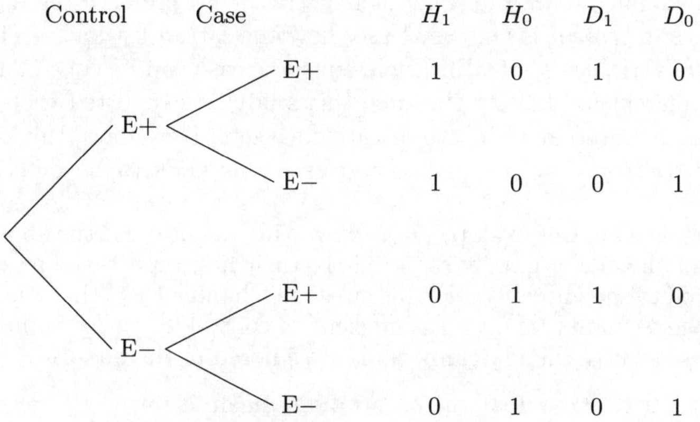

Control	Case		H_1	H_0	D_1	D_0
		E+	1	0	1	0
E+						
		E−	1	0	0	1
		E+	0	1	1	0
E−						
		E−	0	1	0	1

Fig. 19.1. Exposure configurations for 1:1 sets.

branching is according to exposure of the case. The frequencies in Table 19.1 refer to counts of these four configurations.

Exercise 19.1. How often did each of the exposure configurations of Fig. 19.1 occur?

In the analysis of individually matched studies the strata are case-control sets so that, in the notation of Chapter 18, t indexes sets. The number of subjects in each stratum is $N^t = 2$, and since each stratum contains one case and one control, D^t and H^t are always 1. The values of D_1^t, D_0^t, H_1^t, and H_0^t for each exposure configuration are shown in Fig. 19.1. In this figure and henceforth we will omit the superscript t for clarity, and remember that the symbols refer to values in a single case-control set.

Exercise 19.2. What are the contributions of each configuration to Q and R in the Mantel–Haenszel estimate of the odds ratio? Similarly what are the contributions to the score and score variance, U and V? Which configurations contribute to estimation and testing?

It can be seen that only two exposure configurations make any contribution to estimation and testing of the odds ratio. These are the sets in which the exposure status of case and controls differ and are called *discordant* sets. The remaining sets are called *concordant sets*. In our current example, 63 of the case-control sets are concordant and are ignored.

Exercise 19.3. For the tonsillectomy data, what are the values for Q, R, U, V? Using the methods of Chapter 18, estimate the odds ratio, its 90% confidence interval, and a p-value for $\theta = 1$.

The odds ratio estimate is very close to that obtained in the analysis of Chapter 17, but so much data has been lost in this analysis that the result is no longer statistically significant. It is easy to criticize an analysis which discards so much data, but when it is necessary to preserve the matching of controls to cases it is not easy to see how one can adjust for the effects of additional variables by stratification, since the case and its control may fall within different strata. At the time this study was reported there would have been no alternative but to discard such sets. Nowadays, this problem is easily overcome by use of the regression methods to be described in Part II.

Before leaving this example, it is interesting to note that the above analysis is not the one originally reported. In their first report, the researchers subscribed to the misconception discussed in Chapter 18 — that the matching for age, sex, and family was sufficient to control for these variables and that subsequently the matching could be ignored in the analysis.

Exercise 19.4. Show that the odds ratio estimate obtained by ignoring the matching is less than that obtained by the correct analysis.

19.2   The hypergeometric likelihood for 1:1 matched studies

The hypergeometric likelihood is obtained by arguing conditionally upon *both* margins of the 2×2 table, and depends only upon the odds ratio parameter. It is usually difficult to compute, but its use is only necessary when the data within strata are few. This is the case for individually matched studies and the hypergeometric likelihood *must* be used. Luckily in this case the computations are quite easy — particularly in the 1:1 case.

Fig. 19.2 derives the probability of each exposure configuration by multiplying along branches of the tree in the usual way and also lists the total number of *subjects* in the set who were exposed, N_1. The odds that the control in the set was exposed is denoted by Ω_0 and the odds that the case was exposed by Ω_1, and we have written K for the expression

$$\frac{1}{(1 + \Omega_0)(1 + \Omega_1)}$$

which occurs in all four probabilities. To obtain the hypergeometric likelihood we argue conditionally on the number of subjects exposed, N_1. It is clear from the figure that, when $N_1 = 2$, there is only one possible exposure configuration; the *conditional* probability of the observation is 1 and there is no contribution to the log likelihood. Similarly, there is no

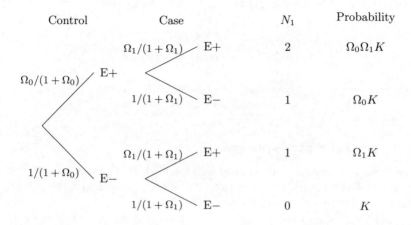

Control		Case	N_1	Probability

Fig. 19.2. Probabilities for a case-control set.

contribution to the log likelihood from sets in which $N_1 = 0$. These configurations correspond to the concordant sets which were also ignored in our previous analysis. However, when $N_1 = 1$ the exposure configuration could be either the second or third. These are the possible configurations of discordant sets. The observed split of discordant sets between the second and third configurations determines the log likelihood.

The conditional probabilities that a discordant set is of the third type (case exposed, control unexposed) and the second type (case unexposed, control exposed) are

$$\frac{\Omega_1 K}{\Omega_0 K + \Omega_1 K} \quad \text{and} \quad \frac{\Omega_0 K}{\Omega_0 K + \Omega_1 K}$$

respectively, and the conditional odds that the case was exposed is the ratio of these, Ω_1/Ω_0. This is the odds ratio parameter θ, assumed in our model to be constant for all the case control sets. The conditional argument therefore leads to a Bernoulli log likelihood based on splits of discordant sets into those in which the case is exposed and those in which the case is unexposed, the odds for such splits being θ. In our data, such sets split 15:7 and the log likelihood is

$$15 \log(\theta) - 22 \log(1 + \theta).$$

Exercise 19.5. Calculate the most likely value of θ, a 90% confidence interval and the score test for the null hypothesis $\theta = 1$. These results of this exercise should agree precisely with those obtained using the Mantel–Haenszel method.

Table 19.2.   Screening history in breast cancer deaths and matched controls

Status of the case	Number of controls screened			
	0	1	2	3
Screened	1	4	3	1
Unscreened	11	10	12	4

19.3   Several controls per case

The arguments outlined above may be extended to the situation in which there are several controls for each case. As before, we start with the Mantel–Haenszel approach.

Table 19.2 shows the results of a case-control study of breast cancer screening. Cases are deaths from breast cancer and each case is matched with three control women.[†] The exposure of interest is attendance for breast cancer screening. If screening is effective in prolonging life, screened women should have lower mortality rates and the odds ratio estimate from the case-control study should be less than 1. Note that as in Table 19.1, the table counts case-control sets and not women.

This study illustrates one of the reasons for matching discussed in Chapter 18. Women who die from breast cancer usually do so some years after initial diagnosis and during the period between diagnosis and death they would not be screened. Thus, controls would have a greater opportunity to be screened than cases. This difficulty was overcome by determining the relevant *exposure window*; the screening history of the controls was assessed over the period up to the time of diagnosis of the case, so that the screening histories of cases and controls are comparable. It was only possible to deal with this problem in this way because the study matched controls to individual cases.

Table 19.2 demonstrates the usual way such data are presented. However, it is very difficult to perceive any pattern — even as to whether or not screening appears to be a protective. To understand the analysis, we shall start by reordering the data as a tree. Fig. 19.3 illustrates the possible exposure configurations. The first three branches represent the exposure status of the three controls, the upper branch representing exposed (E+) and the lower unexposed (E−). Because we do not wish to differentiate between individual controls, this section of the tree may be abbreviated. For the first two controls, we do not need to differentiate between the configurations (E+, E−) and (E−, E+). These are simply grouped together as having 1 control exposed and we write the figure 2 at this point to remind us that branches emanating from this point are *double* branches. Similarly, after consideration of the third control we group together the 3 configu-

---

[†]From Collette, H.J.A. *et al.* (1984) *The Lancet*, June 2, 1984, 1224–1226.

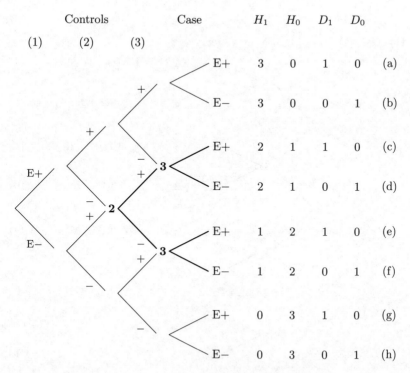

Fig. 19.3.   Exposure configurations for 1:3 sets.

rations with 2 exposed controls and the 3 configurations with 1 exposed control. The final branching represents the exposure status of the case.

Exercise 19.6. In the screening data, how frequently do each of the eight types of exposure configuration occur?

We shall first analyse these data by the Mantel–Haenszel method. In the next section, we shall discuss the likelihood approach and show how it suggests a more useful arrangement of the table.

Exercise 19.7. Tabulate the values of Q, R, U, and V for these eight tables and hence calculate the Mantel–Haenszel significance test, odds ratio estimate and an approximate 90% confidence interval.

This analysis shows that the study finds a substantial and statistically significant reduction in mortality as a result of breast cancer screening.

19.4   The likelihood

The analysis of these data by use of the hypergeometric likelihood method is also quite straightforward. As before we argue conditionally upon the margins. Fig. 19.4 shows the total number of *subjects* exposed, N_1, and the

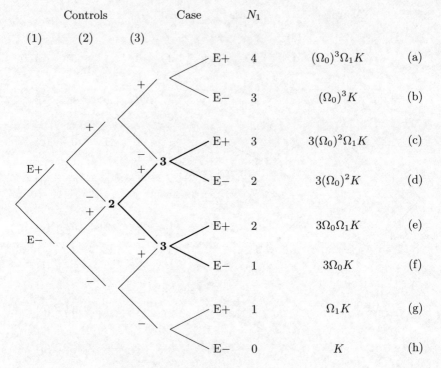

Fig. 19.4. Probabilities for 1:3 sets.

probability of each configuration, again writing K for the common factor, in this case

$$K = \frac{1}{(1 + \Omega_0)^3 (1 + \Omega_1)}.$$

Note that the probabilities for configurations (c) to (f) are multiplied by 3 because each of these represents three paths in the complete tree. Now there are 5 possible values for the total number of subjects exposed. Again there are two *concordant* configurations in which the number of subjects exposed uniquely determines the configuration. $N_1 = 4$ ensures configuration (a) and $N_1 = 0$ ensures configuration (h). These make no contribution to the log likelihood. Each of the other three values of N_1 allows for two possible configurations, one in which the case is exposed and the other in which the case is unexposed. It is the splits of the observed data between these that yield the likelihood.

If the total number of exposed subjects in the set, N_1, is fixed at 3, then the exposure configuration must be either (b) or (c) and the conditional

Table 19.3.   Splits of case-control sets

N_1	Split	Odds	Observed
3	(c):(b)	3θ	3:4
2	(e):(d)	θ	4:12
1	(g):(f)	$\theta/3$	1:10

odds for the split (c):(b) is

$$\frac{3(\Omega_0)^2 \Omega_1 K}{(\Omega_0)^3 K} = \frac{3\Omega_1}{\Omega_0} = 3\theta.$$

Similarly, $N_1 = 2$ implies (d) or (e) and $N_1 = 0$ implies (f) or (g). The odds predicted by the model for these splits are set out in Table 19.3, together with the observed frequencies. By eye we can see that a value of θ of about 0.3 predicts the observed splits very well indeed. More formally, the log likelihood is

$$1\log\left(\frac{\theta}{3}\right) - 11\log\left(1 + \frac{\theta}{3}\right)$$
$$+ \quad 4\log\left(\theta\right) - 16\log\left(1 + \theta\right)$$
$$+ \quad 3\log\left(3\theta\right) - 7\log\left(1 + 3\theta\right).$$

There is no simple expression for the maximum likelihood estimate and it is necessary to use a computer program to search for the maximum. This occurs at $\theta = 0.31$ ($\log(\theta) = -1.18$). The plot of the log likelihood ratio against $\log(\theta)$ is shown in Fig. 19.5. A Gaussian approximation with $S = 0.404$ fits quite closely.

The generalization of this argument to any number of controls per case may be carried out algebraically or by extending our tree. For sets of N_1 exposed subjects and N_0 unexposed subjects, the constant odds ratio model predicts that sets will split between those with an exposed case and those with an unexposed case with odds

$$N_1\theta/N_0.$$

A similar generalization is possible for several *cases* in each set. We will not give the details here, but computer software is readily available. Such analyses do not arise frequently in practice. An exception is family studies in which more than one sibling may be affected by a disease and unaffected siblings are used as controls.

In the examples discussed in this chapter, the Mantel–Haenszel and likelihood methods agree closely. The calculations for the former are rather easier, but the advantage of the likelihood approach lies in its greater generality and possibilities for extension. For example, when there are more

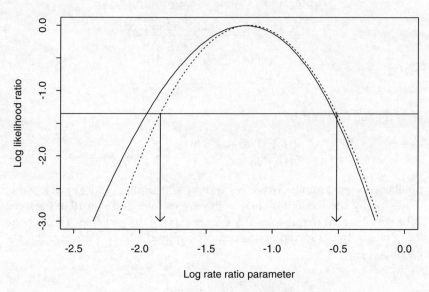

Fig. 19.5. Log likelihood ratio for $\log(\theta)$.

than two exposure categories, there is no simple method analogous to the Mantel–Haenszel approach. We shall defer discussion of such extensions to Part II of the book.

Solutions to the exercises

19.1 In the order in which the exposure configurations are listed in the figure, their frequencies are 26, 7, 15, and 37.

19.2 In the same order as listed,

Q	R	U	V
0	0	0	0
0	1/2	-1/2	1/4
1/2	0	1/2	1/4
0	0	0	0

Only the second and third configurations contribute to Q, R, U, and V.

19.3

$$
\begin{aligned}
Q &= 15 \times (1/2) \\
R &= 7 \times (1/2) \\
U &= 15 \times (1/2) - 7 \times (1/2) = 4
\end{aligned}
$$

$$V \quad = \quad 15 \times (1/4) + 7 \times (1/4) = 5.5$$

The odds ratio estimate is $15/7 = 2.14$. This estimates the underlying rate ratio, so that the suggestion is that tonsillectomy doubles the rate of Hodgkin's disease. Using the expression

$$S = \sqrt{\frac{V}{QR}} = 0.4577,$$

the 90% error factor for the odds ratio is $\exp(1.645 \times 0.4577) = 2.12$. The 90% confidence limits are, therefore, $2.14/2.12 = 1.01$ (lower limit) and $2.14 \times 2.12 = 4.54$ (upper limit). Referring the value $(U)^2/V = 2.91$ to the chi-squared distribution gives $p \approx 0.09$.

19.4 If the matching is ignored, the following 2×2 table is obtained:

History:	Positive	Negative
Cases	41	44
Controls	33	52

The odds ratio in this table is $(41 \times 52)/(33 \times 44) = 1.47$, as compared to the value of 2.14 obtained by the correct analysis.

19.5 The most likely value is $15/7 = 2.14$. To calculate the approximate 90% interval using Gaussian approximation of the log likelihood for $\log(\theta)$ we use

$$S = \sqrt{\frac{1}{15} + \frac{1}{7}} = 0.4577,$$

the same as we obtained with the Mantel–Haenszel method. Under the null hypothesis, the probability for the split is 0.5 so that the expected number of sets with an exposed case is $22 \times 0.5 = 11$. The score and score variance are

$$U \quad = \quad 15 - 11 = 4,$$
$$V \quad = \quad 22 \times 0.5 \times 0.5 = 5.5.$$

Again these are the values we obtained using the Mantel–Haenszel method.

19.6 In the order listed in the figure, the 8 exposure configurations have frequencies 1, 4, 3, 12, 4, 10, 1, 11.

19.7 The contributions to Q, R, U and V are shown below:

	Number of sets	Q	R	U	V
(a)	1	0	0	0	0
(b)	4	0	3/4	−3/4	9/48
(c)	3	1/4	0	1/4	9/48
(d)	12	0	2/4	−2/4	12/48
(e)	4	2/4	0	2/4	12/48
(f)	10	0	1/4	−1/4	9/48
(g)	1	3/4	0	3/4	9/48
(h)	11	0	0	0	0
Total		14/4	46/4	-32/4	354/48

Note that each contribution has to be multiplied by the number of times it occurred so that, for example, the total value of Q is

$$(3 \times 1/4) + (4 \times 2/4) + (1 \times 3/4) = 14/4.$$

The Mantel–Haenszel estimate of θ is $14/46 = 0.30$ and the chi-squared test is $(U)^2/V = 8.68$ ($p < 0.01$). An approximate error factor can be calculated from

$$\exp\left(1.645 \times \sqrt{\frac{V}{QR}}\right) = 2.02$$

so that the 90% confidence interval lies from $\theta = 0.15$ to $\theta = 0.60$.

20
Tests for trend

Up to this point we have dealt exclusively with comparisons of exposed and unexposed groups. Although it is possible that the action of an exposure is 'all or nothing', coming into play only when a threshold dose is exceeded, it is more common to find a dose-response relationship, with increasing dose leading to increasing disease rates throughout the range of exposure. This chapter introduces analyses which take account of the level or *dose* of exposure.

20.1 Dose-response models for cohort studies

The simplest model for dose-response relationship assumes that the effect of a one-unit increase in dose is to multiply the rate (or odds) by θ, where θ is constant across the entire range of exposure. Thus the effect of each increment of dose on the log rate or odds is to add an amount $\beta = \log(\theta)$. This model is called the *log-linear model* and is illustrated in Fig. 20.1. The dose level is denoted by z. The rate at dose $z = 0$ is given by $\log(\lambda_0) = \alpha$, at $z = 1$ by $\log(\lambda_1) = \alpha + \beta$, at $z = 2$ by $\log(\lambda_2) = \alpha + 2\beta$, and so on.

In principle, log-linear models present no new problems. The model describes the rate at different doses z in terms of two parameters α and β. The first of these describes the log rate in unexposed persons and will normally be a nuisance parameter; the second is the parameter β, which describes the effect of increasing exposure. The contribution to the log likelihood from D_z events in Y_z person-years of observation at dose z is

$$D_z \log(\lambda_z) - Y_z \lambda_z$$

and the total log likelihood is the sum of such terms over all levels of exposure observed. This is a function of both α and β but, as before, we can obtain a profile likelihood for the parameter of interest, β, by replacing α by its most likely value for each value of β. This profile likelihood is given by the expression:

$$\sum D_z \log \left(\frac{Y_z \exp(\beta z)}{\sum Y_z \exp(\beta z)} \right),$$

where both summations are over dose levels z. Exactly the same log likeli-

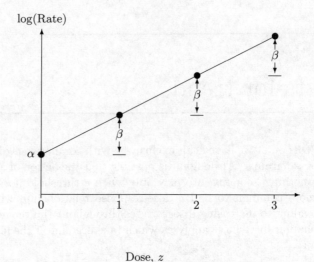

Fig. 20.1.   Log-linear trend.

hood is obtained using the retrospective conditional argument based on the probability that the cases split between exposure categories in the ratios observed.

To find the most likely value of the parameter β requires computer programs for *Poisson regression*, whose use will be discussed in Part II. However, the likelihood can be used to obtain some simpler analytical procedures. Most importantly, a statistical test for the significance of a dose-response effect can be derived by calculating the gradient of the log likelihood at $\beta = 0$. This leads to the score

$$U = D \left(\frac{\sum D_z z}{\sum D_z} - \frac{\sum Y_z z}{\sum Y_z} \right)$$

where summation is over exposure doses z and, as usual, $D = \sum D_z$. The first term within the brackets is the mean exposure for *cases*, while the second is the mean exposure in the entire cohort, using the person-time observation as weights. The weighting ensures that a subject observed for twice as long contributes twice as much to the mean; this is necessary since he or she has twice the chance of becoming a case.

Denoting means of z by $\bar{z}$, the score may be written

$$U = D \left(\bar{z}_{\text{Cases}} - \bar{z}_{\text{Cohort}} \right).$$

The score variance, obtained from the curvature of the log likelihood curve

Table 20.1. Observed and expected deaths from bladder cancer in workers in the nuclear industry

Dose code, z	0	1	2	3	4	5	6
Dose (mSv):	< 10	10–	20–	50–	100–	200–	≥ 400
Observed, D_z	3	2	1	1	3	2	2
Expected, E_z	6.2	1.0	2.2	1.8	1.5	1.0	0.4

at $\beta = 0$, is

$$V = D \left[\frac{\sum Y_z(z)^2}{\sum Y_z} - \left(\bar{z}_{\text{Cohort}} \right)^2 \right].$$

This expression is D times the *variance* of the exposure doses z within the cohort (again weighting by person-time of observation). The calculation of weighted means and variances is easily carried out on scientific calculators which include special keys for these operations.

The same argument applies in the construction of tests for trend in SMR's except that instead of the person-time Y_z we now use E_z, the expected numbers of events obtained by application of age-specific reference rates. The use of this test is illustrated in the following example.

RADIATION AND BLADDER CANCER

Table 20.1 shows observed deaths from carcinoma of the bladder in a cohort of radiation workers, classified according to the radiation dose received. Also shown are the numbers of deaths expected in each category on the basis of England and Wales rates.* The mean dose code for the bladder cancer cases is:

$$\frac{3 \times 0 + 2 \times 1 + 1 \times 2 + \ldots + 2 \times 6}{14} = 2.93$$

The expected mean is obtained by using the expected numbers of cases as weights, is

$$\frac{6.2 \times 0 + 1.0 \times 1 + 2.2 \times 2 + \ldots + 0.4 \times 6}{14.1} = 1.72$$

so the score is

$$U = 14(2.93 - 1.72) = 16.9.$$

The weighted variance of the dose may be calculated using the appropriate calculator key, or from

$$\frac{6.2 \times (0)^2 + 1.0 \times (1)^2 + 2.2 \times (2)^2 + \ldots + 0.4 \times (6)^2}{14.1} - (1.72)^2 = 3.31,$$

---

*From Smith, P.G. and Douglas, A.J. (1986) *British Medical Journal*, **293**, 845–854.

so the score variance is $V = 14 \times 3.31 = 46.4$. The score test is therefore $(16.9)^2/46.4 = 6.16$, which corresponds to a p-value of 0.013. Although in this example, radiation dose was grouped into a few discrete categories, this is not a requirement of the analysis. Dose could be recorded more exactly so that no two individuals share the same dose. Observed and expected mean doses are calculated in the same way.

When the exposure dose is roughly normally distributed within cases, the log likelihood is nearly quadratic and an approximation to the most likely value of β is provided by

$$\frac{U}{V} = \frac{\text{Mean dose (cases)} - \text{Mean dose (cohort)}}{\text{Variance of dose (cohort)}}.$$

The standard deviation of this estimate is approximately $\sqrt{1/V}$.

Exercise 20.1. (a) Calculate a rough estimate of β for the bladder cancer data. (The maximum likelihood estimate is 0.328.)
(b) What is the interpretation of β? How may the effect be expressed in terms of *rate ratios*?
(c) How would the interpretation of the analysis be changed if the calculations had been carried out using the actual radiation dose as z rather than the 0–6 code?

20.2   Stratified analysis of cohort data

The extension of these ideas to stratified analysis involves only a slight extension of the model. Use of either a profile or conditional approach leads to a log likelihood function for β which is simply a sum over strata of contributions of the same form as in the previous section. In consequence, the score and score variances at $\beta = 0$ are simply sums of contributions from each stratum:

$$
\begin{aligned}
U &= \sum U^t \\
&= \sum D^t \left(\bar{z}^t_{\text{Cases}} - \bar{z}^t_{\text{Cohort}} \right),
\end{aligned}
$$

and

$$V = \sum V^t.$$

ENERGY INTAKE AND IHD

An example of the use of this method is shown in Table 20.2. The table is calculated from the same data on energy intake and ischaemic heart disease which has been encountered in previous chapters, and compares observed and expected mean energy intake of heart disease cases. The study cohort was drawn from three rather different occupational groups, bank workers, London bus drivers, and London bus conductors. To control

Table 20.2.   Mean energy intake (kcal/day) of IHD cases

Age	Bank staff		Drivers		Conductors	
	Obs.	Exp.	Obs.	Exp.	Obs.	Exp.
40–49	2769	3015	2918	2853	–	–
		(4)		(2)		(0)
50–59	2514	2894	2808	2838	2515	2845
		(8)		(4)		(5)
60–69	2725	2846	2458	2833	2718	2828
		(7)		(6)		(9)

for confounding by age and occupation, 9 strata are required. Table 20.2 shows the comparisons of means for the 9 strata formed by crossing the three occupational groups by three age bands. The numbers of cases are shown in parentheses.

The most striking feature of this table is the consistency of the finding that energy intake is lower in cases than would be expected under the null hypothesis. This is confirmed by the overall significance test for which

$$
\begin{aligned}
U &= 4 \times (2\,769 - 3\,015) + \cdots + 9 \times (2\,718 - 2\,828) \\
&= -9\,765 \\
V &= 8\,446\,000,
\end{aligned}
$$

so that the score test is $(-9\,765)^2/8\,446\,000 = 11.29$ and $p < 0.001$ (detailed workings for V are not shown).

The use of U and V to obtain a rough estimate of β is exactly the same as in the unstratified case.

Exercise 20.2. Calculate an approximate estimate of β for the energy intake data, using the values of U, V given above. Calculate the change in log rate predicted for a 500 kcal change in energy intake and express this as a rate ratio.

20.3   Dose-response relationships in case-control studies

The extension of these methods to deal with case-control studies requires only the change to an appropriate likelihood. In Chapter 17 we showed that this is the likelihood based upon the split of the N_z subjects observed with exposure level z as D_z cases and H_z controls. If the odds predicted by the model for such a split are ω_z, the log likelihood is

$$
\sum \left[D_z \log(\omega_z) - N_z \log(1 + \omega_z) \right].
$$

The idea that the rate ratio for each dose increment is constant translates, in the case-control study, to a constant *odds ratio* for each one unit change

Table 20.3. Screening histories in breast cancer deaths and controls

| | \multicolumn{4}{c}{Negative screens} | |
	0	1	2	3	Total
Cases	29	22	3	3	57
Controls	99	122	40	24	285
Subjects	128	144	43	27	442

in dose. Thus the model for the log odds takes the same form as Fig. 20.1:

$$\log(\omega_z) = \alpha + \beta z.$$

This is a *logistic regression* model. Computer programs for estimating β are widely available and their use will be discussed in Part II, but a score test of the null hypothesis $\beta = 0$ requires only simple tabulations and a hand calculator. The nuisance parameter, α, is removed either by a profile likelihood approach, or by a conditional argument leading to the hypergeometric likelihood. In either case, the score test given by the gradient of the log likelihood curve turns out to be:

$$U = \frac{DH}{N}\left(\frac{\sum D_z z}{D} - \frac{\sum H_z z}{H}\right).$$

$$= \frac{DH}{N}\left(\bar{z}_{\text{Cases}} - \bar{z}_{\text{Controls}}\right)$$

The score variance is obtained from the curvature of the log likelihood and, as in section 17.3, the profile and the conditional approaches lead to slightly different expressions. For the conditional approach,

$$V = \frac{DH}{N}\frac{\sum N_z(z)^2 - N(\bar{z})^2}{(N-1)},$$

where $\bar{z}$ is the overall mean dose $(\sum N_z z)/N$. Apart from the factor DH/N, this is the usual estimate of the variance of dose in the study when cases and controls are combined. The profile likelihood argument leads to the same expression, but with $(N-1)$ replaced by N.

Exercise 20.3. In Chapter 19, a case control study of the efficacy of a radiographic breast cancer screening programme was discussed. Table 20.3 shows data drawn from a similar study concerning the number of times women had been screened (with negative result).[†]
(a) By calculating case/control ratios, examine the data for evidence of decreasing risk with increasing numbers of negative screens.
(b) The mean number of screens for cases is 0.649, and for controls is 0.961. The

---

[†]From Palli, D. *et al.* (1986) *International Journal of Epidemiology*, **38**, 501–504.

overall variance of the number of screens is 0.810. Calculate the score and score
variance and the corresponding chi-squared value.

Extension of these results to stratified and matched case-control studies
follows along familiar lines. Each stratum (or case-control set) provides its
own contribution to the score:

$$U^t = \frac{D^t H^t}{N^t} \left(\bar{z}^t_{\text{Cases}} - \bar{z}^t_{\text{Controls}} \right).$$

The overall score is the sum of these contributions and the score variance
(using the hypergeometric conditional argument) is the sum contributions:

$$V^t = \frac{D^t H^t}{N^t} \frac{\sum_z N^t_z(z)^2 - N^t(\bar{z}^t)^2}{N^t - 1}.$$

This stratified version of the score test for $\beta = 0$ is often called the *Mantel
extension* test.

Under the log-linear model, if the dose is normally distributed in controls then it will also be normally distributed in cases, but with a different
mean value. In those circumstances, an estimate of β will be provided by
U/V as in earlier sections.

When there are only two dose levels ($z = 0$ and $z = 1$), it can be shown
that the tests set out in this chapter are identical to those discussed in
previous chapters. It follows from this equivalence that all the score tests
discussed in this book may be thought of as comparisons of mean exposures.
This insight makes possible the use of standard computer programs for
summary tabulations of large bodies of data. This is particularly valuable
for preliminary analysis and for demonstrating the consistency of a finding
over subgroups.

Exercise 20.4. If you are undeterred by algebra, you might like to try and prove
this equivalence.

Solutions to the exercises

20.1 The rough estimate of β is $16.9/46.4 = 0.36$. This is the log of the
rate ratio for one unit change in dose score. The rate ratio is $\exp 0.36 = 1.4$.
The dose code is constructed so that one unit change in z represents a
doubling of the radiation dose, so that the approximately fitted model
suggests that doubling the radiation dose multiplies the bladder cancer rate
by approximately 1.4. If the analysis had been carried out by calculating
means of radiation dose itself rather than mean dose code, the implied
model would have been rather different — that the *addition* of a given
radiation dose would multiply the rate by some constant amount.

20.2 The rough estimate of β is $-9\,765/8\,446\,000 = -1.16 \times 10^{-3}$. This is the change in the log rate for one unit change in energy intake. For 500 kcal change, the change in log rate is $-1.16 \times 10^{-3} \times 500 = -0.58$. This corresponds to a rate ratio of $\exp -0.58 = 0.56$. The study therefore indicates that an increase of 500 kcal in daily energy intake is associated with an approximate halving of the incidence rate of IHD.

20.3 The case/control ratios for 0, 1, 2 and 3 previous negative screens are 0.29, 0.18, 0.08 and 0.13 respectively, suggesting that mortality rates from breast cancer fall with increasing numbers of previous negative screens. The score is

$$U = \frac{57 \times 285}{342}(0.649 - 0.961) = -14.82$$

and the score variance is

$$V = \frac{57 \times 285}{342} \times 0.810 = 38.47,$$

so that the score test is $(-14.82)^2/38.47 = 5.71$, corresponding to a p-value of 0.017. The use of this test in this case is debatable, since it is not by any means clear that a simple linear or log-linear dose-response relationship should apply. The true relationship between screening history and subsequent mortality depends in a complex way upon the sensitivity of the test, the speed of growth of tumours, the relationship between prognosis and tumour stage at start of treatment, together with the time interval between screens. Most of the evidence for trend comes from the higher case/control ratios in the *never* screened group, rather than from a gradient with increasing number of screens. We must be careful not to interpret a significant trend test as indicating evidence for dose-response as such.

20.4 For cohort studies, the equivalence follows from the fact that $\bar{z}_{\text{Cases}}$ is the proportion of cases exposed, D_1/D. Similarly $\bar{z}_{\text{Cohort}}$ is the proportion of person-time exposed, Y_1/Y. The variance of a binary z in the cohort is

$$\frac{Y_1}{Y} - \left(\frac{Y_1}{Y}\right)^2 = \frac{Y_0 Y_1}{(Y)^2}$$

and substitution of these expressions into the formulas given in section 20.1 gives the same test as Chapter 13.

For case-control studies, the means of z in cases and in controls are the corresponding proportions exposed, D_1/D and H_1/H. The variance of z in the study is

$$\frac{N_1 - N(N_1/N)^2}{N - 1} = \frac{N_0 N_1}{N(N - 1)}.$$

Substitution of these values into the formulas of section 20.3 gives the test discussed in Chapter 17.

21
The size of investigations

Before embarking on an epidemiological study, it is important to ensure that the study will be large enough to answer the questions it addresses. Calculation of the required study size is often regarded as rather difficult, but in fact requires no new methods.

The problem is usually presented as if the scientist comes to the statistician with a clearly formulated hypothesis and the simple question 'How large should my study be?'. This is rarely the case. More usually the investigator has a very clear idea of the size of study proposed, this being determined by budgetary and logistic constraints, and requires an answer to the question 'Is my proposed study large enough?'. All too often calculations show the answer to be no! The investigator then needs to know how much larger the study needs to be.

This chapter will address the problem of study size from this standpoint. In addition to being more realistic, it follows more naturally from earlier chapters since the first stage of the calculation is to guess the results of the proposed study and analyse these. It will be convenient to develop the argument in the simplest case — the comparison of incidence in a cohort with that in a standard reference population. Generalization to other study designs is straightforward and will be discussed towards the end of the chapter.

21.1 The anticipated result

In order to answer the question 'Is my proposed study large enough?', we need to put ourselves in the position of having carried it out. To do this, it will be necessary to make some guesses about how things will turn out. A careful calculation of study size may involve a range of guesses. The most important thing to guess is the size of the effect of primary interest.

We shall take as an example a cohort study to investigate an occupational risk of lung cancer. In the proposed study, a cohort of industrial workers will be traced, and all deaths from lung cancer counted. This number will be compared with the expected number of deaths obtained by applying national age- and period-specific mortality rates to the table of person-time observation for the cohort. The first stage of the calculation will be to guess this person-time table, allowing for mortality in the cohort.

Let us assume that this has been done and that it leads to an expected number of lung cancer deaths of $E = 12.5$.

Exercise 21.1. What is the anticipated outcome of the study when θ, the rate ratio parameter for occupational exposure, is (a) 1.4, (b) 1.7, (c) 2.0, and (d) 5.0. In each case calculate the logarithm of θ and calculate the anticipated standard deviation for the log SMR (which estimates $\log(\theta)$). Is the study large enough to detect these rate ratios?

It is clear that the study would not be large enough to detect a rate ratio of 1.4, since the anticipated result would yield a 90% confidence interval which includes the null hypothesis $\theta = 1$ ($\log(\theta) = 0$). It should be equally clear that the study will almost certainly detect a rate ratio of 5, since in that case the size of effect is very large in comparison with its standard deviation. The two intermediate values for θ are more problematic and in such cases it is useful to further quantify the chances that the study will detect the effect.

21.2   Power

The *power* of a study is defined as the probability that it will yield a significant result when the true size of effect is as specified. The power is different for each size of effect considered, being greater for larger effects. Thus the power of a study is not a single number, but a whole range of values. The plot of power against size of effect is called a *power curve*. Two such curves for studies of different sizes are illustrated in Fig. 21.1. In practice it is rare for the entire power curve to be presented; more usually a few points in the range of effects are tabulated.

Exercise 21.2. Which curve corresponds to the larger study?

A significant result is defined as a result where the p-value for the null hypothesis is below a specified threshold (the *significance* level). Alternatively (and equivalently) it may be thought of as a result in which the null hypothesis falls outside a specified confidence interval. To calculate the power, it will be necessary to specify the significance (confidence) level to be used to categorize the result as significant. A study will have a higher power to detect a finding at the 5% level of statistical significance (95% confidence) than at the 1% level (99% confidence).

21.3   Calculating the power

It has already been stated that study size calculations require some guess-work. There is therefore little point in calculating power to a high order of accuracy. In this section we outline approximate power calculations which are accurate enough for all practical purposes.

Fig. 21.2 sets out our notation. The study aims to estimate an effect

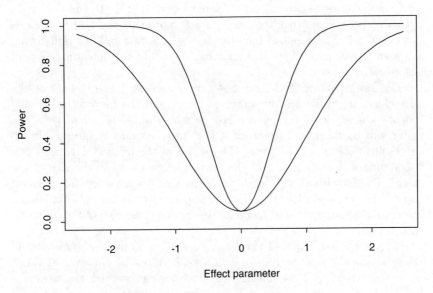

Fig. 21.1. Power curves for two studies.

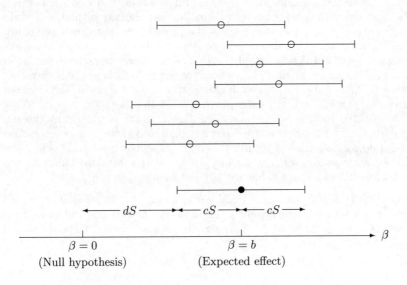

Fig. 21.2. Calculating the power of a study.

parameter, β,* and we assume that the log likelihood may be approximated by a Gaussian log likelihood with standard deviation S. To simplify notation, we also assume that the point $\beta = 0$ represents the null hypothesis (no effect). For example, β may be the log of a rate ratio or odds ratio. We wish to calculate the probability that the study will detect an effect of size $\beta = b$.

The lower part of the figure shows the anticipated result of the study. The black disc indicates the expected effect and the lines to either side indicate the expected confidence interval which would be calculated. The result will be taken as significant if the entire confidence interval lies to the right of the null hypothesis. The width of the interval depends upon the standard deviation S, and this in turn depends upon the size of the study. The interval also depends upon the significance or confidence level chosen. For example, for a 5% significance level we use the 95% confidence interval, which extends 1.96 standard deviations either side of the estimate, so $c = 1.96$.

If the expected value of the lower confidence limit lies above $\beta = 0$, the study would be expected to yield a positive result. However, it is not *guaranteed* to do so. If we imagine the study being repeated, the estimates obtained will vary from occasion to occasion. These estimates are indicated on the diagram by open circles.

The variation of estimates around the expected value is approximately Gaussian with standard deviation S. Ignoring the slight dependence of S upon the estimated value, the lower confidence limit will also vary around its expected value according to a Gaussian distribution with standard deviation S. The power of the study is the probability that this lower bound falls above zero. This depends upon the number of standard deviations between zero and the expected position of the lower bound. Referring to this number as d, the probability that the lower limit is above zero is then given by the probability that an observation in a standard Gaussian distribution exceeds $-d$. For example, if $d = 1.645$, the power is 0.95. When the expected location of the lower confidence limit is exactly at the null hypothesis, so that $d = 0$, the power is 0.50 and there is an even chance of obtaining a significant result. When the expected position is below zero $d < 0$, the power is less than 0.50. (Tables of the standard Gaussian distribution are widely available and are not included in this book.)

Exercise 21.3. For the study discussed in Exercise 21.1, calculate d for each value of the log rate ratio, assuming that a 5% significance level will be used (i.e. $c = 1.96$). Using tables of the Gaussian distribution, obtain the power in each case.

---

*We use this letter as it is the usual symbol for an effect parameter in regression models. It should not be confused with the 'type II error probability', for which it stands in some texts.

Table 21.1. Choice of c and d

Significance	c	Power	d
0.10	1.645	0.95	1.645
0.05	1.960	0.90	1.282
0.01	2.576	0.75	0.674

21.4 Increasing the power

If the results of the power calculations are disappointing, it will be necessary to increase the study size in some way. In this section we show how to determine by how much the study size must be increased to achieve the desired power.

Predetermining the significance level fixes the value of c. Similarly, predetermining the *power* fixes d. Since we require the distance $(c+d)S$ to equal the expected effect, b, we must choose the size of the study so that

$$S = \frac{b}{c+d}.$$

Table 21.1 lists some common requirements for significance and power. Note that, in each row of the Table, $(c+d)$ is between 3.2 and 3.3 so that these choices of significance and power suggest designing the study so that the expected effect, b, is just over 3 standard deviations.

Exercise 21.4. Calculate the value of the S which must be achieved if there were to be a power of 0.90 to detect a rate ratio $\theta = 1.7$ at the $p = 0.05$ significance level.

If the value of S required to achieve the desired power is smaller than that we expected to achieve with the study as originally proposed, then the study size must be increased. In general the factor by which the study size must be increased is

$$\left(\frac{\text{Current value of } S}{\text{Required value of } S} \right)^2$$

Exercise 21.5. Carrying on from the previous exercise, by what factor must the study be increased to achieve the required power? How could this be done in practice?

21.5 Application to other study designs

The extension of the above argument to different study designs introduces no serious new problems, although the first stage of the process — calculating the expected study result — may be more difficult.

COHORT STUDIES

When comparing exposed and unexposed groups in a cohort study, the standard deviation of the estimate of $\log \theta$ is

$$S = \sqrt{\frac{1}{D_0} + \frac{1}{D_1}}.$$

In order to predict the value of S, we need to be able to predict the values of D_0 and D_1. This can be done by using the total person-time of observation in the proposed cohort study, Y, and a guess for the disease rate in this population, λ. The total number of events we expect to observe is given by

$$D = \lambda Y.$$

If the proportion of the study cohort who will have been exposed is P, the person-time observed in the exposed and unexposed groups will be approximately PY and $(1 - P)Y$ respectively. When the anticipated rate ratio is θ, the odds that a case was exposed will be

$$\theta \frac{PY}{(1 - P)Y} = \theta \frac{P}{1 - P},$$

and it follows that the D cases we anticipate are expected to split between exposed and unexposed as

$$D_1 = D \frac{\theta P}{1 - P + \theta P}, \qquad D_0 = D \frac{1 - P}{1 - P + \theta P}.$$

The expected value of S for the estimated log rate ratio can then be calculated and the power calculated as before.

Exercise 21.6. You plan a cohort study of ischaemic heart disease in middle-aged men. The proposed size of the cohort is 10 000 men and a 5-year follow up period is envisaged. The estimated incidence rate in the study population is 10 per thousand person-years. What is the power of the study to detect a rate ratio of 1.5 for a risk factor to which 10% of the population is exposed?

CASE CONTROL STUDIES

Similar calculations are involved in the calculation of the power of a case control study. If it is planned to study D cases and H controls, and if the proportion of the population thought to be exposed to the factor of interest is P, we would expect the D cases to split between exposed and unexposed groups as above, and we expect the H controls to split as

$$H_1 = PH, \qquad H_0 = (1 - P)H.$$

We are then in a position to calculate the expected standard deviation for the log odds ratio estimate, by the usual formula:

$$S = \sqrt{\frac{1}{D_0} + \frac{1}{D_1} + \frac{1}{H_0} + \frac{1}{H_1}}.$$

The calculation of the power follows as before.

Exercise 21.7. What is the power of a study of 100 cases and 200 controls to detect an odds ratio of 2.0 for an exposure present in 25% of the population?

STRATIFICATION AND MATCHING

Extension of these ideas to allow for stratification is straightforward in principle. In practice the difficulty is that the standard deviation of the effect of interest depends in a rather complicated way upon the strength of relationship between the exposure of interest and the stratifying variable(s). The same is true of matched case-control studies. It is particularly easy to see the difficulty in the case of the 1:1 design, since only case-control pairs which are discordant in exposure status contribute to the estimation of exposure effect. In such cases it will often be necessary to carry out a small pilot study, to provide estimates of the quantities necessary to calculate power.

DOSE-RESPONSE RELATIONSHIPS

If the level of exposure is graded, the log-linear model described in Chapter 20 allows an anticipated slope of a dose-response curve to be translated into a predicted increase in mean exposure of cases. If the standard deviation of the level of exposure in the study group is known, sample size calculations are then straightforward.

Solutions to the exercises

21.1 The anticipated number of deaths will be $D = \theta E$ and the corresponding standard deviation for the estimate of $\log \theta$ will be

$$\sqrt{\frac{1}{D}}.$$

For our four values of θ,

θ	1.4	1.7	2.0	5.0
D	17.5	21.25	25.0	62.5
$\log(\theta)$	0.336	0.531	0.693	1.609
S (estimated)	0.239	0.217	0.200	0.126

21.2   The larger study would correspond to the inner curve. For any size of effect, this curve predicts a higher probability of obtaining a significant result.

21.3   In each case, dS is obtained by subtracting $1.96S$ from the value of $\log(\theta)$. Thus, d is obtained by dividing this difference by S:

θ		d	Power
1.4	$(0.336 - 1.96 \times 0.239)/0.239 = -0.55$		0.29
1.7	$(0.531 - 1.96 \times 0.217)/0.217 = 0.49$		0.69
2.0	$(0.693 - 1.96 \times 0.200)/0.200 = 1.51$		0.93
5.0	$(1.609 - 1.96 \times 0.126)/0.126 = 10.81$		1.00

There is a slight chance of detecting a rate ratio of $\theta = 1.4$, quite a good chance for $\theta = 1.7$, a very good chance at $\theta = 2.0$ and the probability of failing to obtain a significant result at $\theta = 5.0$ is negligible.

21.4   The expected result at $\theta = 1.7$ is $b = 0.531$. By reference to Table 21.1 we see that $c = 1.960$ and $d = 1.282$ so that we need the standard deviation for the effect estimate to be:

$$S = \frac{0.531}{1.960 + 1.282} = 0.164.$$

21.5   The current standard deviation is 0.217 and it must be reduced to 0.164. The study must therefore be scaled up by a factor of

$$\left(\frac{0.217}{0.164}\right)^2 = 1.75.$$

The study must be increased so as to yield 75% more deaths. This can be achieved in practice either by increasing the size of the cohort or by extending the follow-up period.

21.6   The proposed study would accumulate $5 \times 10\,000 = 50\,000$ person-years of observations. At the anticipated incidence rate we would expect to observe $D = 10 \times 50 = 500$ disease events. If a proportion $P = 0.1$ of the total person-time is of exposed subjects and $(1 - P) = 0.9$ is of unexposed subjects, and if the rate ratio is $\theta = 1.5$, the expected number of exposed and unexposed cases is

$$
\begin{aligned}
D_1 &= 500 \times \frac{1.5 \times 0.1}{0.9 + 1.5 \times 0.1} \\
&= 71.4 \\
D_0 &= 500 \times \frac{0.9}{0.9 + 1.5 \times 0.1}
\end{aligned}
$$

$$= 428.6$$

The expected standard deviation for $\log(\theta)$ is

$$S = \sqrt{\frac{1}{71.4} + \frac{1}{428.6}} = 0.128$$

and $b = \log(1.5) = 0.405$. Thus, the number of standard deviations between expected result and null hypothesis, $(c + d)$, is $0.405/0.128 = 3.164$. For a 5% significance level, $c = 1.960$ so that $d = 3.164 - 1.960 = 1.204$. The power is the probability of exceeding -1.204 in a standard Gaussian distribution, given by tables as 0.885. The study has slightly less than 90% power to detect a rate ratio of 1.5.

21.7 Since the exposure is present in 25% of the population, we would expect the 200 controls to split as $H_1 = 50$ exposed, and $H_0 = 150$ unexposed. For $\theta = 2.0$, the expected split of the 100 cases is

$$
\begin{aligned}
D_1 &= 100 \times \frac{2.0 \times 0.25}{0.75 + 2.0 \times 0.25} \\
&= 40, \\
D_0 &= 60.
\end{aligned}
$$

The expected standard deviation of the estimate of $\log(\theta)$ is

$$S = \sqrt{\frac{1}{50} + \frac{1}{150} + \frac{1}{40} + \frac{1}{60}} = 0.261$$

and $b = \log(2.0) = 0.693$. The number of standard deviations between expected result and null hypothesis is 2.65. If a 5% significance level is to be used, $d = 2.65 - 1.96 = 0.69$. By referring -0.69 to the table of the standard Gaussian distribution, the power is 0.755 — just over 75%.

Part II

Regression models

22
Introduction to regression models

One of the main problems discussed in Part I was how to compare two rate parameters, λ_0 and λ_1, using their ratio λ_1/λ_0. To do this the log likelihood for the parameters λ_0 and λ_1 was re-expressed in terms of λ_0 and θ, where $\theta = \lambda_1/\lambda_0$. This technique was then extended to deal with comparisons stratified by a confounding variable by making the assumption that the parameter θ was constant over strata. In this second part of the book, the technique will be further extended to deal with the joint effects of several exposures and to take account of several confounding variables.

A common theme in all these situations is a change from the original parameters to new parameters which are more relevant to the comparisons of interest. This change can be described by the equations which express the old parameters in terms of the new parameters. These equations are referred to as *regression* equations, and the statistical model is called a *regression model*. To introduce regression models we shall first express some of the comparisons discussed in Part I in these terms. We use models for the rate parameter for illustration, but everything applies equally to models for the odds parameter.

22.1 The comparison of two or more exposure groups

When comparing two rate parameters, λ_0 and λ_1, the regression equations which relate the original parameters to the new ones are

$$\lambda_0 = \lambda_0, \qquad \lambda_1 = \lambda_0\theta,$$

where the first of these simply states that the parameter λ_0 is unchanged.

When there are three groups defined by an exposure variable with three levels, corresponding (for example) to no exposure, moderate exposure, and heavy exposure, the original parameters are λ_0, λ_1, and λ_2, and there are now more ways of choosing new parameters. The most common choice is to change to

$$\lambda_0, \qquad \theta_1 = \lambda_1/\lambda_0, \qquad \theta_2 = \lambda_2/\lambda_0.$$

With this choice of parameters the moderate and heavy exposure groups

Table 22.1. A regression model to compare rates by exposure levels

Age	Exposure 0	Exposure 1
0	λ_0^0	$\lambda_0^0 \theta$
1	λ_0^1	$\lambda_0^1 \theta$
2	λ_0^2	$\lambda_0^2 \theta$

are compared to the unexposed group. The regression equations are now

$$\lambda_0 = \lambda_0, \qquad \lambda_1 = \lambda_0 \theta_1, \qquad \lambda_2 = \lambda_0 \theta_2.$$

22.2 Stratified comparisons

When the comparison between exposure groups is stratified by a confounding variable such as age the change to new parameters is first made separately for each age band; for two exposure groups the regression equations for age band t are

$$\lambda_0^t = \lambda_0^t \qquad \lambda_1^t = \lambda_0^t \theta^t.$$

The parameter θ^t is age-specific and to impose the constraint that it is constant over age bands it is set equal to the constant value θ, in each age band. The regression equations are now

$$\lambda_0^t = \lambda_0^t \qquad \lambda_1^t = \lambda_0^t \theta.$$

This choice of parameters is the same as for the proportional hazards model, introduced in Chapter 15. The model is written out in full in Table 22.1 for the case of three age bands.

Although our main interest is whether the rate parameter varies with exposure, within age bands, we might also be interested in investigating whether it varies with age, within exposure groups. The parameter θ does not help with this second comparison because it has been chosen to compare the exposure groups. When making the comparison the other way round the age bands are the groups to be compared and the exposure groups are the strata. To combine the comparison across these strata requires the assumption that the rate ratios which compare levels 1 and 2 of age with level 0 are the same in both exposure groups. This way of choosing parameters is shown in Table 22.2, where the parameters ϕ^1 and ϕ^2 are the rate ratios for age, assumed constant within each exposure group. Note that there are two parameters for age because there are three age bands being compared.

Putting these two ways of choosing parameters together gives the regression model shown in Table 22.3. The parameter λ_0^0 has now been written as λ_C, for simplicity and to emphasize that it refers to the (top left-hand)

Table 22.2. A regression model to compare rates by age bands

Age	Exposure 0	1
0	λ_0^0	λ_1^0
1	$\lambda_0^0\phi^1$	$\lambda_1^0\phi^1$
2	$\lambda_0^0\phi^2$	$\lambda_1^0\phi^2$

Table 22.3. A regression model for exposure and age

Age	Exposure 0	1
0	λ_C	$\lambda_C\theta$
1	$\lambda_C\phi^1$	$\lambda_C\theta\phi^1$
2	$\lambda_C\phi^2$	$\lambda_C\theta\phi^2$

corner of the table. Both sorts of comparison can now be made in the same analysis. It is no longer necessary to regard one variable as the exposure, and the other as a confounder used to define strata; the model treats both types of variable symmetrically. To emphasize this symmetry the term *explanatory* variable is often used to describe both exposures and confounders in regression models. Although this is useful in complex situations where there are many variables, there are also dangers. Although it makes no difference to a computer program whether an explanatory variable is an exposure or confounder it makes a great deal of difference to the person trying to interpret the results. Perhaps the single most important reason for misinterpreting the results of regression analyses is that regression models can be used without the user thinking carefully about the status of different explanatory variables. This will be discussed at greater length in Chapter 27.

Exercise 22.1. Table 22.4 shows a set of values for the rate parameters (per 1000 person-years) which satisfy exactly the model shown in Table 22.3. What are the corresponding values of $\lambda_C, \theta, \phi^1, \phi^2$?

Exercise 22.2. When the model in Table 22.3 is fitted to data it imposes the constraint that the rate ratio for exposure is the same in all age bands, and equally, that each of the two rate ratios for age is constant over both levels of exposure. Is the constraint on the rate ratios for age a new constraint, or does it automatically follow whenever the rate ratio for exposure is the same in all age bands?

Table 22.4. Parameter values (per 1000) which obey the constraints

Age	Exposure 0	Exposure 1
0	5.0	15.0
1	12.0	36.0
2	30.0	90.0

Table 22.5. A regression model using names for parameters

Age	Exposure 0	Exposure 1
0	Corner	Corner × Exposure(1)
1	Corner × Age(1)	Corner × Age(1) × Exposure(1)
2	Corner × Age(2)	Corner × Age(2) × Exposure(1)

22.3 Naming conventions

Using Greek letters for parameters is convenient when developing the theory but less so when applying the methods in practice. With many explanatory variables there will be many parameters and it is easy to forget which letter refers to which parameter. For this reason we shall now move to using names for parameters instead of Greek letters.

The first of the parameters in Table 22.3, λ_C, is called the Corner. The θ parameter, which is the effect of exposure controlled for age, is referred to as Exposure(1); when the exposure variable has three levels there are two effects and these are referred to as Exposure(1) and Exposure(2), and so on. When the exposure variable is given a more specific name such as Alcohol then the effects are referred to as Alcohol(1) and Alcohol(2). The ϕ parameters, which are the effects of age controlled for exposure, are referred to as Age(1) and Age(2). The model in Table 22.3 is written using names in Table 22.5.

Because writing out models in full is rather cumbersome, particularly when using names for parameters, we shall use a simple abbreviated form instead. The entries in Tables 22.3 and 22.5 refer to the right-hand sides of the regression equations; the left-hand sides are the original rate parameters which are omitted. Such a set of regression equations is abbreviated to

$$\text{Rate} = \text{Corner} \times \text{Exposure} \times \text{Age}.$$

It is important to remember that this abbreviation is not itself an equation (even though it looks like one!); it represents a set of equations and is shorthand for tables like Table 22.5. The regression model is sometimes

Table 22.6.   Energy intake and IHD incidence rates per 1000 person-years

| | Unexposed (≥ 2750 kcals) | | | Exposed (< 2750 kcals) | | | Rate |
Age	Cases	P-yrs	Rate	Cases	P-yrs	Rate	ratio
40–49	4	607.9	6.58	2	311.9	6.41	0.97
50–59	5	1272.1	3.93	12	878.1	13.67	3.48
60–69	8	888.9	9.00	14	667.5	20.97	2.33

Table 22.7.   Estimated values of the parameters for the IHD data

Parameter	Estimate
Corner	0.00444
Exposure(1)	×2.39
Age(1)	×1.14
Age(2)	×2.00

abbreviated even further and referred to simply as a *multiplicative model* for exposure and age.

22.4 Estimating the parameters in a regression model

Table 22.6 shows the data from the study of ischaemic heart disease and energy intake. There are two explanatory variables, age with three levels and exposure with two. The two levels of exposure refer to energy intakes above and below 2750 kcals per day.

Although the rate ratio for exposure is rather lower in the first age band than in the other two age bands, it is based on only 6 cases, and a summary based on the assumption of a common rate ratio seems reasonable. In the new terminology this means fitting the regression model

$$\text{Rate} = \text{Corner} \times \text{Exposure} \times \text{Age}.$$

The most likely values of the parameters in this model, obtained from a computer program, are shown in Table 22.7. Note that the most likely value of the Exposure(1) parameter is the same, to two decimal places, as the Mantel–Haenszel estimate of the common rate ratio, given in Chapter 15.

Exercise 22.3. Use the most likely values of the parameters in the regression model, shown in Table 22.7, to predict the rates for the six cells in Table 22.6.

Computer programs differ in the precise details of how the output is

Table 22.8.   Estimated parameters and SDs on a log scale

Parameter	Estimate (M)	SD (S)
Corner	−5.4180	0.4420
Exposure(1)	0.8697	0.3080
Age(1)	0.1290	0.4753
Age(2)	0.6920	0.4614

labelled. In particular you may see the word *variable* where we have used *parameter*, and the word *coefficient* where we have used *estimate*. We have used the term *corner* for the parameter which measures the level of response in the first age band of the unexposed group but several other terms are in widespread use, for example *constant*, *intercept*, *grand mean*, and (most cryptically of all) the number 1. We have numbered strata and exposure categories starting from zero, but some programs start numbering from one.

22.5   Gaussian approximations on the log scale

Gaussian approximations to the likelihood are used to obtain approximate confidence intervals for the parameter values. For the simple multiplicative models discussed so far the approximation is always made on the log scale, and in many programs the output is also in terms of logarithms. Table 22.8 shows the output on a log scale for the ischaemic heart data; the second column shows the most likely values (M) of the logarithms of the parameters and exponentials of these give the values on the original scale. For example,

$$\exp(0.8697) = 2.39,$$

which is the rate ratio for exposure. The third column shows the standard deviations (S) of the estimates, obtained from Gaussian approximations to the profile log likelihoods for each parameter. The standard deviation of the effect of exposure, on the log scale, is 0.3080, so the error factor for a 90% confidence interval for this parameter is $\exp(1.645 \times 0.3080) = 1.66$, and the limits are from $2.39/1.66 = 1.44$ to $2.39 \times 1.66 = 3.96$.

Exercise 22.4. Use Table 22.8 to calculate the 90% confidence limits for the first effect of age.

When the regression model is fitted on a log scale it is written in the form

$$\log(\text{Rate}) = \text{Corner} + \text{Exposure} + \text{Age}.$$

Table 22.9.   A more complete description of the age effects

Parameter	Estimate	SD
Age(1)	0.1290	0.4753
Age(2)	0.6920	0.4614
Age(2) − Age(1)	0.5630	0.3229

Table 22.10.   An abbreviated table for the age effects

Parameter	Estimate	SD	
Age(1)	0.1290	0.4753	0.3229
Age(2)	0.6920	0.4614	

Strictly speaking, the parameters on the right-hand side of this expression should be written as log(Corner) etc., but in practice the log on the left-hand side is enough to signal the fact that the parameter estimates will be on a log scale.

For variables with more than two categories, comparisons other than those with the first category are sometimes of interest. Taking the variable age in the ischaemic heart disease data as an example, the effect of changing from level 1 to level 2 of age is the difference between the two age effects, namely $0.6920 - 0.1290 = 0.5630$. Because the two age effects are based on some common data the standard deviation of their difference cannot be obtained from the simple formula

$$\sqrt{0.4753^2 + 0.4614^2} = 0.6624,$$

which was used in Chapter 13. To obtain the correct standard deviation we usually need to resort to a trick, such as recoding age so that the corner parameter refers to the *second* age band rather than the first. Table 22.9 shows how a fuller analysis of age effects could be reported; an option to obtain output in this form would be a useful feature not currently available in most computer programs.

An abbreviated way of conveying the same information is shown in Table 22.10. This provides the standard deviations for all three comparisons but leaves the user to do the subtraction to find the effect of changing from level 1 to level 2. The method extends naturally for factors with more than three levels; for example, a four-level factor would need a triangular array of 6 standard deviations for the six possible pairwise comparisons.

22.6   Additive models

When comparing two groups, in the first section of this chapter, the two parameters λ_0 and λ_1 were replaced by λ_0 and $\theta = \lambda_1/\lambda_0$. This change of parameters made it possible to estimate the rate ratio θ along with its standard deviation. The parameters could equally well have been changed to λ_0 and $\theta = \lambda_1 - \lambda_0$, thus making it possible to estimate the rate difference instead of the rate ratio.

The choice between the rate ratio and the rate difference is usually an empirical one, depending on which of the two is more closely constant over strata. In the early years of epidemiology, when age was often the only explanatory variable apart from exposure, methods of analysis were all based (implicitly) on multiplicative models. This is because most rates vary so much with age that the rate ratio is almost always more closely constant over age bands than the rate difference. More recently, particularly when investigating the joint effects of several exposures, epidemiologists have shown a greater interest in rate differences.

To impose the constraint that the rate difference is constant over age strata, the regression model

$$\text{Rate} = \text{Corner} + \text{Exposure} + \text{Age}$$

is fitted. This is called an *additive model* for exposure and age. Note that it is the rate and not the log rate which now appears on the left-hand side. The same likelihood techniques are used as with the additive model as with the multiplicative model, but because the estimated values of the parameters in the additive model must be restricted so that they predict positive rates, it is much harder to write foolproof programs to fit these models. We shall return to additive models in Chapter 28.

22.7   Using computer programs

There is a certain amount of specialized terminology connected with computer programs which we shall introduce briefly in this section.

VARIABLES AND RECORDS

The information collected in a study is best viewed as a rectangular table in which the columns refer to the different kinds of information collected for each subject, and the rows to the different subjects. In computer language the columns are called *variables* and the rows are called *records*. Variables such as age and observation time are called *quantitative* because they measure some quantity. Variables such as exposure group are called *categorical* because they record the category into which a subject falls. The different categories are called the *levels* of the variable. Another name for a categorical variable is *factor*. Categorical variables with only two categories (or levels) are also known as *binary* variables.

DERIVED VARIABLES

The raw data which is collected in a study may not be in exactly the right form for analysis. For example, in a follow-up study the observation time will usually be recorded as date of entry to the study and date of exit. The computer can be instructed to derive the observation time from these two dates by subtraction. Another example is where the grouped values of a quantitative variable are required in an analysis; it is then convenient to derive a new categorical variable which records the group into which each subject falls.

VARIABLE NAMES

In order to give instructions to a computer program each of the variables needs a name. These can usually be at least eight characters long and it is a good idea to make full use of this and to choose names which will mean something to you (and someone else) in a year's time.

SUMMARY TABLES

It is always important when using computer programs to keep in close touch with the data you are analyzing. The simplest way of doing this is to start by looking at tables which show the estimated rate or odds parameters for different combinations of the values of the explanatory variables. When there are two explanatory variables the table is called two-way, and so on. Three-way tables are presented as a series of two-way tables. When an explanatory variable is quantitative it will usually be necessary to group the values of the variable before using it to define a table. Only after inspecting various summary tables to get some feel for the main results should you use regression models to explore the data more fully.

FREQUENCY OR INDIVIDUAL RECORDS

Computer programs are generally able to accept either *individual records* or *frequency records* based on groups of subjects. For example, in the ischaemic heart disease study, we could use the data records for each subject, or frequency records showing the number of subjects in each combination of age band and exposure group. Entering a frequency record for 25 subjects has exactly the same effect as entering 25 identical individual records.

When an explanatory variable is quantitative its values must be grouped before frequency records can be formed, while the actual values can be used with individual records. Frequency records can be stored more compactly than individual records, and log likelihood calculations are correspondingly faster, but using frequency records requires two computer programs — one

to compute the frequency records and one to carry out the regression analysis — and communication between these programs may be inconvenient.
For case-control studies the number of subjects is usually relatively small
and the data are usually entered as individual records. For cohort studies
there may be tens of thousands of individual records, possibly further subdivided between time-bands, so the data are usually entered as frequency
records.

MISSING VALUES

Most studies contain records which have some missing values, and it is
essential to have some way of indicating this to the computer program.
The most convenient code for a missing value is the character *, but when
a program insists on a numeric code it is best to choose some large number
like 9999. When there are many variables in a study the analyses are usually
on some subset of the variables, and the program will automatically include
those records with complete data on the subset being used.

Solutions to the exercises

22.1 $\lambda_C = 5.0$ per 1000, $\theta = 3.0$, $\phi^1 = 2.4$, $\phi^2 = 6.0$.

22.2   It is not a new constraint. Table 22.1 shows that when the rate
ratio for exposure is constant over age bands then the rate ratios for age
will automatically be constant over exposure groups.

22.3   The predicted rates for the six combinations of age and exposure
are

Age	Unexposed	Exposed
40 – 49	4.44	10.61
50 – 59	5.06	12.10
60 – 69	8.88	21.22

22.4   The effect of age level 1 is $\exp(0.1290) = 1.14$. The 90% confidence
interval for this effect is

$$1.14 \overset{\times}{\div} \exp(1.645 \times 0.4753)$$

which is from 0.52 to 2.49.

23
Poisson and logistic regression

In principle the way a computer program goes about fitting a regression model is simple. First the likelihood is specified in terms of the original set of parameters. Then it is expressed in terms of the new parameters using the regression equations, and finally most likely values of these new parameters are found. In studies of event data the two most important likelihoods are Poisson and Bernouilli, and the combinations of these with regression models are called *Poisson* and *logistic* regression respectively. Gaussian regression is the combination of the Gaussian likelihood with regression models and will be discussed in Chapter 34.

23.1 Poisson regression

When a time scale, such as age, is divided into bands and included in a regression model, the observation time for each subject must be split between the bands as described in Chapter 6. This is illustrated in Fig. 23.1, where a single observation time ending in failure (the top line) has been split into three parts, the last of which ends in failure. These parts can then be used to make up frequency records containing the number of failures and the observation time, as was done for the ischaemic heart disease data in Table 23.1, or they can be analysed as though they were individual records.

If they are to be analysed as though they were individual records then each of these new records must contain variables which describe which time band is being referred to, how much observation time is spent in the time band, and whether or not a failure occurs in the time band. Values of

Table 23.1. The IHD data as frequency records

Cases	Person-years	Age	Exposure
4	607.9	0	0
2	311.9	0	1
5	1272.1	1	0
12	878.1	1	1
8	888.9	2	0
14	667.5	2	1

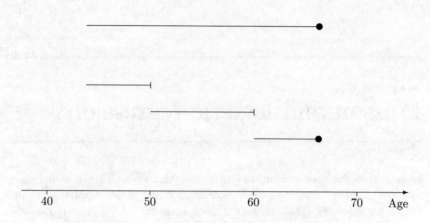

Fig. 23.1.   Splitting the follow-up record.

other explanatory variables, such as exposure, must also be included. The idea extends to more than one time scale — each record then refers to an observation of a subject through one cell of a Lexis diagram — but the number of new records can then be many times the number of subjects and analysis becomes cumbersome.

To instruct a computer program to fit a Poisson regression model to the frequency records in Table 23.1 it is first necessary to enter the names of the variables which contain the observation time for the record, the number of failures, the exposure level and the age band. When the Poisson regression option is selected the program automatically assumes that the regression model is of the form

$$\log(\text{Rate}) = \text{Corner} + \text{A} + \text{B} + \ldots,$$

where A, B, etc., are explanatory variables. It is therefore only necessary to instruct the program that the rate for each record is to be calculated from the person-years variable and the number of failures variable, and that exposure and age are to be included in the model as explanatory variables.

The log likelihood for each combination of age band and exposure takes the standard Poisson form. For example when age is at level 2 and exposure is at level 1 the rate parameter is λ_1^2. There are 14 failures and 667.5 person-years so the log likelihood for λ_1^2 is

$$14 \log(\lambda_1^2) - 667.5 \lambda_1^2.$$

The total log likelihood (in terms of the original parameters) is equal to the sum of the separate log likelihoods for the six cells of the table. This total is expressed (by the computer program) in terms of the four new parameters Corner, Age(1), Age(2), and Exposure(1), using the information provided by the regression model. As usual the most likely values of the log parameters are found on the log scale and some programs leave the user to convert these back to the original scale.

The same log likelihood is obtained from individual records as from frequency records, provided the explanatory variables in the individual records take discrete values in the same way as for the frequency records. For example, the contribution to the log likelihood from a subject with exposure at level 1, age band at level 2, and observation time y, is

$$d\log(\lambda_1^2) - y\lambda_1^2,$$

where d takes the value 1 if the subject fails in this age band and 0 otherwise. Adding this log likelihood over all subjects contributing to the frequency record with exposure at level 1 and age at level 1 gives

$$14\log(\lambda_1^2) - 667.5\lambda_1^2,$$

which is the same as the log likelihood for this frequency record.

A computer program for Poisson regression can also be used after the confounding effect of age has been allowed for by indirect standardization, that is by calculating the expected number of failures using standard reference rates. This is because the log likelihood for the parameter representing the (common) ratio of age-specific rates in a study group to the age-specific reference rates has the same algebraic form as the log likelihood for a rate parameter; one is obtained from the other by exchanging the person-years and the expected number of failures. With this exchange, the original parameters are now rate ratios expressing age-controlled comparisons of different sections of the study group to the reference rates. The regression model relates these to a smaller number of parameters in the same way as with rates. Note that the parameter estimates in such models are, in effect, ratios of SMRs. For the reasons discussed in Chapter 15, they can be misleading if an inappropriate set of reference rates is used.

23.2 Logistic regression

In logistic regression the original parameters are odds parameters and these are expressed in terms of new parameters in the same way as for the rate parameter. The most important application of logistic regression is to case-control studies and we shall use the study of BCG and leprosy as an illustration.

For convenience the data from this study are repeated in Table 23.2, which shows the numbers of cases and controls by age and BCG vaccination. Taking a prospective view the response parameter is the odds of being a case rather than a control, so a useful way of summarizing these data is to

Table 23.2. Cases of leprosy and controls by age and BCG scar

Age	Leprosy cases		Healthy controls	
	Scar −	Scar +	Scar −	Scar +
0–4	1	1	7 593	11 719
5–9	11	14	7 143	10 184
10–14	28	22	5 611	7 561
15–19	16	28	2 208	8 117
20–24	20	19	2 438	5 588
25–29	36	11	4 356	1 625
30–34	47	6	5 245	1 234

Table 23.3. Case/control ratio ($\times 10^3$) by age and BCG scar

	BCG scar	
Age	Absent	Present
0–4	0.13	0.08
5–9	1.54	1.37
10–14	4.99	2.91
15–19	7.25	3.45
20–24	8.20	3.40
25–29	8.26	6.77
30–34	8.96	4.86

show the estimated value of this parameter, which is the case/control ratio, for different levels of age and BCG vaccination. This summary is given in Table 23.3 and shows a consistently lower case/control ratio for those with a BCG scar than for those without. It also shows that the case/control ratio increases sharply with age in both groups.

Because there are many subjects in this study the data are entered to the computer program as frequency records. Table 23.4 shows the data as an array of frequency records ready for computer input. Programs often require the data to be entered as the number of cases and the total number of subjects for each record, rather than as the number of cases and the number of controls. The change is easily made by deriving a new variable equal to the variable for the number of cases plus the variable for the number of controls.

The log likelihood contribution for a frequency record in which N subjects split as D cases and H controls takes the Bernoulli form

$$D \log(\omega) - N \log(1 + \omega),$$

where ω is the odds, given by the model, that a subject in that frequency

Table 23.4.   The BCG data as frequency records

Cases	Total	Scar	Age
1	7594	0	0
1	11720	1	0
11	7154	0	1
14	10198	1	1
28	5639	0	2
22	7583	1	2
16	2224	0	3
28	8145	1	3
20	2458	0	4
19	5607	1	4
36	4392	0	5
11	1636	1	5
47	5292	0	6
6	1240	1	6

record is a case rather than a control. When fitting a regression model the total log likelihood is expressed in terms of new parameters using the regression equations and most likely values of the new parameters are found. For individual records the log likelihood is

$$d \log(\omega) - \log(1 + \omega),$$

where $d = 1$ for a case and $d = 0$ for a control. The sum of the log likelihoods for all subjects contributing to a frequency record is equal to

$$D \log(\omega) - N \log(1 + \omega),$$

which is the same as the log likelihood for the frequency record.

The regression model

$$\log (\text{Odds}) = \text{Corner} + \text{Age} + \text{BCG},$$

expresses the constraint that the odds ratio for BCG vaccination is constant over age groups. Apart from the corner, all the parameters in this model are odds ratios. The BCG parameter compares the odds of being a case for subjects who are BCG positive to the odds of being a case for subjects who are BCG negative. The six age parameters compare the odds of being a case for subjects in the age groups 1–6 to the odds of being a case in age group 0. The most likely values of these parameters (on a log scale) are shown in Table 23.5.

Exercise 23.1. What is the most likely value of the odds ratio for BCG vac-

Table 23.5.   Output from a logistic regression program

Parameter	Estimate	SD
Corner	−8.880	0.7093
Age(1)	2.624	0.7340
Age(2)	3.583	0.7203
Age(3)	3.824	0.7228
Age(4)	3.900	0.7244
Age(5)	4.156	0.7224
Age(6)	4.158	0.7213
BCG(1)	−0.547	0.1409

cination? Does this seem about right, from Table 23.3? Compare this estimate with the Mantel–Haenszel estimate given in Chapter 18.

The parameters in the model

$$\log (\text{Odds}) = \text{Corner} + \text{Age} + \text{BCG},$$

apart from the corner, refer to changes in the log odds of being a case. From Chapter 16 we know that the odds of being a case is proportional to the odds of being a failure in the study base, provided the selection of cases and controls is independent of both age and BCG status. More precisely,

$$\text{Odds of being a case} = K \frac{\pi}{1 - \pi}$$

where

$$K = \frac{\text{Probability that a failure is sampled as a case}}{\text{Probability that a survivor is sampled as a control}}.$$

On a log scale

$$\log(\text{Odds}) = \log(K) + \log \left(\frac{\pi}{1 - \pi} \right),$$

so a change in the log odds of being a case is equal to the corresponding change in the log odds of failure in the study base. It follows that estimates of the effects of age and BCG on the log odds of being a case also estimate the effects of age and BCG on the log odds of failure in the study base. This argument does not apply to the corner (which is not a change in log odds) so unless K is known the corner parameter in the study base cannot be estimated.

Table 23.6. A simulated group-matched study

| | BCG scar | | | |
| | Cases | | Controls | |
Age	Absent	Present	Absent	Present
0–4	1	1	3	5
5–9	11	14	48	52
10–14	28	22	67	133
15–19	16	28	46	130
20–24	20	19	50	106
25–29	36	11	126	62
30–34	47	6	174	38

When the disease is rare the probability of failure in the study base is small and the odds of failure are related to the rate λ by

$$\frac{\pi}{1-\pi} \approx \lambda T,$$

where T is the duration of the study. Thus

$$
\begin{aligned}
\log(\text{Odds}) &= \log(K) + \log\left(\frac{\pi}{1-\pi}\right), \\
&\approx \log(K) + \log(T) + \log(\lambda),
\end{aligned}
$$

and the same argument shows that effects estimated from a logistic regression model are also estimates of effects on the log rate in the study base.

23.3   Matched case-control studies

In Chapter 18 we presented a simulated group-matched case-control study, based on the BCG study, in which the age distribution of controls is made equal to that of the cases by taking four times as many controls as cases in each age stratum. The results from this study are shown again in Table 23.6.

When estimating the effect of BCG the matching variable, age, cannot be ignored, so the appropriate model to fit is

$$\log(\text{Odds}) = \text{Corner} + \text{Age} + \text{BCG},$$

even though the effects of age in this model may be close to zero. The results of fitting this model are shown in Table 23.7. As expected the estimate of the BCG effect is virtually unchanged, although it has a slightly larger standard deviation because it is based on a smaller number of controls.

Table 23.7.   Regression output for the group-matched study

Parameter	Estimate	SD
Corner	−1.0670	0.800
Age(1)	−0.0421	0.827
Age(2)	0.0119	0.812
Age(3)	0.0713	0.814
Age(4)	0.0244	0.816
Age(5)	−0.1628	0.814
Age(6)	−0.2380	0.813
BCG(1)	−0.5721	0.155

However, the age effects are very different from the previous output for the whole data set in Table 23.5. They are now all close to zero but this does not mean that age can be omitted from the model. To do so would produce a biased estimate of the BCG effect. Variables which have been used in the matching must be included in the model used to estimate the effects of interest. The same point was made in Chapter 18 where matched case-control studies were analysed by stratifying on the matching variable and using the Mantel–Haenszel method to combine the separate estimates of the effect of interest over strata.

Exercise 23.2. Explain the large differences in the age effects between the two outputs. You may find it helps to make a summary table of case/control ratios based on the data in Table 23.6.

Using a computer program for logistic regression is a convenient way of analyzing group-matched case-control studies and gives correct estimates of odds ratios, at least for variables not used in the matching, provided there are not too many matching strata. However, in individually matched case-control studies each new case introduces its own stratum and, therefore, a new nuisance parameter. This turns out to be one of the situations in which replacing the nuisance parameters by their most likely values and using profile likelihood to estimate the parameters of interest gives the wrong answer. For individually matched studies the likelihood argument of Chapter 19 can be extended to cover regression models. This new method is called *conditional* logistic regression analysis, and will be discussed in Chapter 29.

⋆ **23.4   Modelling risk and prevalence**

The prospective approach to the regression analysis of case-control studies regards the case/control status as the outcome variable. In Chapter 1 we discussed other epidemiological studies in which the outcome of interest is binary. Most important are studies of risk(sometimes called *cumulative incidence* studies) in which each subject is studied for a fixed period, the outcome being failure or survival, and cross sectional *prevalence studies* in which each subject's present state is recorded as diseased or healthy.

In both these types of study the original parameters are probabilities. For case-control studies, we choose to model odds rather than probabilities because odds ratios are independent of the sampling fractions used and have a ready interpretation as risk or rate ratios in the study base. For risk and prevalence studies there is no such compelling reason to use the odds, although it often proves useful to do so because the log odds is unconstrained and models for the log odds are likely to describe the data better than models for π or $\log(\pi)$.

An alternative to the log odds may be derived from the relationship between π, the probability of failure in a time interval of length T, and λ, the failure rate for this interval. This relationship is given by

$$\text{Cumulative survival probability} = \exp(-\text{ Cumulative failure rate})$$

that is,

$$1 - \pi = \exp(-\lambda T),$$

so

$$\log(1 - \pi) = -\lambda T$$

and

$$\log(-\log(1 - \pi)) = \log(T) + \log(\lambda).$$

Thus models for $\log(-\log(1 - \pi))$ may be interpreted as models for $\log(\lambda)$, apart from the corner parameter, and parameters which are estimated from such models may be interpreted as the logarithms of rate ratios. The function $\log(-\log(1 - \pi))$ is called the *complementary log-log* transformation of π and some programs allow regression models to be fitted on this scale. Provided π is less than about 0.2 the complementary log-log function does not differ appreciably from the log odds, so in this case regression models for the log odds can also be interpreted as regression models for $\log(\lambda)$.

For diseases in which mortality (and migration) of subjects is unaffected by their contracting the disease, there is a similar relationship between age-specific prevalence and the age-specific incidence rate. In this case, parameters of complementary log-log models for prevalence are identical to parameters of an underlying model for log incidence rates. However in general such an assumption cannot be made and the relationship between effects on prevalence and effects on incidence is complicated.

Solutions to the exercises

23.1 The most likely value of the log of the BCG parameter is -0.547. This corresponds to an odds ratio of $\exp(-0.547) = 0.579$. We therefore estimate that vaccination with BCG reduces the incidence rate of leprosy in the base study to about 58% of what it would be without vaccination. From Chapter 18 the Mantel–Haenszel estimate of the BCG parameter is 0.587.

23.2 The discrepancies between the two outputs is due to the age matching of controls to cases in the second analysis. In the first analysis there is no such matching, and the age parameters refer to the underlying relationship between age and leprosy incidence (incidence increases with age). Matching controls to cases with respect to age has the effect that the sampling probabilities for controls differ between age strata so that K, the constant of proportionality between the odds of being a case and the odds of failure in the study base, now varies between age bands. It follows that the age parameters of the model now include the effect of variation in sampling probabilities, and are not interpretable.

24
Testing hypotheses

The scientific imagination knows no bounds in the creation of theories and interesting models, but when should such elaboration end? The principle which is invoked to deal with this problem is *Occam's razor*. This principle holds that we should always adopt the simplest explanation consistent with the known facts. Only when the explanation becomes inconsistent are we justified in greater elaboration. Occam's razor has much in common with statistical tests of null hypotheses. Statisticians erect null hypotheses and seek positive evidence against them before accepting alternative explanations. This philosophical position should not be taken to imply that the absence of evidence against a null hypothesis establishes the null hypothesis as being true.

24.1 Tests involving a single parameter

An explanatory variable with two levels requires only one parameter to make a comparison between them. When the comparison is made using a rate ratio (or an odds ratio) the null value is 1.0, or zero on the log scale. The simplest way of testing for a zero null value is to use the Wald test, based on the profile log likelihood for the parameter being tested. This involves referring

$$\left(\frac{M-0}{S}\right)^2$$

to tables of the chi-squared distribution on one degree of freedom, where M is the most likely value of the log of the parameter and S is its standard deviation. These quantities are the ones listed in the computer output under estimate and standard deviation.

Exercise 24.1. Table 24.1 repeats the results of the regression analysis of the ischaemic heart disease data. Carry out the Wald test of the hypothesis of no effect of exposure on IHD incidence.

A log likelihood ratio test based on the profile likelihood for the exposure parameter can also be used to test the hypothesis in Exercise 24.1. The profile log likelihood ratio for a zero exposure effect is the difference between two log likelihoods: (a) the log likelihood when the exposure parameter is

Table 24.1.   Program output for the ischaemic heart disease data

Parameter	Estimate	SD
Corner	−5.4180	0.4420
Exposure(1)	0.8697	0.3080
Age(1)	0.1290	0.4753
Age(2)	0.6920	0.4614

zero and the age parameters take their most likely values given that there is no exposure effect, and (b) the log likelihood evaluated when all parameters take their most likely values. The former is obtained by fitting a model which includes age but not exposure, and the latter is obtained by fitting a model which includes both age and exposure. The difference between these two log likelihoods gives the profile log likelihood ratio, and the test is carried out by referring minus twice this value to the chi-squared distribution with one degree of freedom. Some programs report the *deviance*, a quantity closely related to the log likelihood which we shall discuss in a later section of this chapter.

Exercise 24.2. The log likelihoods for the models

$$\log(\text{Rate}) = \text{Corner} + \text{Age} + \text{Exposure}$$
$$\log(\text{Rate}) = \text{Corner} + \text{Age}$$

for the ischaemic heart disease data, are −247.027 and −251.176. How can you tell which likelihood was obtained for which model? Carry out the likelihood ratio test for a zero exposure effect and compare it with the Wald test calculated in the previous exercise.

The score test for a zero exposure effect is found from a quadratic approximation which has the same gradient and curvature as the profile log likelihood at the null value. Since the log likelihood ratio test is easy to obtain using a computer program the score test is rarely carried out, although some programs do offer this option.

24.2   Tests involving several parameters

When a variable has three levels two parameters are required to make comparisons between the levels. A test that just one of these parameters takes its null value is rarely of interest. The hypothesis that both take their null values is usually more relevant, because this corresponds to the variable having no effect on the response. We shall now consider the extension of the likelihood ratio test to cover this situation. A convenient example is provided by the problem of testing the effect of age in the analysis shown in Table 24.1, although this is a hypothesis of no scientific interest!

The same general principle as for one parameter is used: the log likelihood for the model

$$\text{Corner} + \text{Age} + \text{Exposure}$$

which includes the two age parameters, is subtracted from the log likelihood for the model

$$\text{Corner} + \text{Exposure},$$

in which the two age parameters are zero. This gives the log likelihood ratio for testing the hypothesis that both age parameters take their null values. Minus twice the log likelihood ratio is referred to the chi-squared distribution with *two* degrees of freedom, because two parameters have been set to their null values. In this case minus twice the log likelihood ratio is equal to 4.016, and the p-value is 0.134, showing that there is no significant effect of age on ischaemic heart disease in this study.

Exercise 24.3. Does the fact that there is no significant effect of age on incidence in this study mean that there is no need to control for age when comparing exposure groups?

There is some temptation to scan the output for the model which includes both age and exposure and to try to interpret the separate tests of the two parameters for age, rather than making a joint test. Using the Wald test with the results in Table 24.1 shows that the data support both null values for age when tested separately, but it would be unwise to deduce from this that there is no effect of age. This is because both age effects are rather imprecisely estimated, due to the fact that only 6 heart attacks were observed in the first age band. When the corner is located where there is very little data it is common to see effects for both levels 1 and 2 which are small compared to their standard deviations, yet a highly significant effect from level 1 to level 2. The only safe way of testing the effect of age is to make a test of the joint hypothesis that both age effects take their null value. The Wald test can be generalized to do this (as can the score test), but the easiest test to use is the log likelihood ratio test.

24.3   Testing for interaction

The regression model used in the test for an exposure effect imposes the constraint that the effect of exposure is constant over age bands. Similarly for the test for age effects. An important question to ask is whether it is reasonable to impose these constraints, or whether the data better support different exposure effects in each age band, and different age effects in each exposure group. When the effects of exposure vary with age there is said to be *interaction* between exposure and age. Interaction between exposure and age automatically implies interaction between age and exposure and vice versa.

Table 24.2. Definition of interactions in terms of exposure

		Exposure	
		0	1
	0	5.0	15.0
Age	1	12.0	42.0
	2	30.0	135.0
	0	5.0	5.0×3.0
Age	1	12.0	12.0×3.5
	2	30.0	30.0×4.5
	0	5.0	5.0×3.0
Age	1	12.0	$12.0 \times 3.0 \times 1.167$
	2	30.0	$30.0 \times 3.0 \times 1.5$

To test for interaction it is necessary to choose new parameters in a way that allows for separate effects of exposure in the different age bands. This is done by choosing one parameter to measure the effect of exposure in the first age band and two to measure the extent to which the effects of exposure in the other two age bands differ from the effect in the first age band. The way this is done is best illustrated using numerical values for the parameters.

A set of illustrative values for the 6 rate parameters are shown at the top of Table 24.2. The rate ratios for exposure by levels of age are 3.0, 3.5, and 4.5, shown in the middle part of the table, so these rate parameters do not obey a multiplicative model. The extent of the departure from the multiplicative model can be measured by expressing 3.5 and 4.5 as ratios relative to 3.0, as shown in the third part of the table. These ratios, which take the values 1.167 and 1.5 in this case, are called *interaction* parameters.

Table 24.3 shows the same thing in terms of the rate ratios for age by levels of exposure. These rate ratios are 2.4 and 6.0 when exposure is at level 0 but 2.8 and 9.0 when exposure is at level 1. The extent to which these differ, measured as ratios relative to the rate ratios at level 0 of exposure, are again equal to 1.167 and 1.5. Thus the interaction parameters are symmetric in exposure and age.

Tables 24.2 and 24.3 are combined in Table 24.4. Using the terminology of regression models, the 6 original rate parameters are re-expressed in terms of the corner, the rate ratio for exposure when age is at level 0, the rate ratio for age when exposure is at level 0, and the two interaction parameters. This way of re- expressing the original rate parameters has not resulted in any reduction in the number of parameters; its sole purpose is to assess the extent of the departures from the multiplicative model. We

Table 24.3. Definition of interactions in terms of age

		Exposure	
		0	1
	0	5.0	15.0
Age	1	12.0	42.0
	2	30.0	135.0
	0	5.0	15.0
Age	1	5.0×2.4	15.0×2.8
	2	5.0×6.0	15.0×9.0
	0	5.0	15.0
Age	1	5.0×2.4	$15.0 \times 2.4 \times 1.167$
	2	5.0×6.0	$15.0 \times 6.0 \times 1.5$

Table 24.4. Definition of interactions in terms of exposure and age

Age	Exposure	
	0	1
0	5.0	5.0×3.0
1	5.0×2.4	$5.0 \times 3.0 \times 2.4 \times 1.167$
2	5.0×6.0	$5.0 \times 3.0 \times 6.0 \times 1.5$

shall write the model with interaction in one or other of the forms

$$\text{Rate} \quad = \quad \text{Corner} \times \text{Exposure} \times \text{Age} \times \text{Exposure·Age}$$
$$\log(\text{Rate}) \quad = \quad \text{Corner} + \text{Exposure} + \text{Age} + \text{Exposure·Age}.$$

To test for interaction it is necessary to fit the model with and without interaction parameters and to measure the log likelihood ratio for these two models. Minus twice this log likelihood ratio is then referred to tables of chi-squared on two degrees of freedom. The chi-squared has two degrees of freedom because the hypothesis being tested is that two interaction parameters take their null values. The instruction to include interaction parameters is done by including the term Age·Exposure in the model description. When this is done the output will include estimated values for the interaction parameters, but these are rarely of much use because they are chosen specifically to make the test for no interaction. If there is interaction then it will usually be best to report the effects of exposure separately for each age band. If there is no interaction then the effects of exposure and age should be obtained from the model without interaction parameters. Further details on how to report interactions are given in Chapter 26.

Table 24.5.   Estimates of parameters in the model with interaction

Parameter	Estimate	SD
Corner	−5.0237	0.500
Exposure(1)	−0.0258	0.866
Age(1)	−0.5153	0.671
Age(2)	0.3132	0.612
Age(1)·Exposure(1)	1.2720	1.020
Age(2)·Exposure(1)	0.8719	0.973

Table 24.5 shows the output for the ischaemic heart disease data when fitting the model which includes the interaction between exposure and age. The interaction parameters are given names like Age(1)·Exposure(1) and Age(2)·Exposure(1). In general the number of interaction parameters between a variable on a levels and one on b levels is $(a-1)(b-1)$.

Exercise 24.4. Verify from Table 24.5 that the estimated corner parameter in the model with interaction is now the log of the observed rate for unexposed subjects in age band 0, and the estimated Exposure(1) parameter is now the observed rate ratio (exposed/unexposed) in age band 0. (The observed rates are in Table 22.6.)

24.4 Deviance

The log likelihood for a regression model, evaluated at the most likely values of the parameters, is a measure of *goodness-of-fit* of the model — the greater the log likelihood, the better the fit. Since the absolute value of the log likelihood is not itself of interest there is some advantage in always reporting a log likelihood ratio, compared to some other model. A convenient choice is the *saturated* which includes the maximum possible number of parameters. The output would then include the log likelihood ratio between the model being fitted and the saturated model. For use with tables of chi-squared it is slightly more convenient to report minus twice the log likelihood ratio, a quantity which is called the *deviance* for the model being fitted. Each deviance has degrees of freedom equal to the difference between the number of parameters in the model and the number in the saturated model.

The deviance is a measure of badness of fit; the larger the deviance the worse the fit. Two models are compared by comparing their deviances. The change in deviance is minus twice the log likelihood ratio for the two models because the log likelihood for the saturated model occurs in both deviances and cancels (see Fig. 24.1.) The degrees of freedom for this test are found by subtracting the degrees of freedom for the two deviances. For

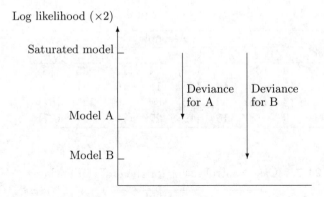

Fig. 24.1. Relationship between deviance and log likelihood

example, when fitting the models

$$\log(\text{Rate}) \; = \; \text{Corner} + \text{Age} + \text{Exposure}$$
$$\log(\text{Rate}) \; = \; \text{Corner} + \text{Exposure},$$

to the ischaemic heart disease data the corresponding values for the two deviances were 1.673 and 5.689. The difference between these is 4.016 which is the same as the result obtained earlier in the chapter for minus twice the log likelihood ratio.

Exercise 24.5. How do you know which deviance was obtained for which model? How many degrees of freedom do the two deviances have?

When the data are entered as frequency records the saturated model has the same number of parameters as there are frequency records. In the case of the ischaemic heart disease data there are six records so the saturated model has 6 parameters. All models with six parameters are saturated and have the same log likelihood. The model which includes the interaction parameters between age and exposure has six parameters, and is saturated, so it follows that the deviance for the model

$$\log(\text{Rate}) = \text{Corner} + \text{Age} + \text{Exposure}$$

provides a test of no interaction between age and exposure. It may be referred directly to a chi-squared distribution with two degrees of freedom.

When the data are entered as individual records the saturated model has the same number of parameters as the number of individual records and the deviance measures minus twice the difference between the log likelihood for the fitted model and this saturated model. This is not a test of anything useful. There is no short cut for making a test of no interaction using individual records: it is necessary to obtain the deviances for the models

Table 24.6. Cases (controls) for oral cancer study

Tobacco	Alcohol							
	0		1		2		3	
0	10	(38)	7	(27)	4	(12)	5	(8)
1	11	(26)	16	(35)	18	(16)	21	(20)
2	13	(36)	50	(60)	60	(49)	125	(52)
3	9	(8)	16	(19)	27	(14)	91	(27)

Table 24.7. Case/control ratios for the oral cancer data

Tobacco	Alcohol			
	0	1	2	3
0	0.26	0.26	0.33	0.63
1	0.42	0.46	1.13	1.05
2	0.36	0.83	1.22	2.40
3	1.12	0.84	1.93	3.37

with and without the interaction parameters.

24.5 Models with two exposures

Because regression models treat all explanatory variables in the same way, models for studies with two exposures look very similar to models for studies with one exposure and one confounder. However, there are some differences in the way different hypotheses are interpreted.

Table 24.6 repeats the study of oral cancer introduced in Chapter 16, in which the numbers of cases and controls are tabulated by two exposures, alcohol consumption (on four levels) and tobacco consumption (also on four levels). For alcohol the levels are 0, 0.1–0.3, 0.4–1.5, and 1.6+ ounces per day (coded as 0, 1, 2, and 3). For tobacco the levels are 0, 1–19, 20–39, and 40+ cigarettes per day (also coded as 0, 1, 2, and 3). A summary table of case/control ratios by alcohol and tobacco is shown in Table 24.7. Because the frequencies in the table are small, there is a lot of random variation, but there is an overall tendency for the ratios to increase both from left to right along rows, and from top to bottom down columns. This indicates that *both* variables have an effect on cancer incidence; there is an effect of tobacco when alcohol intake is held constant, and vice versa.

An important question is whether the two exposures act independently of one another. In other words, are the effects of tobacco the same at all levels of alcohol, and are the effects of alcohol the same at all levels of tobacco? This question is answered by testing for no interaction between alcohol and tobacco, but it must be emphasized that the test depends on how the effect parameters are defined. When they are defined as ratios the interaction parameters are also ratios and measure departures from a model in which the two exposures combine multiplicatively. By choosing to measure effects as ratios we have therefore chosen to interpret independent action as meaning that the two exposures act multiplicatively. In Chapter 28 we show how the effects can be defined as differences, in which case the interaction parameters are also differences and measure departures from a model in which the two exposures combine additively. In this case we have chosen to interpret independent action as meaning the two exposures act additively.

If there is a significant interaction then it will be necessary to report the effects of alcohol separately as odds ratios for each level of tobacco consumption, and the effects of tobacco separately as odds ratios for each level of alcohol. On the other hand, if there is no significant interaction then the two exposures may be assumed to act independently and we can estimate the effects of alcohol controlled for tobacco and the effects of tobacco controlled for alcohol. Note that even when the two exposures act independently it is still necessary to control each for the other. This is because people's drinking and smoking habits are not independent so ignoring one when studying the other could lead to biased estimates.

The test for no interaction is carried out by comparing the fit of the multiplicative model

$$\log(\text{Odds}) = \text{Corner} + \text{Alcohol} + \text{Tobacco},$$

with that of the model which includes the interaction parameters,

$$\log(\text{Odds}) = \text{Corner} + \text{Alcohol} + \text{Tobacco} + \text{Alcohol} \cdot \text{Tobacco}.$$

Since the second of these models is saturated the test can be based directly on the deviance for the multiplicative model. Provided the data support the hypothesis of no interaction it is then possible to test for an effect of alcohol, controlled for tobacco, by comparing the models

$$\log(\text{Odds}) = \text{Corner} + \text{Alcohol} + \text{Tobacco}$$
$$\log(\text{Odds}) = \text{Corner} + \text{Tobacco}.$$

Similarly the test for an effect of tobacco is made by comparing the models

$$\log(\text{Odds}) = \text{Corner} + \text{Alcohol} + \text{Tobacco}$$
$$\log(\text{Odds}) = \text{Corner} + \text{Alcohol}.$$

In each of these tests the smaller of the two models being compared is obtained from the larger by setting some parameters to zero. The smaller

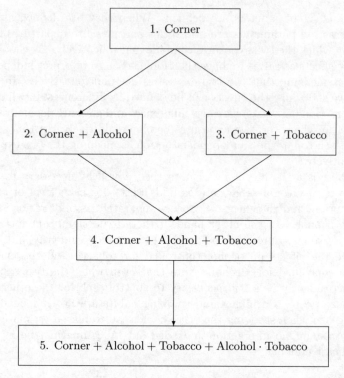

Fig. 24.2.   Nesting of models.

model is then said to be *nested* in the larger model. Comparisons between models where neither is nested in the other are not allowed since they do not correspond to a hypothesis in which some parameter values are set equal to zero. Fig. 24.2 shows the five possible models which could be fitted to the alcohol and tobacco data. The arrows indicate nesting so any two models joined by an arrow correspond to a hypothesis which can be tested. For example, a comparison of models 4 and 5 is a test of no interaction, and a comparison of models 4 and 2 is a test of no effect of tobacco (controlling for alcohol). In model 1 both alcohol and tobacco parameters are set to zero so it is nested in all of the other models.

Exercise 24.6. For the models set out in Fig. 24.2, the deviances are (1) 132.561, (2) 37.951, (3) 61.880, and (4) 6.689. What are the degrees of freedom associated with each of these deviances? Carry out the four tests corresponding to the arrows in the figure. What is the interpretation of these tests?

24.6   Goodness-of-fit tests

A question which is often asked is whether a model provides an adequate fit to the data. Because the absolute value of the log likelihood has no meaning this question can only be answered by comparing the model with other more complicated models and asking whether the extra complication is justified. The saturated model represents the most complicated model which could be used and the deviance automatically provides a comparison of the model currently being fitted with the saturated model. For this reason the deviance for a model is often put forward as a test of goodness of fit (really badness-of-fit) of the model. There are several cautions which need to be borne in mind when interpreting the deviance in this way.

1. Comparisons with the saturated model are meaningless when the data are entered as individual records.

2. Comparisons with the saturated model which are on many degrees of freedom will lack power to discriminate; in this case it will be better to make comparisons with models which are less complicated than the saturated model.

3. The deviance is only approximately distributed as chi-squared and this approximation gets worse as the degrees of freedom increase.

24.7 Collinearity

In a study in which tobacco and alcohol consumption were very highly associated it would be very difficult to make an estimate of the effects of alcohol controlled for tobacco (or of the effects of tobacco controlled for alcohol). This is because controlling for tobacco involves fixing the level of tobacco consumption and then estimating the effects of alcohol from subjects whose tobacco consumption is at this level. If alcohol and tobacco are highly associated then nearly all subjects at a fixed tobacco level will have the same level of alcohol consumption and it will therefore be difficult to estimate the effects of alcohol. In extreme cases fixing the level of tobacco might fix the level of alcohol completely, in which case it would be impossible to estimate the effects of alcohol. In such a case the two variables are said to be *collinear*. This situation is not uncommon, particularly when working with derived variables.

Solutions to the exercises

24.1 In the Wald test $(0.8697/0.3080)^2 = 7.97$ is referred to the chi-squared distribution with one degree of freedom, giving a p-value of 0.005.

24.2 The larger likelihood, -247.027, corresponds to the first model because this has more parameters than the second. The log likelihood ratio for the two models is $-251.176 - (-247.027) = -4.149$. Minus twice this is 8.298 which is quite close to the Wald chi-squared value obtained in the

previous exercise. Referring 8.30 to the chi-squared distribution with one
degree of freedom gives $p = 0.004$.

24.3 No. When taking account of confounding variables it is best to
play safe and to control for them regardless of whether their effects are
significant or not. Very little is lost by doing this.

24.4 The Corner, Exposure(1), Age(1) and Age(2) parameters are

$$
\begin{aligned}
\log(6.580/1000) &= -5.0237 \\
\log(6.412/6.580) &= -0.0258 \\
\log(3.931/6.580) &= -0.5153 \\
\log(9.00/6.58) &= 0.3132.
\end{aligned}
$$

24.5 The smaller deviance corresponds to the larger model since this will
be a better fit. The degrees of freedom are 2 and 4 respectively.

24.6 The number of parameters in models 1 to 5 are 1, 4, 4, 7, and
16, respectively. The number of parameters in the saturated model is 16,
so the degrees of freedom for the deviances are $16 - 1 = 15$, $16 - 4 = 12$,
$16 - 4 = 12$, $16 - 7 = 9$, and $16 - 16 = 0$ respectively. Note that model 5 has
16 parameters so it is saturated. The table below shows the comparisons
of models in terms of the change in deviance.

Comparison	Change in deviance	Change in df
(1) vs (2)	$132.56 - 37.95 = 94.61$	$15 - 12 = 3$
(1) vs (3)	$132.56 - 61.88 = 70.68$	$15 - 12 = 3$
(2) vs (4)	$37.95 - 6.69 = 31.26$	$12 - 9 = 3$
(3) vs (4)	$61.88 - 6.69 = 55.19$	$12 - 9 = 3$
(4) vs (5)	$6.69 - 0 = 6.69$	$9 - 0 = 9$

The last of these comparisons shows that there is no significant interaction.
This means that the next two comparisons (working up from the bottom)
make sense. The change in deviance from model 3 to model 4 shows that
there is a significant effect of alcohol after controlling for tobacco; similarly
the change in deviance from model 2 to model 4 shows that there is a
significant effect of tobacco after controlling for alcohol. All of the models
can be compared with model 1, but these comparisons have little interest.
For example, a comparison of model 1 with model 2 is a test of the alcohol
effects (ignoring tobacco) while a comparison of model 1 with model 4 is
a joint test of the alcohol effects (controlling for tobacco) *and* the tobacco
effects (controlling for alcohol).

25
Models for dose-response

When the subjects in a study receive different levels of exposure, measured on a quantitative or ordered scale, it is likely that any effect of exposure will increase (or decrease) systematically with the level of exposure. This is known as a dose-response relationship, or trend. The existence of such a relationship provides more convincing evidence of a causal effect of exposure than a simple comparison of exposed with unexposed subjects. Some simple procedures for testing for trend were introduced in Chapter 20. These tests are based on a log-linear dose-response relationship, that is, a linear relationship between the log rate parameter (or log odds parameter) and the level of exposure. We now return to this topic and show how such dose-response relationships are easily described as regression models.

25.1 Estimating the dose-response relationship

To illustrate the use of regression models when exposure is measured on a quantitative scale we shall use the case-control study of alcohol and tobacco in oral cancer in which there are two exposure variables, both with four levels. The model

$$\log(\text{Odds}) = \text{Corner} + \text{Alcohol} + \text{Tobacco},$$

in which alcohol and tobacco are categorical variables each with four levels, makes no assumption about dose-response; there are three alcohol parameters and three tobacco parameters. The estimated values of these parameters are shown in Table 25.1. If we were able to assume simple dose-response relationships for these two exposures, we could concentrate the available information into fewer parameters and, as a result, gain power.

To study the dose-response for tobacco consumption it helps to change from the parameters Tobacco(1), Tobacco(2), and Tobacco(3), which are chosen to compare each level of exposure with level 0, to

Tobacco(1) ,   Tobacco(2)−Tobacco(1) ,   Tobacco(3)−Tobacco(2) ,

which are chosen to compare each level with the one before.

Exercise 25.1. Use the results of Table 25.1 to write down the estimated values of these new parameters. Repeat the exercise for alcohol.

Table 25.1. Alcohol and tobacco treated as categorical variables

Parameter	Estimate	SD
Corner	−1.6090	0.2654
Alcohol(1)	0.2897	0.2327
Alcohol(2)	0.8437	0.2383
Alcohol(3)	1.3780	0.2256
Tobacco(1)	0.5887	0.2844
Tobacco(2)	1.0260	0.2544
Tobacco(3)	1.4090	0.2823

Table 25.2. The linear effect of tobacco consumption

Alcohol	Tobacco	log(Odds) = Corner + $\cdots$
0	0	–
0	1	1×[Tobacco]
0	2	2×[Tobacco]
0	3	3×[Tobacco]
1	0	Alcohol(1)
1	1	Alcohol(1) + 1×[Tobacco]
1	2	Alcohol(1) + 2×[Tobacco]
1	3	Alcohol(1) + 3×[Tobacco]
2	0	Alcohol(2)
2	1	Alcohol(2) + 1×[Tobacco]
2	2	Alcohol(2) + 2×[Tobacco]
2	3	Alcohol(2) + 3×[Tobacco]
3	0	Alcohol(3)
3	1	Alcohol(3) + 1×[Tobacco]
3	2	Alcohol(3) + 2×[Tobacco]
3	3	Alcohol(3) + 3×[Tobacco]

The simplest possible dose-response model would assume that each step in tobacco consumption, from one level to the next, produces the same change in the log odds. This model requires only one parameter for tobacco, namely the common change in log odds per change in level. This parameter is called the *linear effect* of tobacco and we shall write it as [Tobacco], where the brackets are used to distinguish the linear effect parameter from the separate effect parameters for each level. The model is written in full in Table 25.2.

The data from this study are in the form of frequency records containing the number of cases, the total number of cases and controls, alcohol

Table 25.3.   Linear effect of tobacco per level

Parameter	Estimate	SD
Corner	−1.5250	0.219
Alcohol(1)	0.3020	0.232
Alcohol(2)	0.8579	0.237
Alcohol(3)	1.3880	0.225
[Tobacco]	0.4541	0.083

consumption coded as 0, 1, 2, 3, and tobacco consumption coded as 0, 1, 2, 3. We shall write the model of Table 25.2 in the abbreviated form:

$$\log(\text{Odds}) = \text{Corner} + \text{Alcohol} + [\text{Tobacco}].$$

The regression program output for this model is illustrated in Table 25.3.

Exercise 25.2. How would you report the meaning of the number 0.4541 in Table 25.3?

A more accurate scale for tobacco consumption would be to use the midpoints of the ranges of tobacco use at each level, namely 0, 10, 30, and (say) 50 cigarettes per day. If the tobacco variable were coded in this way then the parameter [Tobacco] would refer to the linear effect per extra cigarette rather than per change of level. If the data were entered as individual records then the individual values for consumption could be used. In view of the uncertainties in measuring tobacco use there is something to be said for sticking to the scale 0, 1, 2, 3.

The reparametrization of the alcohol effects carried out in Exercise 25.1 also suggests a constant effect with increasing level of alcohol consumption. This allows the model to be further simplified to

$$\log(\text{Odds}) = \text{Corner} + [\text{Alcohol}] + [\text{Tobacco}],$$

where the parameter [Alcohol] is the common effect of an increase of one level in alcohol consumption. The regression output for this model is shown in Table 25.4.

Exercise 25.3. Use the output in Table 25.4 to work out what the model predicts for the combined effect of level 3 for tobacco and level 3 for alcohol compared to level 0 for both. Use the output in Table 25.1 to work out the same prediction when tobacco and alcohol are both treated as categorical.

For comparison we also show, in Table 25.5, the regression output for the model where alcohol consumption is measured in approximate mean ounces of alcohol per day for each category (0.0, 0.2, 1.0 and 2.0), and

Table 25.4.   Linear effects of alcohol and tobacco per level

Parameter	Estimate	SD
Corner	−1.6290	0.1860
[Alcohol]	0.4901	0.0676
[Tobacco]	0.4517	0.0833

Table 25.5.   Alcohol in ounces/day and tobacco in cigarettes/day

Parameter	Estimate	SD
Corner	−1.2657	0.1539
[Alcohol]	0.6484	0.0881
[Tobacco]	0.0253	0.0046

tobacco consumption is measured in approximate cigarettes per day for
each category (0, 10, 30, or 50). The [Alcohol] and [Tobacco] parameters
now look quite different from those in Table 25.4, but this is because they
are measured per ounce of alcohol and per cigarette respectively.

TESTING FOR TREND

Comparison of log likelihoods for the models

$$\log(\text{Odds}) = \text{Corner} + \text{Alcohol} + [\text{Tobacco}]$$

and

$$\log(\text{Odds}) = \text{Corner} + \text{Alcohol}$$

yields a one degree of freedom test for the effect of tobacco controlled for
the effect of alcohol. The Mantel extension test described in Chapter 20 is
the corresponding score test, which tests the hypothesis that the [Tobacco]
parameter takes the value zero.

TESTING FOR DEPARTURE FROM LINEARITY

To test for departures from linearity in the dose-response for tobacco, the
models

$$\log(\text{Odds}) = \text{Corner} + \text{Alcohol} + \text{Tobacco}$$
$$\log(\text{Odds}) = \text{Corner} + \text{Alcohol} + [\text{Tobacco}],$$

can be compared. In the first model Tobacco refers to the three effects
of a categorical variable with 4 levels, while in the second [Tobacco] refers

Table 25.6. A quadratic dose-response relationship for tobacco

z	$(z)^2$	$\log(\text{Odds}) = \text{Corner} + \cdots$
0	0	–
1	1	$1 \times [\text{Tobacco}] + 1 \times [\text{Tobsq}]$
2	4	$2 \times [\text{Tobacco}] + 4 \times [\text{Tobsq}]$
3	9	$3 \times [\text{Tobacco}] + 9 \times [\text{Tobsq}]$

Table 25.7. Predictions from a quadratic relationship

Effect	Predicted from model
Tobacco(1)	$[\text{Tobacco}] + 1 \times [\text{Tobsq}]$
Tobacco(2) − Tobacco(1)	$[\text{Tobacco}] + 3 \times [\text{Tobsq}]$
Tobacco(3) − Tobacco(2)	$[\text{Tobacco}] + 5 \times [\text{Tobsq}]$

to the effect of a change of one level in tobacco consumption. The second model is a special case of the first, so they can be compared using a log likelihood ratio test.

Exercise 25.4. (a) How many parameters are there in the two models? (b) Reparametrize the models so that the second model is a special case of the first, with two parameters set to zero. (c) How would you interpret a significant difference between the fit of these two models?

25.2 Quadratic dose-response relationships

The simplest departure from a log-linear dose relationship is a log-quadratic relationship. To fit this model it is necessary to create a new dose variable which takes the values 0, 1, 4, 9, that is the squares of the values used to code tobacco consumption. We shall call this new variable 'tobsq'. The model is then fitted by including both tobacco and tobsq and declaring them as quantitative variables. The regression equations for this model are given in Table 25.6 and these show that when [Tobsq] is zero the dose-response is log-linear. Table 25.7 shows the tobacco effects for each level relative to the previous one, predicted from the quadratic model, and these show that the parameter [Tobsq] measures the degree to which the dose-response relationship departs from linearity.

The log-quadratic model also provides another way of testing for departures from a log-linear dose-response relationship, by comparing the models

$$\log(\text{Odds}) = \text{Corner} + \text{Alcohol} + [\text{Tobacco}]$$
$$\log(\text{Odds}) = \text{Corner} + \text{Alcohol} + [\text{Tobacco}] + [\text{Tobsq}].$$

The comparison of these two models provides a test (on one degree of freedom) which will be sensitive to a departure from linearity in which the effect of tobacco increases with level ([Tobsq]> 0), or decreases with level ([Tobsq]< 0).

25.3   How many categories?

When collecting data, exposure is often measured as accurately as possible for individuals and only later are the observed values grouped into a relatively small number of categories. For example, the number of previous births would be recorded exactly, but might then be grouped as

$$0, \quad 1-3, \quad 4-6, \quad 7-9, \quad 10+ \ .$$

When the variable is to be treated as categorical it is best to keep the number of categories small; three may be enough, and five is usually a maximum number. For exploratory analyses the use of just two categories has the advantage that there is only one effect to interpret, and it can often be easier to see what is going on.

The number of subjects in each category should be roughly the same, and to achieve this tertiles, quartiles or quintiles of the distribution of exposure are often used. Tertiles define three equal-sized groups, quartiles define four equal-sized groups, and quintiles define five such groups. This is quite a sensible way of choosing the grouping intervals provided the actual intervals are reported. A serious disadvantage is that such grouping intervals will vary from study to study, thus making it harder to compare findings.

When the variable is to be treated as quantitative there is no penalty in taking a larger number of categories. In the extreme case the original values are used. However, it is best to avoid the situation where one or two of the subjects have much higher values than all the rest. This can occur with an exposure like the number of previous sexual partners, which might lie between 0 and 10 for most subjects but reach numbers in excess of 100 for a few. In such a case the few subjects with high values can dominate the fit of a model, and it will be best to group the values so that all the high ones fall into a group such as 15 or more.

⋆ 25.4   Indicator variables

In order to fit a model to data the computer program must use the abbreviated description of the model to form the regression equations. These express the log rate (or log odds) parameter for each record as a linear combination of new parameters. For example, when the variable alcohol is entered in a model as categorical with levels coded 0, 1, 2, and 3, the regression equations include the parameter Alcohol(1) for records in which alcohol is at level 1, the parameter Alcohol(2) for records in which alcohol is at level 2, and the parameter Alcohol(3) for records in which alcohol is

Table 25.8. Indicator variables for the three alcohol parameters

A_1	A_2	A_3	Level	log(Odds) = Corner + $\cdots$
0	0	0	0	–
1	0	0	1	Alcohol(1)
0	1	0	2	Alcohol(2)
0	0	1	3	Alcohol(3)

at level 3. The way the program does this is to create an *indicator* variable for each parameter. These variables are coded 1 for records which include the parameter and 0 otherwise. The indicator variables A_1, A_2, A_3 for the three alcohol parameters are shown in Table 25.8 alongside the levels of alcohol. Note that A_1, which indicates when Alcohol(1) should be included, takes the value 1 when alcohol is at level 1, and so on.

Exercise 25.5. Repeat Table 25.8 to show indicator variables for the case where both alcohol and tobacco have four levels.

A variable which is treated as quantitative acts as its own indicator since the way the variable is coded indicates what multiple of the linear effect parameter is to be included in the regression equations. For example, when tobacco is included as a quantitative variable, coded 0, 1, 2, and 3, the equations include the parameter [Tobacco] when tobacco is at level 1, twice the parameter [Tobacco] when tobacco is at level 2, and three times the parameter [Tobacco] when tobacco is at level 3. The coding of the tobacco variable thus indicates which multiple of the parameter is to be included in the model.

INTERACTION PARAMETERS

When interaction terms are included in the model, indicator variables are again used to form the regression equations. For simplicity we shall consider the situation where tobacco has only two levels, 0 for non-smokers and 1 for smokers. The model in which both alcohol and tobacco are categorical, and which contains interaction terms, is shown in full in Table 25.9. Indicator variables A_1, A_2, A_3 have been used for alcohol, and the indicator variable T has been used for tobacco. Note that when tobacco has only two levels, coded 0 and 1, it serves as its own indicator variable.

The indicator variable for Alcohol(1)·Tobacco(1) takes the value 1 when both alcohol and tobacco are at level 1, and 0 otherwise. The indicator variable for Alcohol(2)·Tobacco(1) takes the value 1 when alcohol is at level 2 and exposure is at level 1, and 0 otherwise, and so on. The most convenient way of generating these interaction indicator variables is by multiplying together pairs of the original indicator variables for alcohol and tobacco. This is shown in Table 25.10: the indicator for Alcohol(1)·Tobacco(1) is found from the product of A_1 and T; the indicator for Alcohol(2)·Tobacco(1) is

Table 25.9. The model with interaction between alcohol and tobacco

Alc.	Tob.	$\log(\text{Odds}) = \text{Corner} + \cdots$
0	0	–
0	1	Tobacco(1)
1	0	Alcohol(1)
1	1	Alcohol(1) + Tobacco(1) + Alcohol(1)·Tobacco(1)
2	0	Alcohol(2)
2	1	Alcohol(2) + Tobacco(1) + Alcohol(2)·Tobacco(1)
3	0	Alcohol(3)
3	1	Alcohol(3) + Tobacco(1) + Alcohol(3)·Tobacco(1)

Table 25.10. Indicator variables for interaction parameters

A_1	A_2	A_3	T	$A_1 \cdot T$	$A_2 \cdot T$	$A_3 \cdot T$
0	0	0	0	0	0	0
0	0	0	1	0	0	0
1	0	0	0	0	0	0
1	0	0	1	1	0	0
0	1	0	0	0	0	0
0	1	0	1	0	1	0
0	0	1	0	0	0	0
0	0	1	1	0	0	1

made up from product of A_2 and T, and so on. When the categorical variables are on a and b levels respectively there are $(a-1)(b-1)$ new indicators for the interaction parameters.

In the first regression programs it was left to the user to create indicator variables for all parameters other than those referring to quantitative variables. Although it is rarely necessary to do this today, indicator variables are still important when we wish to use a non-standard parametrization of a regression model.

★ **25.5   The zero level of exposure**

The level of exposure which is coded zero is often qualitatively different from the other levels. For example, zero previous births represents a very different biological experience from any other point on this scale. In such cases it may be better to omit the zero level when estimating the dose-response relationship, by allowing the response of at zero dose to differ from the general relationship (see Fig. 25.1). A parameter for each of these comparisons can be included in a model by using the indicator variable for

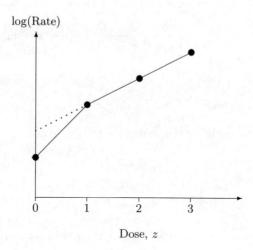

Fig. 25.1. Separating zero exposure from the dose-response.

Table 25.11. Separating zero exposure from the dose-response

Tobacco	Non-smoker	$\log(\text{Odds}) = \text{Corner} + \cdots$
0	1	[Non-smoker]
1	0	$1 \times$ [Tobacco]
2	0	$2 \times$ [Tobacco]
3	0	$3 \times$ [Tobacco]

non-smokers to fit the model

$$\log(\text{Odds}) = \text{Corner} + [\text{Non-smoker}] + [\text{Tobacco}].$$

The regression equations for all four dose levels are shown in Table 25.11. The parameter [Non-smoker] measures the discrepancy between the log odds for non-smokers and that predicted by extrapolation of the dose-response line to zero dose.

25.6 Using indicators to reparametrize the model

Indicator variables provide a convenient way of changing from one set of parameters to another. We shall give one example, namely changing from parameters which compare each level with level 0, to parameters which compare each level with the one before. Using tobacco as an example, the first set of parameters are Tobacco(1), Tobacco(2), and Tobacco(3). We shall call the new parameters Tobdiff(1), Tobdiff(2), and Tobdiff(3). The

Table 25.12. Indicators to compare each level with the one before

Tobacco	D_1	D_2	D_2
0	0	0	0
1	1	0	0
2	1	1	0
3	1	1	1

relationship between the new parameters and the old is

$$
\begin{aligned}
\text{Tobdiff}(1) &= \text{Tobacco}(1) \\
\text{Tobdiff}(2) &= \text{Tobacco}(2) - \text{Tobacco}(1) \\
\text{Tobdiff}(3) &= \text{Tobacco}(3) - \text{Tobacco}(2).
\end{aligned}
$$

This relationship may be inverted to give the old in terms of the new as

$$
\begin{aligned}
\text{Tobacco}(1) &= \text{Tobdiff}(1) \\
\text{Tobacco}(2) &= \text{Tobdiff}(1) + \text{Tobdiff}(2) \\
\text{Tobacco}(3) &= \text{Tobdiff}(1) + \text{Tobdiff}(2) + \text{Tobdiff}(3)
\end{aligned}
$$

Let the indicator variables for Tobdiff(1), Tobdiff(2), Tobdiff(3), be denoted by D_1, D_2, D_3. The first of these should indicate Tobdiff(1) when tobacco is at level 1, 2, or 3; the second should indicate Tobdiff(2) when tobacco is at level 2 or 3; and the third should indicate Tobdiff(3) when tobacco is at level 3. Their values are shown in Table 25.12.

Solutions to the exercises

25.1 The estimates of the new parameters will be

Tobacco(1)	0.5887
Tobacco(2)−Tobacco(1)	0.4373
Tobacco(3)−Tobacco(2)	0.3830

and

Alcohol(1)	0.2897
Alcohol(2)−Alcohol(1)	0.5540
Alcohol(3)−Alcohol(2)	0.5343

25.2 The parameter represents the change in log odds for each increase in level of tobacco consumption.

25.3 The combined effect on the log odds is

$$+(3 \times 0.4901) + (3 \times 0.4517) = 2.8254.$$

This corresponds to a multiplicative effect of $\times 16.87$ on the odds. When alcohol and tobacco are both treated as categorical the combined effect on the log odds is

$$+1.3780 + 1.4090 = 2.7870$$

which corresponds to a multiplicative effect of $\times 16.23$ on the odds.

25.4 (a) The first model has 7 parameters, the second has 5. (b) Starting with Tobacco(1), Tobacco(2), and Tobacco(3), change to the parameters New(1), New(2), and New(3), where

$$
\begin{aligned}
\text{New}(1) &= \text{Tobacco}(1) \\
\text{New}(2) &= \{\text{Tobacco}(2) - \text{Tobacco}(1)\} - \text{Tobacco}(1) \\
\text{New}(3) &= \{\text{Tobacco}(3) - \text{Tobacco}(2)\} - \text{Tobacco}(1).
\end{aligned}
$$

Then New(1) measures the effect of changing level from 0 to 1; New(2) measures the difference between this and the effect of changing level from 1 to 2; New(3) measures the difference between this and changing level from 2 to 3. The model with all three parameters allows separate effects of changing level while the model with New(2) and New(3) equal to zero imposes the constraint that there is a common effect of changing level.
(c) When the first model is a significantly better fit than the second model it means that there is a significant departure from linearity in the dose-response.

25.5 Let $A_1, A_2, A_3, T_1, T_2, T_3$ be the indicator variables for alcohol and tobacco. The table below shows how these variables are coded and the regression model which is fitted when all the indicators are included.

A_1	A_2	A_3	T_1	T_2	T_3	log(Odds) = Corner + $\cdots$
0	0	0	0	0	0	–
0	0	0	1	0	0	Tobacco(1)
0	0	0	0	1	0	Tobacco(2)
0	0	0	0	0	1	Tobacco(3)
1	0	0	0	0	0	Alcohol(1)
1	0	0	1	0	0	Alcohol(1) + Tobacco(1)
1	0	0	0	1	0	Alcohol(1) + Tobacco(2)
1	0	0	0	0	1	Alcohol(1) + Tobacco(3)
0	1	0	0	0	0	Alcohol(2)
0	1	0	1	0	0	Alcohol(2) + Tobacco(1)
0	1	0	0	1	0	Alcohol(2) + Tobacco(2)
0	1	0	0	0	1	Alcohol(2) + Tobacco(3)
0	0	1	0	0	0	Alcohol(3)
0	0	1	1	0	0	Alcohol(3) + Tobacco(1)
0	0	1	0	1	0	Alcohol(3) + Tobacco(2)
0	0	1	0	0	1	Alcohol(3) + Tobacco(3)

26
More about interaction

In this chapter we draw together some of the ideas of the previous chapters, particularly those relating to interaction, and consider studies with several explanatory variables. The first stage in the analysis of such studies is to classify the explanatory variables into those whose effects are of interest (the exposures), and those whose effects are of no interest, but which must be included in the model (the confounders). In order to illustrate the problems which arise with several confounders we introduce a new example in Table 26.1* This shows the proportion of subjects with monoclonal gammapathy by age, sex, and work. Work can be agricultural or non-agricultural and is the exposure of interest. Age and sex are confounders.

26.1 Interaction between confounders

To control for the confounding effect of both age and sex using stratification it would be necessary to form $5 \times 2 = 10$ age– sex strata. The separate estimates of the effect of work for each stratum would then be pooled over strata using the Mantel–Haenszel method. The same thing can be done by fitting the model

$$\log(\text{Odds}) = \text{Corner} + \text{Age} + \text{Sex} + \text{Age} \cdot \text{Sex} + \text{Work},$$

which includes age–sex interaction parameters. The total number of parameters for the corner, age, sex, and the age–sex interaction is $1+4+1+4 = 10$, which is the same as the number of the age–sex strata. Fitting the model with interaction does the same job as age–sex stratification, which has one parameter for each of the 10 strata.[†]

It is also possible to control for age and sex by omitting the interaction term and fitting the model

$$\log(\text{Odds}) = \text{Corner} + \text{Age} + \text{Sex} + \text{Work}.$$

---

*From Healy, M. (1988) *GLIM. An Introduction*, Oxford Science Publications.

[†]The abbreviation Age⋆Sex is sometimes used for the group of terms

$$\text{Age} + \text{Sex} + \text{Age} \cdot \text{Sex}$$

Table 26.1. Prevalence of monoclonal gammapathy

| | Agricultural (0) | | Non-agricultural (1) | |
Age	Male (0)	Female (1)	Male (0)	Female (1)
< 40 (0)	1/1590	1/1926	2/1527	0/712
40–49 (1)	12/2345	7/2677	3/854	0/401
50–59 (2)	24/2787	15/2902	5/675	4/312
60–69 (3)	53/2489	38/3145	3/184	1/80
70+ (4)	95/2381	63/2918	2/75	0/20

The estimated effect of work is -0.134 with standard deviation 0.244 in the model with interaction and -0.136 with standard deviation 0.243 in the model without. In this case, therefore, omitting the interaction term makes almost no difference.

Exercise 26.1. How should the effect of work be interpreted in terms of disease prevalence?

When using stratification or logistic regression to control for confounders it is best to keep the number of parameters in the model as low as possible. This is because both techniques are based on profile likelihood which can be unreliable when there are too many parameters to eliminate. Including interactions can require a lot of extra parameters, possibly too many to deal with by using profile likelihood. For example, if one confounder has 45 levels and another has 6 levels, then the model with interaction requires $5 \times 44 = 220$ extra parameters. Even when none of the confounders has a large number of levels it will still take many extra parameters to include interactions when there are a lot of them. For example, 10 confounders each with 3 levels require 180 extra parameters to include interactions between all possible pairs. In the monoclonal gammapathy example the model with interaction has 11 parameters while the model without interaction has only 7. By fitting a model without interaction we have reduced the number of parameters from 11 to 7. This is not a great saving and little is lost in this case by playing safe and fitting a model with the interaction.

It is possible, of course, to test for interaction between any pair of confounders. For the monoclonal example the deviance for the model with age–sex interaction is 6.771 on 9 degrees of freedom, and the deviance for the model without interaction is 7.649 on 13 degrees of freedom. The difference between these two deviances is only $7.649 - 6.771 = 0.878$, on 4 degrees of freedom, so the interaction is not significant. Unfortunately such a test has only sufficient power to be useful when based on a few degrees of freedom, and these are just the situations where nothing much is gained by omitting interactions. Thus the decision about whether or not to include interactions must usually be taken on other grounds. As a general rule, interactions between a confounder with many levels, and any other confounder, are omitted. For confounders with fewer levels it is only necessary to consider interaction between those pairs in which both are known to be very strongly related to the outcome. It is then probably best to include the interaction term for such pairs as a matter of course. Age and sex often form such a pair, and are usually controlled for by using a model which includes the age–sex interaction.

It can happen that a confounding variable has too many levels to be included into a logistic regression model, even before considering interactions. This occurs with matched case-control studies in which controls are individually matched to each case. Each case-control set then corresponds to a level of the categorical variable which defines the sets. The effects of this variable are of no interest but they must be included in the model when estimating the effects of other more interesting variables. The way out of this dilemma is to use conditional logistic regression (see Chapter 29) which uses a conditional likelihood in place of the profile likelihood.

26.2 Interaction between exposure and confounders

When controlling the effect of an exposure for the confounding effects of other variables there is a basic assumption that there is no interaction between exposure and the confounding variables. This assumption can be tested by comparing the model without interaction with a model containing the appropriate interaction term.

For example, when using the model

$$\log(\text{Odds}) = \text{Corner} + \text{Age} + \text{Sex} + \text{Work}$$

to control the effect of work for age and sex, there is an assumption of no interaction between work and age and no interaction between work and sex. To test the work and age interaction we compare the model without interactions with the model

$$\log(\text{Odds}) = \text{Corner} + \text{Age} + \text{Sex} + \text{Work} + \text{Work} \cdot \text{Age}.$$

To test the work and sex interaction we compare the model without interactions with

$$\log(\text{Odds}) = \text{Corner} + \text{Age} + \text{Sex} + \text{Work} + \text{Work} \cdot \text{Sex}.$$

Exercise 26.2. Use the deviances in Table 26.2 to test for interaction between work and the other two variables.

Table 26.2.   Testing for interaction

Model	Deviance
Corner + Age + Sex + Work	7.65
Corner + Age + Sex + Work + Work·Age	5.81
Corner + Age + Sex + Work + Work·Sex	7.24

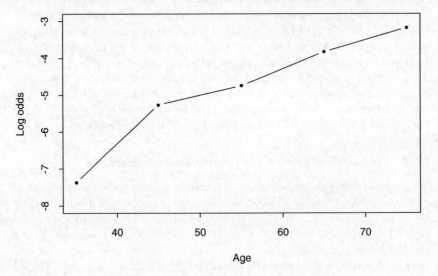

Fig. 26.1.   Log prevalence odds by age

26.3   Confounders measured on a quantitative scale

The variable age in Table 26.1 is measured on a quantitative scale (years) which has been divided into five groups. When controlling for age we have the choice between treating it as categorical with five levels, treating it as quantitative with values equal to the mid- points of the five age groups, or treating it as quantitative with values on the original scale. The last of these alternatives is only possible when the data are in the form of individual records.

Fig. 26.1 shows a plot of the log of the prevalence odds against the mid-points of the age bands (35, 45, 55, 65, and 75 years) for male agricultural workers. The plot shows that the log odds increases approximately linearly with age. Plots for the other three groups in the study also show a roughly log-linear relationship with age.

Exercise 26.3. From Fig. 26.1 make a rough estimate by eye of the gradient of the line relating log odds to age. Express your answer per 10 years of age.

The model which assumes a log-linear relationship between odds and

Table 26.3.   A quadratic relationship with age

Parameter	Estimate	SD
Corner	−6.682	0.344
Work(1)	−0.148	0.243
[Age]	1.204	0.264
[Agesq]	−0.084	0.049
Sex(1)	−0.583	0.115

age for each work–sex combination has fewer parameters than the model which ignores the quantitative nature of the age scale, and this suggests that there may be some advantage in treating age as quantitative with values equal to mid-points of the five age groups. Making this modification to the model with age, sex, and work, we obtain

$$\log(\text{Odds}) = \text{Corner} + [\text{Age}] + \text{Sex} + \text{Work},$$

where [Age] refers to the effect for a change in age of one year. There are now only 4 parameters in this model and the work effect is −0.186 compared to −0.134 using the model in which age was treated as a categorical variable. This difference is large in comparison with the size of the effect, even though in neither analysis does the effect achieve statistical significance. The reason for the difference is that the relationship with age is not entirely linear.

We can test for linearity using a log-quadratic model for the relationship between log odds and age. The parameters in this model are estimated by fitting the model

$$\log(\text{Odds}) = \text{Corner} + [\text{Age}] + [\text{Agesq}] + \text{Sex} + \text{Work},$$

where the variable agesq takes as values the squares of the values of age. The results are shown in Table 26.3. When both [Age] and [Agesq] are included the deviance is 8.93 on 15 degrees of freedom — 3.13 less than when only [Age] is included. Referring this difference to the chi-squared distribution on 1 degree of freedom shows it to be significant at the 0.10 level. This would not normally be considered very convincing evidence of departure from linearity, but note that the estimate of the work effect is now in rather better agreement with earlier values.

The important lesson to be learned from this example is that the effect of a strong confounder such as age must be properly modelled, and that the yardstick of statistical significance may not be adequate for deciding upon the appropriate level of complexity. When the data are grouped in frequency records it is best to treat the variable as categorical; when using

Table 26.4. Interaction between age (quantitative) and work

Parameter	Estimate	SD
Corner	−6.211	0.201
Work(1)	−0.299	0.471
[Age]	0.763	0.058
Sex(1)	−0.584	0.115
[Age]·Work(1)	0.053	0.188

individual records it is best to err on the side of over-detailed modelling and to fit quadratic or even cubic dose-response relationships.

26.4 Interaction between categorical and quantitative variables

One situation where it can be valuable to treat a variable as quantitative is when testing for interaction; the resulting reduction in the number of parameters needed to measure interaction means that the test will be more powerful.

We have seen how to test for interaction between age and work when both are categorical variables, but what if age is a quantitative variable? The model without interaction, in which age is quantitative, is

$$\log(\text{Odds}) = \text{Corner} + [\text{Age}] + \text{Sex} + \text{Work}.$$

To test for interaction between work and quantitative age this is compared with

$$\log(\text{Odds}) = \text{Corner} + [\text{Age}] + \text{Sex} + \text{Work} + [\text{Age}] \cdot \text{Work}.$$

The model without interaction assumes that the gradient of the log-linear relationship of log odds with age is the same in both work groups, while the model which contains the interaction term allows for different gradients in the two work groups. The [Age].Work parameter measures the extent to which the gradient in the second work group differs from the gradient in the first, and its null value, corresponding to no interaction, is zero. Output for the model which includes the interaction between the linear effect of age and work is shown in Table 26.4.

Exercise 26.4. Use the output in Table 26.4 to test for interaction between age as a quantitative variable and work.

Exercise 26.5. How many parameters would there be for the interaction term [Age]·Work if there were three categories of work?

For a variable which is very strongly related to the response, such as

Table 26.5.   Interaction between [Age] and Work

Parameter	Estimate	SD
Corner	−7.064	0.553
Age(1)	1.666	0.567
Age(2)	2.394	0.562
Age(3)	3.239	0.562
Age(4)	3.860	0.559
Sex(1)	−0.585	0.115
Work(1)	0.046	0.544
[Age]·Work(1)	−0.083	0.220

age in this example, it may be necessary to model the relationship with age more closely than by using a linear relationship. Even so, the linear part of any new relationship will be the main part and it is worth testing for interaction just with this linear part. For example, if a quadratic relationship with age is used, as in the model

$$\log(\text{Odds}) = \text{Corner} + [\text{Age}] + [\text{Agesq}] + \text{Sex} + \text{Work},$$

then the interaction of work with the linear effect of age is tested by including the term [Age]·Work in the model. It is also possible to test for the interaction of work with the linear effect of age when the effect of age is modelled by a categorical variable. This is done by comparing

$$\log(\text{Odds}) = \text{Corner} + \text{Age} + \text{Sex} + \text{Work}.$$

with

$$\log(\text{Odds}) = \text{Corner} + \text{Age} + \text{Sex} + \text{Work} + [\text{Age}] \cdot \text{Work}.$$

This is a more powerful way of testing for interaction than including the term Age·Work (which has four parameters), provided the relationship with age is predominantly linear. Table 26.5 shows the results of this analysis, with quantitative age coded 0 to 4. The deviance for this model is 7.51, which is only a little smaller than the deviance for the model without interaction. Thus there is no evidence that the work effect varies with age. The same conclusion is reached by comparing the estimate of the interaction parameter with its standard deviation. Since the estimate of the work effect in the model without interaction is also not significant, it seems clear that these data provide no evidence for a relationship between agricultural work and the prevalence of monoclonal gammapathy.

Table 26.6.   Model in terms of separate work parameters

Age	Work	$\log(\text{Odds}) = \text{Corner} + \cdots$
0	0	–
1	0	Age(1)
2	0	Age(2)
3	0	Age(3)
4	0	Age(4)
0	1	Wbyage(1)
1	1	Wbyage(2) + Age(1)
2	1	Wbyage(3) + Age(2)
3	1	Wbyage(4) + Age(3)
4	1	Wbyage(5) + Age(4)

⋆ 26.5   What to do when there is interaction

Interaction parameters are chosen specifically to test for interaction; their estimated values are of no use in themselves. When there is interaction it is necessary to reparametrize so that the new parameters provide a satisfactory summary of the data in this situation. Indicator variables are a useful way of doing this.

Suppose, for example, that in a study of work and age there was an interaction between them. The most sensible way of reporting the results would be to estimate the effect of work separately for each level of age, but few packages allow this as a standard option. One way of doing it is by separating the data into age groups and analyzing these separately. Another is to reparametrize so that instead of one work parameter and four work·age parameters, we use five work parameters, one for each age group. Writing these separate work parameters as Wbyage, short for work by age, the model is shown in Table 26.6.

The values taken by the indicator variables for the age parameters are the same as before. The indicator variable for Wbyage(1) takes the value 1 when work is at level 1 and age is at level 0, and 0 otherwise; the indicator for Wbyage(2) takes the value 1 when work is at level 1 and age is at level 1, and 0 otherwise; and so on. One advantage of using indicator variables is that it is then possible to include another variable in the model with the indicators. This model imposes the constraint that the indicator effects are the same within the levels of this extra variable and provides estimates of their common values. It would not be possible to do this if the data were subdivided on age because subdividing on age is equivalent to fitting interaction terms of all variables with age.

When there is interaction between two exposures it is commonly reported by creating a new categorical variable with a level for each combination of the levels of the two exposures. For two exposures, each on four

Table 26.7.   Rate parameters per 100 000 person-years

	A	
B	0	1
0	5.0	15.0
1	20.0	λ

levels, the new variable would have 16 levels, with level 0 corresponding to
level zero on both exposures and level 16 corresponding to level 3 on both
exposures. There are 15 parameters for this new variable, measuring the
ratio of the rate (or odds) for each one of the levels relative to the zero
level. These are entered in the model in place of the 6 parameters for the
two exposures and the 9 parameters for their interaction. The estimated
parameters would be displayed in a four by four table, with the levels of
one exposure determining the rows and the levels of the other determining
the columns.

26.6   Interaction is scale-dependent   ★

Interaction parameters are chosen to measure departures from a model.
When the effects of variables are measured as ratios interaction parameters are ratios, chosen to measure departures from a multiplicative model.
When the effects of variables are measured as differences (see Chapter 28)
interaction parameters are differences chosen to measure departures from
an additive model. Thus interaction depends on how the effects are measured. For example, consider two explanatory variables, A and B, each
with two levels. Values for three of the parameters involved are shown in
Table 26.7. For the moment the fourth parameter, λ, is left unspecified.
When effects are measured as ratios the effect of A when B is at level 0 is
$15/5 = 3$, and the effect of A when B is at level 1 is $\lambda/20$. The interaction
parameter is the ratio of these two effects which is $\lambda/60$. When effects are
measured as differences the effect of A when B is at level 0 is $15 - 5 = 10$,
and the effect of A when B is at level 1 is $\lambda - 20$. The interaction parameter is now the difference between these two effects, which is $\lambda - 30$. It
follows that if $\lambda = 60$ there is no departure from the multiplicative model
but there is a departure from the additive model. Similarly if $\lambda = 30$ there
is no departure from the additive model but there is a departure from the
multiplicative model.

The choice between measuring effects as ratios or differences is usually
an empirical one, with the investigator preferring to measure effects in such
a way as to minimize the interaction, but there are sometimes biological
grounds for preferring one method to the other.

Solutions to the exercises

26.1 The multiplicative effect of work is the ratio of the prevalence odds for non-agricultural workers to the prevalence odds for agricultural workers.

26.2 The degrees of freedom for the deviances are

$$
\begin{aligned}
20 - (1 + 4 + 1 + 1) &= 13 \\
20 - (1 + 4 + 1 + 1 + 4) &= 9 \\
20 - (1 + 4 + 1 + 1 + 1) &= 12
\end{aligned}
$$

The change of deviance with inclusion of the Work.Age interaction is 1.84 with 4 degrees of freedom, and for the Work.Sex interaction it is 0.41 with 1 degree of freedom. Neither is significant.

26.3 The change in log odds over the age range of 35 to 75 is approximately +4. The gradient is therefore approximately +1 per 10 year age band.

26.4 The Wald test for interaction between the linear effect of age and work is

$$
\left(\frac{0.053}{0.188} \right)^2 = 0.079,
$$

which is not significant.

26.5 There would be two parameters for this interaction term.

27
Choice and interpretation of models

Previous chapters have illustrated the use of regression models using simple bodies of data containing relatively few variables. More commonly, we are faced with large data files containing many variables. Sometimes derived variables such as Quetelet's weight-for-height index are included in the model in addition to or in place of the original variables. In such situations it can be difficult to know where to begin, and all too easy to lose one's way. This chapter offers some guidance towards the sensible use of regression methods.

27.1 Variable selection strategies

A lot has been written about the process of finding the 'best' regression model in problems involving many variables. Much of this activity has been concerned with the search for an optimal strategy, and the relative merits of different approaches have been hotly debated. Many computer programs implement one or more of these strategies in an automatic model selection option called *stepwise regression*. These programs usually work by a combination of the *step-up* strategy (examining the effect of inclusion of variables not yet in the model) and the *step-down* strategy (examining the effect of of removing variables currently in the model). With the recent increased speed and reduced cost of computers, some programs now offer an exhaustive search of *all subsets* from a list of possible explanatory variables.

In assessing the value of such procedures it is important to note that regression models have two very different uses in epidemiology. Historically they were first used to derive *risk scores* designed to classify subjects into graded categories with respect to risk of developing disease. Later, when attention turned to interpretation of the parameter estimates and the close relationship between regression and stratification methods became apparent, regression models became important tools for analyses whose aim was the advancement of scientific knowledge. For convenience we refer to these two uses as *prediction* and *explanation*, respectively.

When the aim is prediction, the best model is the one which best predicts the fate of a future subject. This is a well defined task and automatic strategies to find the model which is best in this sense are potentially useful. However, when used for explanation the best model will depend on the scientific questions being asked, and automatic selection strategies have no place.

An important tool for assessing how well a model predicts the fate of a future subject is *cross-validation* — a technique in which each subject in turn is removed from the dataset and the actual outcome for that subject is compared with the predicted outcome using the model based on the remaining observations. The deviance for a model will always decrease with the introduction of more parameters, but prediction of future observations is not always improved. There comes a point at which increasing the complexity of the model to gain a slightly better fit to the observed data will reduce the accuracy of its predictions. Cross-validation measures the predictive properties of the model directly and therefore reflects the adverse consequences of fitting too many parameters.

Cross-validation is potentially expensive in computer time, but simple approximate criteria have been developed which allow the assessment of whether any step up or down in an automatic model selection procedure would be expected to improve prediction. The best known is *Akaike's information criterion*, namely

(Reduction in deviance) $- 2 \times$ (Increase in number of parameters).

If this is positive the increased complexity would be expected to improve prediction and if negative, to degrade prediction.

27.2   Explanatory variables and natural experiments

This book has been entirely concerned with the use of models whose aim is explanation. In such analyses there is a clear distinction between the roles of exposures and confounders but this distinction is lost when using regression models — both become explanatory variables. Ignoring the distinctions between different types of explanatory variable is appropriate when using regression models for prediction, since all variables have the same role, but in a scientific analysis of data different explanatory variables may play quite different roles.

The distinction between exposure and confounder, as described in this book, relies heavily on the idea of experiments of nature. An exposure is something which we can intervene to change while a confounder is a variable which we would have held constant had we designed the experiment rather than leaving it to nature. It is helpful to think of regression analysis as simulating an experiment, in the same way. For example, the effects of A in the model

$$\log(\text{Rate}) = \text{Corner} + A + B + C$$

are the effects of changing the level of A in a simulated experiment in which B and C are held constant. Similarly, the effects of B are the effects of changing the level of B in a simulated experiment in which the levels of A and C are held constant. Thus regression analysis does not simulate a single experiment but many. This flexibility of the regression approach is undoubtedly useful, but in practice it can also become its most serious weakness. To extend our analogy, the data analyst is in a position like that of an experimental scientist who has the capability to plan and carry out many experiments within a single day. Not surprisingly a cool head is required! Before embarking on a regression analysis it is essential to spend an hour or so, preferably away from the computer, to list the main scientific questions and to think how these can be answered by fitting a series of models. Analyses which follow such thought are always simpler and more incisive than those which are born of uncritical use of the computer or worse, of a stepwise regression program.

It will rarely be necessary to include a large number of variables in the analysis, because only a few exposures are of genuine scientific interest in any one study, and there are usually very few variables of sufficient *a priori* importance for their potential confounding effect to be controlled for. Most scientists are aware of the dangers of analyses which search a long list of potentially relevant exposures. These are known as *data dredging* or *blind fishing* and carry a considerable danger of false positive findings. Such analyses are as likely to impede scientific progress as to advance it. There are similar dangers if a long list of potential confounders is searched, either with a view to explaining the observed relationship between disease and exposure or to enhancing it — findings will inevitably be biased. Confounders should be chosen *a priori* and not on the basis of statistical significance. In particular, variables which have been used in the design, such as matching variables, must be included in the analysis.

Recently there has been some dispute between 'modellers', who support the use of regression models, and 'stratifiers' who argue for a return to the methods described in Part I of this book. Logically this dispute is based on a false distinction — there is no real difference between the methods. In practice the difference lies in the inflexibility of the older methods which thereby imposes a certain discipline on the analyst. Firstly, since stratification methods treat exposures and confounders differently, any change in the role of a variable requires a new set of computations. This forces us to keep in touch with the underlying scientific questions. Secondly, since strata must be defined by cross classification, relatively few confounders can be dealt with and we are forced to control only for confounders of *a priori* importance. These restraints can be helpful in keeping a data analysis on the right tracks but once the need for such discipline is recognized, there are significant advantages to the regression modelling approach.

EXAMPLE: DIETARY FAT AND TOTAL ENERGY INTAKE

The analogy between regression models and imaginary experiments is very useful in making decisions about whether to include a variable in a regression model or not. An interesting illustration arises in nutritional epidemiology when considering the relationship between total energy intake and the incidence of coronary heart disease. This relationship was first detected because relationships were observed between intake and disease risk for a large number of nutrients — the more that was eaten, the lower the risk. A relationship with total energy intake, possibly reflecting energy expenditure, was considered the most likely explanation.

However, once this relationship is recognized, how should the relationship between risk and other aspects of the diet, notably fat intake, be analysed? One way is to measure *nutrient density*, which is the ratio of daily intake of fat to the total energy intake. This approach is open to the criticism that such nutrient densities are not usually independent of total energy intake — subjects with high energy intakes typically have a different pattern of nutrient densities from subjects with low energy intakes.

If energy intake is to be regarded as a confounder, then it should be controlled for, either by stratification or with a regression model. In the latter case we fit a model such as

$$\log(\text{Rate}) = \text{Corner} + \text{Fat} + \text{Energy}$$

and interpret the parameters representing the effect of fat in terms of an experiment in which fat intake is varied but the total energy content of the diet is held constant. Of course, such an experiment would require other constituents of the diet such as carbohydrate to vary in order to maintain the total energy intake and this must be born in mind when interpreting parameters.

Exercise 27.1. How would you interpret the effect of fat in the model

$$\log(\text{Rate}) = \text{Corner} + \text{Fat} + \text{Carbohydrate} + \text{Energy}?$$

Other authors have approached the problem of allowing for total energy expenditure by dividing total calories between calories from fat and calories from other sources, and fitting the model

$$\log(\text{Rate}) = \text{Corner} + \text{Fat-calories} + \text{Other-calories}.$$

The parameters representing the effect of fat intake must now be interpreted in terms of an experiment in which fat intake is varied while intake of other calories is held constant. In this experiment a reduction of fat intake would result in a reduction of total energy intake. Such an experiment would be difficult to interpret, even if it could be carried out.

Finally we should point out that a real public health intervention to reduce dietary fat intakes would be unlikely to mimic either of the above imaginary experiments. When dietary fat intake is reduced in free–living subjects, some of the energy intake is made up from other sources, but typically there is a net reduction in energy intake. This demonstrates that the use of models to predict the effect of intervention usually requires considerable extra knowledge. In particular, we need to have some understanding of the mechanism by which change will be effected.

27.3 Endogenous and exogenous explanatory variables

The 'effects' of an explanatory variable are defined in terms of differences in log rate (or log odds) between groups of subjects with different levels of the variable. Thus the effect of cigarette smoking is defined by contrasting rates in smokers and non-smokers, and the effect of serum cholesterol concentration (classified as high or low) is defined as the difference in log rate between subjects with high cholestrol concentration and subjects with low cholesterol concentration. This language encourages people to interpret 'effects' as the change in rates to be expected as a result of intervention to change the level, but this is a big step. How are the subjects to alter their level? For a variable like serum cholesterol there is no direct way to alter its level and any intervention would have to be indirect, for example by change of diet or by cholesterol lowering drugs. However, there is no guarantee that such mechanisms will bear any relationship to the mechanism which led the the study subjects to have different levels in the first place. The effect of indirectly changing the levels of serum cholesterol in a group of subjects may be completely different from that estimated by comparing groups of subjects who just happen to have different levels of cholesterol.

The same problem arises in an even more acute form when studying the effects of two or more interrelated variables, such as blood pressure and obesity in relation to the incidence of coronary disease. The effect of blood pressure controlled for obesity might now be interpreted as the expected effect of changing blood pressure while keeping obesity constant. However, is it be possible to intervene to change blood pressure while keeping obesity constant? While this could be achieved, for example by using drug treatment, this method of intervention would bear little relation to the mechanism that led subjects to their current levels in the first place, and it might have different effects. Intervention aimed at life style changes are more likely to duplicate these conditions, but might be expected to change both blood pressure and obesity simultaneously. In this case the estimated effects of blood pressure controlled for obesity, or obesity controlled for blood pressure could be poor predictors of the effect of the intervention.

The position is much clearer when considering environmental exposures, such as radiation dose, occupational exposure to toxic chemicals, and even cigarette smoking. In such cases, it is entirely reasonable to imagine an experiment in which exposure of groups is directly varied without any consequent change in other variables, and the parameters of regression models are easier to interpret.

Variables such as cholesterol concentration, blood pressure, and obesity are called *endogenous*. The word endogenous means 'growing from within'. Variables such as smoking, diet and occupation are called *exogenous*. The distinction between endogenous and exogenous variables is borrowed from the behavioural sciences and, although the distinction is not hard and fast, is useful in drawing attention to the different assumptions which it is necessary to make for the two kinds of variable when interpreting the parameters of regression models as expected effects following intervention.

27.4   Interpretation of interaction

An underlying theme of this chapter is that while distinctions between different types of explanatory variable are not relevant to the mechanical process of estimating the parameters of a regression model, they are essential to the strategy adopted in the analysis and to the interpretation of results. This is particularly true when dealing with interaction. The word describes a purely mathematical concept in regression models. Its relationship to the scientific language of epidemiology requires further consideration of the nature of the variables involved.

We shall first consider interaction between two confounders. There seems to be no word to describe this in epidemiology, almost certainly because the phenomenon is of no scientific interest. Whether we include such terms in a model or not is a purely technical matter of trading the number of parameters against freedom from assumptions. Usually if there are two strong confounders such as age and sex, the gain in efficiency from assuming no interaction between them is extremely modest and it will usually be safer to include an interaction term regardless of its significance. However, if we are worried about the aggregate effect of five or six weak confounders, then omission of interaction terms is unlikely to have a major effect on estimates of parameters of interest.

Interaction between a confounder and an exposure of interest is known in epidemiology as *effect modification* and is clearly of considerable scientific importance, since the *consistency* of an effect in diverse study groups would usually be considered relevant to labelling a relationship as 'causal', in the sense of predicting the effect of future interventions. The ease with which we can test for such interaction in the framework of regression models represents a clear advance over earlier stratification methods in which the absence of such interaction is a hidden assumption.

Finally, the question of interaction between two exposures of interest is usually of considerable importance, both for the scientific interpretation of

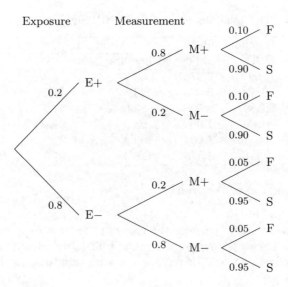

Fig. 27.1.   Misclassification of exposure.

an analysis and for its implications for preventive intervention. We shall deal with this in more detail in Chapter 28.

27.5   Errors of measurement of explanatory variables

In the models discussed in this book it is assumed that explanatory variables are correctly measured. This assumption is often unjustified in practice, but epidemiologists have generally been prepared to ignore measurement errors. Some have believed that to do so is justifiable providing there is no relationship between errors of measurement of exposure and disease outcome, that is if there is no *differential misclassification*. This is now known to be false.

To illustrate the effect of ignoring measurement error we consider the hypothetical situation illustrated in Fig. 27.1, in which exposure E is measured imperfectly by measurement M. As a result of this misclassification there is a probability of 0.2 that an exposed subject is misclassified as unexposed, and a probability of 0.2 that an unexposed subject is misclassified as exposed. The probability of failure depends only on true exposure, taking the value 0.1 for exposed subjects and 0.05 for unexposed subjects. An epidemiological study observes only the marginal relationship between measured exposure and failure.

Exercise 27.2. Calculate probabilities for each of the eight tips of the tree in Fig. 27.1. By collapsing over exposure categories, calculate the probabilities for each of the four possible combination of measured exposure and disease (failure) status. Hence derive the probability tree expressing the probability of failure

Table 27.1.   Diastolic blood pressure (DBP) and rate ratios for stroke

Baseline DBP	Rate ratio	Mean DBP	
		at baseline	after 2 years
≤ 69	0.276	63.6	72.7
70–79	0.395	73.8	77.0
80–89	0.595	83.6	83.0
90–99	1.000	93.5	91.2
100–109	1.904	103.4	99.2
≥ 110	3.875	116.4	107.3

conditional upon measured exposure.

It is clear from this exercise that the effect of exposure is decreased by the measurement error: whereas the risk ratio for true exposure is 2, the risk ratio for measured exposure is only 1.42. It is worth noting that 20% misclassification would be regarded as acceptable in many branches of epidemiology.

Similar considerations apply when exposure takes on more than two levels. The observed dose-response relationship between measured exposure and disease outcome is less steep than the underlying relationship with true exposure, under any realistic assumptions about the dose-response relationship. This is illustrated by the data of Table 27.1 which concern the relationship between diastolic blood pressure and subsequent incidence of stroke.* These data are taken from a re-analysis of seven cohort studies, and the first two columns of the table summarize the relationship between diastolic blood pressure at a single initial visit (the 'baseline' measurement) and subsequent incidence. Note that in the rate ratios the fourth category is taken as reference. These were obtained by fitting the model

$$\log(\text{Rate}) = \text{Corner} + \text{Study} + \text{DBP}$$

where study is a categorical variable with one level for each study, so that confounding of the relationship due to differences between the study cohorts is eliminated. The third column shows the mean of the baseline diastolic pressures for each of the five categories. The log rate ratios are plotted against the mean baseline values in Fig. 27.2 (solid line). This line represents the apparent dose-response relationship between a single measurement of diastolic blood pressure and the incidence of stroke. It is approximately log-linear, so that essentially the same relationship would have been obtained by fitting the model

$$\log(\text{Rate}) = \text{Corner} + \text{Study} + [\text{DBP}],$$

---

*From Macmahon, S. *et al.* (1990), *The Lancet*, **335**, 765–774.

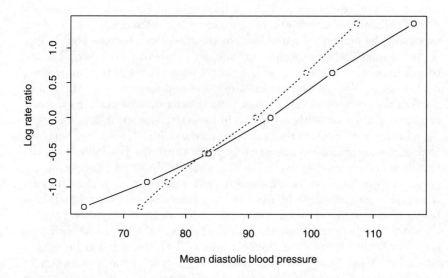

Fig. 27.2. Apparent and true dose-response relationships.

where [DBP] is measured per mm Hg. However, this line is a poor representation of the true relationship between blood pressure and the incidence of stroke. Blood pressure is subject to both short-term fluctuations and to measurement errors, neither of which will be reflected in the risk of stroke which is determined by the longer-term average level of blood pressure. The final column of Table 27.1 shows the mean blood pressure taken two years later in representative samples taken from each of the five groups. These figures provide a better estimate of long-term average blood pressure in the six groups as the short-term fluctuations and measurement errors are washed out. Plotting the rate ratios for stroke against these new values for mean diastolic blood pressure provides a truer estimate of the relationship between stroke incidence and the long- term average level of diastolic pressure. This plot is shown in Fig. 27.2 as a broken line and clearly represents a stronger relationship than the apparent relationship based on a single baseline measurement. This finding is true in general. When an explanatory variable suffers from measurement error or within subject variability the linear effects of this variable will be closer to zero than when there is no error or variability. This is known as *regression dilution*

This second example demonstrates both the attenuation of relationships owing to exposure measurement error and one of the methods which has been suggested for correcting for it. An alternative approach is to formally adopt probability models such as that illustrated in Fig. 27.1 and to estimate the conditional probabilities for every branch of the tree. Validation substudies are required in order to estimate the misclassification probabilities. A difficulty with this approach is that when there are several levels of exposure, the number of parameters in the model can become very large.

In summary, when exposures are subject to measurement error, the apparent exposure effects will be less pronounced than the true underlying relationships. When confounders are measured inaccurately, the consequences are even more serious. Since the relationship between disease and confounder is not correctly estimated in these circumstances, it follows that the analysis will not properly control for confounding. If both exposure and confounder are measured inaccurately, there exists the possibility that the two sets of errors may be interrelated, so that the apparent relationship between exposure and confounder may be quite different from that between the underlying variables. In these circumstances models for relationships between measured exposure, measured confounder, and response have no interpretation in terms of an imaginary experimental intervention and may be scientifically meaningless. Such might well be the position in our example involving dietary fat and total energy intake. Measured intakes of total energy and of each specific nutrient are usually derived from the same dietary records, taken over a period of several days. Not only are such measurements very imperfect measures of long-term intake, but it is reasonable to believe that errors in the measured fat intake will be closely related to errors in measured energy intake, since the former is an important contributor to the latter. Regression models which include total energy as well specific nutrients may, therefore, not be interpretable in practice.

Solutions to the exercises

27.1 The parameter(s) measure the effect of changes in fat intake while holding both total energy intake and carbohydrate intake constant. To reduce fat intake while holding both total energy and carbohydrate intake constant would be very difficult for an individual to do and would require large changes in other components of the total energy intake, such as protein.

27.2 From top to bottom the probabilities are 0.016, 0.144, 0.004, 0.036, 0.008, 0.152, 0.032, and 0.608. The remaining calculations are shown in Fig. 27.3. The probability of failure conditional upon having been measured as exposed is 0.075, while the failure probability conditional upon having been measured as unexposed is 0.053.

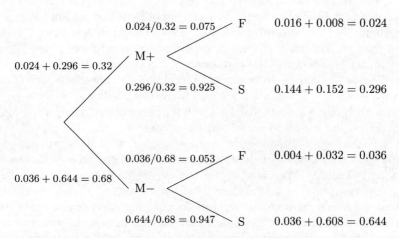

Fig. 27.3. Failure probabilities conditional upon measured exposure.

28
$\boxed{\star}$ Additivity and synergism

When discussing the way two exposures combine to influence the risk of disease the word interaction is used to refer to departures from either multiplicative or additive models. In general these models have no biological basis and interaction is therefore a purely statistical concept. The interaction parameters are chosen solely to test hypotheses and are not useful for describing the data when there is interaction. The word *synergism* is often used, in a similar sense, to refer to departures from a biological model for the independent action of two exposures. When the joint effect of two exposures is greater than would be expected from the separate effects, according to such a model, the exposures are said to display positive synergism. Synergism is therefore a particular kind of interaction but precisely what kind depends on the biological model for independent action.

Epidemiologists often use the word synergism without specifying precisely what they mean by independent action. In other words they use it in a statistical sense. When used in this way synergism is generally measured as a departure from an additive model. This suggests an ill-defined biological model which predicts that the rate for the joint effect of two exposures is the sum of the rates for the separate effects. An example of such a model is shown in Fig. 28.1 which refers to a situation where disease is caused by one or other of two *precipitating* events. Exposure A influences the chance of the first event occurring, while exposure B influences the chance of the second event occurring. When A and B act independently their effects on the rate will be additive because

$$\text{Rate(Event 1 } or \text{ 2)} = \text{Rate(Event 1)} + \text{Rate(Event 2)}.$$

In cases like this it makes sense to fit an additive model so that departures from this model can be measured and used to test whether the two exposures act independently. In this chapter we consider some of the special problems which arise when using additive regression models.

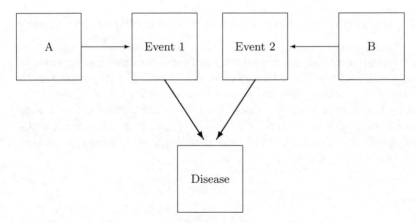

Fig. 28.1.   Two precipitating events for disease.

28.1   Fitting additive models

With additive models effects are measured as differences between rates (or odds) parameters rather than as ratios. The use of stratification to control the additive effects of an exposure for confounding would be based on the assumption that the difference between the rate parameters for the different levels of exposure is constant over the strata. Formulating the same problem in terms of regression models the effects of an exposure controlled for a confounder are found by fitting the additive model for the rate,

$$\text{Rate} = \text{Corner} + \text{Exposure} + \text{Confounder}.$$

The assumption that the additive effect of the exposure is the same for all strata formed by the confounder is expressed by the fact that the model is additive, with no interaction terms.

Additive models are fitted to data by choosing parameters to maximize the log likelihood in the same way as for multiplicative models, but the calculations are different and require different computer programs. Similarly log likelihood ratios are used to test hypotheses in the same way as for multiplicative models. In practice additive models can be more troublesome to fit than multiplicative models because the most likely parameter values do not *necessarily* predict rates which are greater than zero. It is then rather difficult to know what to do. Should one treat this as evidence that the additive model is a poor fit, or should one find most likely values subject to the constraint that they predict positive rates? Generally the latter policy is followed, but it can be difficult to implement.*

---

*This problem does not arise with multiplicative models because these are fitted as additive models for the log rate and the log rate is not constrained to be positive.

28.2   Discriminating between additive and multiplicative models

When there are rival biological grounds for choosing an additive model and a multiplicative model the investigator will wish to discriminate between the two models by seeing which fits the data best. The deviances for the two models provide an informal way of looking at this but they cannot be compared in a formal test because the additive and multiplicative models are not nested. The solution to this technical problem is to find an *extended model* which contains both additive and multiplicative models as special cases. One such model is

$$\frac{(\text{Rate})^{\rho} - 1}{\rho} = \text{Corner} + \text{A} + \text{B},$$

where ρ is a parameter yet to be determined. In this model A and B refer to parameters which measure differences in the value of

$$\frac{(\text{Rate})^{\rho} - 1}{\rho}.$$

As ρ approaches 1 the model reduces to

$$\text{Rate} - 1.0 = \text{Corner} + \text{A} + \text{B}$$

in which the A and B parameters measure differences in the rate. As ρ approaches zero, the left-hand side of the model approaches the log of the rate [†] , so the model reduces to

$$\log(\text{Rate}) = \text{Corner} + \text{A} + \text{B},$$

in which the A and B parameters measure differences in the log rate. The two extremes of the extended model therefore correspond to an additive model ($\rho = 0$) and a multiplicative model ($\rho = 1$). When this extended model is fitted for a range of values for ρ, including $\rho = 1$ and $\rho = 0$, a comparison of the log likelihoods for the different values of ρ will indicate which is the most likely value for ρ and whether the additive or multiplicative model is preferred. It may turn out, of course, that both models provide an adequate fit, or that neither model is acceptable. We do not advocate the use of the model with values of ρ other than zero or one, because effect parameters measured as differences in the value of

$$\frac{(\text{Rate})^{\rho} - 1}{\rho}$$

[†]This follows because, for small ρ,

$$R^{\rho} = [\exp(\log(R))]^{\rho} = \exp[\rho \log(R)] \approx 1 + \rho \log(R).$$

would be hard to interpret. The sole purpose of the extended model is to provide a framework in which to choose between additive and multiplicative models.

Using the extended model to discriminate between multiplicative and additive models involves fitting a non-standard regression model for each of a range of values of ρ. Even with software which allows non-standard models this can be quite a lot of work.

28.3   Additive models with case-control studies

There are some special problems which arise when trying to fit additive models to data from case-control studies. To illustrate these we shall consider a case-control study of the joint effect of two exposures A and B in which the ratio of sampling probabilities is

$$K = \frac{\text{Probability of selecting a failure as a case}}{\text{Probability of selecting a survivor as a control}}.$$

We showed in Chapter 23 that parameters which are defined as ratios of the odds of being a case are also ratios of the corresponding odds of failure in the study base. Unfortunately this does not apply to additive models. Parameters which are defined as differences in the odds of being a case are K times the corresponding differences in the odds of being a failure in the study base. The factor K, which relates the odds of being a case to the odds of faliure, cancels in ratios but not in differences. It follows that fitting an additive model to case-control data tells us nothing about the additive effects on the odds of failure in the study base except in those rare cases where the value of K is known. It is still possible, of course, to test hypotheses about zero parameter values since a zero additive effect on the odds of being a case corresponds to a zero additive effect on the odds of being a failure in the study base.

Although it is not possible to estimate the additive effects of A and B on the odds of failure in the study base it is still possible to estimate the ratio of these effects to the corner. This is less satisfactory than estimating differences in the odds themselves, but better than nothing. These new parameters are estimated by fitting the model

$$\text{Odds} = \text{Corner} \times (1.0 + A + B).$$

When the model is written in this way the corner parameter is still the odds of being a case when A and B are at level zero, but the A and B parameters are now differences in the ratio

$$\frac{\text{Odds}}{\text{Corner}}.$$

Table 28.1. Estrogen replacement, weight, and endometrial cancer

Weight (kg)	No		Yes	
	Cases	Controls	Cases	Controls
< 57	12	183	20	61
57–75	45	378	37	113
> 75	42	140	9	23

This model can be fitted to data using likelihood in the same sort of way as for conventional models but special software is required.

Exercise 28.1. Table 28.1 shows results of a case-control study relating endometrial cancer incidence to use of estrogen therapy and body weight. Calculate odds ratios for each category of weight and estrogen use relative to the corner (top left corner cell). Obtain differences in these odds ratios for estrogen replacement yes compared to estrogen replacement no, at each level of weight. Do the data appear consistent with an additive model?

When a case-control study is stratified by age at time of diagnosis, and controls are sampled separately in each age stratum, there will be a different value of K for each stratum. To make sure the A and B parameters do not depend on these K's the parameters must now be defined as differences in the value of

$$\frac{\text{Odds}}{\text{Age specific corner}},$$

where the age specific corners are the odds in each age stratum when A and B are both at level 0. The A and B parameters will then equal the corresponding differences in the ratio of the odds of failure to the age specific corners in the study base.

Assuming that the new A and B parameters are constant over age strata, their common value can be estimated by fitting the model

$$\text{Odds} = \text{Corner} \times \text{Age} \times (1.0 + A + B).$$

where age is a categorical variable with one level for each age stratum. The $\boxed{\text{Corner} \times \text{Age}}$ part of the model corresponds to fitting separate corner parameters for each age stratum. This model again requires special software.

28.4 Discriminating between models using case-control studies

The extended model containing the extra parameter ρ can also be used to compare the fit of a multiplicative model with an additive model using data from a case-control study. The two models we wish to compare are

$$\text{Odds} = \text{Corner} \times A \times B,$$

in which A and B parameters are ratios of odds, and

$$\text{Odds} = \text{Corner} \times (1.0 + A + B),$$

in which the A and B parameters are differences in the ratios of odds to the corner. The multiplicative model can also be written in the form

$$\log(\text{Odds}) = \text{Corner} + A + B,$$

in which the A and B parameters are defined as differences in log odds. The extended model is now

$$\frac{(\text{Odds}/\text{Corner})^\rho - 1.0}{\rho} = A + B.$$

As ρ approaches 0 this model approaches

$$\log(\text{Odds}/\text{Corner}) = A + B,$$

which simplifies to

$$\log(\text{Odds}) = \log(\text{Corner}) + A + B.$$

This is the multiplicative model written in log form, apart from the fact that because the corner parameter is on the original scale in the extended model it appears as log(Corner). As ρ approaches 1, the extended model approaches

$$\text{Odds} = \text{Corner} \times (1.0 + A + B),$$

which is the additive model.

The procedure for comparing the fit of a multiplicative and an additive model is illustrated by fitting the extended model to the data in Table 28.1 for a range of values of ρ. To actually do this involved fitting a non-standard model for each of these values. The resulting log likelihood ratios are shown in Fig. 28.2. At $\rho = 0$ the log likelihood ratio is -2.774 and at $\rho = 1$ it is -0.408. To test for the adequacy of the multiplicative model we take $\rho = 0$ as the null value. Minus twice the log likelihood ratio for $\rho = 0$ is 5.548 ($p \approx 0.02$), so the data do not support this model. To test for the adequacy of the additive model we take $\rho = 1$ for the null value. Minus twice the log likelihood ratio for $\rho = 1$ is 0.816 ($p > 0.10$) so the data are consistent with the additive model.

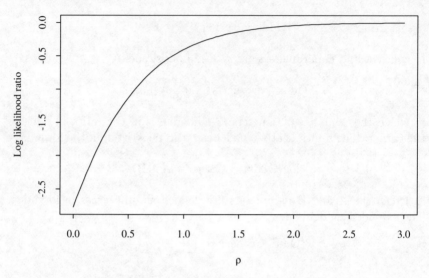

Fig. 28.2.   The log likelihood ratio for ρ.

The most frequent outcome when comparing the fit of multiplicative and additive models is that both provide an acceptable description of the data. This has been taken by some epidemiologists as a serious flaw in the modern modelling approach to statistical analysis, since additive and multiplicative models have radically different public health implications (notably in relation to the targeting of interventions). This difficulty is indeed serious, but it is attributable more to an attempt to extrapolate beyond the data than to any shortcomings in statistical methodology.

A good example of this arises in attempts to study the implication of different dose-response relationships for the carcinogenic effect of ionizing radiation. The public health problem (if there is one) is one of relatively large populations exposed to low doses, but the available epidemiological studies have concentrated upon high exposure groups — A-bomb survivors, irradiated patient groups and so on. Additive and multiplicative dose-response models make similar predictions at high doses so these studies are poorly discriminated. However, they make very different predictions for subjects receiving low dose exposure. If data were available for subjects receiving low dose exposure the two models would be easily discriminated; the problem lies in trying to discriminate between them using data from a range of dose levels for which the two models make the same predictions.

Exercise 28.2. We plan to reduce the total burden of disease in a community by attempting to eliminate exposure A but another explanatory variable, B, is also known to be important. Should the intervention be targeted on individuals whose exposure to B is greatest? Consider how the answer to this question depends on whether the effects of A and B on the rate are additive or multiplicative.

Solutions to the exercises

28.1 The odds ratios are shown below.

Weight	Estrogen replacement		
(kg)	No	Yes	Difference
< 57	1.00	5.00	4.00
57–75	1.82	4.99	3.17
> 75	4.58	5.97	1.39

The additive model does not appear to fit particularly well as the differences between the odds ratios for the two estrogen groups seems to fall with increasing weight. Further examination of the table suggests the possibility that there is only a relationship with weight when there is no estrogen replacement.

28.2 Consider a population classified according to the two factors A and B. When these act additively or multiplicatively, the rates follow one of the following patterns:

	Additive model			Multiplicative model		
	A		Potential	A		Potential
B	No	Yes	reduction	No	Yes	reduction
No	1	3	2	1	3	2
Yes	3	5	2	3	9	6

When the multiplicative model holds the reduction in rates by eliminating exposure A is greater in the B-Yes group than in the B-No group. It would therefore be cost effective to target intervention at the high- risk section of the population. When the additive model holds this is no longer the case — there is an equal potential reduction in both sections of the population, and targeted intervention makes little sense.

29
Conditional logistic regression

In an individually matched case-control study, it is necessary to introduce a new parameter for every case-control set, if the matching is to be preserved in the analysis. This means that the number of parameters in the model exceeds the number of cases and in this case the profile likelihood does not lead to sensible estimates. Instead the nuisance parameters must be eliminated using a conditional likelihood. In Chapter 19 we indicated how this is done for a simple binary exposure. In this chapter we show how to use a conditional likelihood with the logistic regression model.

29.1 The logistic model

Suppose we wish to fit a logistic regression model which contains parameters for the case-control sets in addition to parameters for the effects of two explanatory variables A and B. Using a categorical variable to define the set to which each subject belongs, the model would be written

$$\log(\text{Odds}) = \text{Corner} + \text{Set} + \text{A} + \text{B}.$$

The model can also be written in the multiplicative form as

$$\text{Odds} = \text{Corner} \times \text{Set} \times \text{A} \times \text{B}.$$

For the case where A has three levels and B has two levels, the parameters in this model are Corner, A(1), A(2), B(1), together with

$$\text{Set}(1), \ \text{Set}(2), \ \cdots, \ \text{Set}(N-1)$$

where N is the number of case-control sets. These set parameters are those used in standard logistic regression models, but they are no longer the most convenient choice. It is now more convenient to choose a separate corner for each set, namely the odds parameter for each set when A and B are at level 0. The corner for the first case-control set is the corner parameter referred to above, the corner for the second case-control set is

$$\text{Corner} \times \text{Set}(1),$$

and so on. This corresponds to splitting the terms in the model into two groups, as follows:

$$\text{Odds} = \boxed{\text{Corner} \times \text{Set}} \times \boxed{\text{A} \times \text{B}}.$$

The first part of the model contains the separate corners, and these are the nuisance parameters to be eliminated, while the second part contains the effects of interest. When a conditional logistic program is used to fit this model the nuisance parameters are eliminated using conditional likelihood and estimates of the effects of A and B are reported. No estimates of either the corner or the set parameters are obtained in this method, so none can be reported.

To see how the nuisance parameters are eliminated using conditional likelihood it is convenient to return to the algebraic notation for parameters using Greek letters. For any particular case-control set let the corner parameter be ω_C. Let the odds for any subject in the set be ω_i, where $i = 1, 2, \ldots$, indexes the subjects within the case-control set, and write

$$\omega_i = \omega_C \theta_i,$$

so that θ_i is the ratio of the odds for subject i to the corner odds. The way θ is related to the effects of A and B is determined by the $\boxed{\text{A} \times \text{B}}$ part of the model. The corner parameter refers to subjects within the set with both A and B at level 0, so that the value of θ for such subjects is 1. For subjects with A at level 1 and B at level 0,

$$\theta = \text{A}(1),$$

for subjects with A at level 1 and B at level 1,

$$\theta = \text{A}(1) \times \text{B}(1),$$

and so on.

To be specific about which case-control set is being referred to, the parameters should be written with superscripts t, as in

$$\omega_i^t = \omega_C^t \theta_i^t.$$

where $t = 0, 1, 2, \ldots$ refers to the levels of the variable defining set membership. The parameters ω_C^t correspond to the

$$\boxed{\text{Corner} \times \text{Set}}$$

part of the model, and are the nuisance parameters to be eliminated. In the rest of this chapter we shall derive the contribution to the conditional

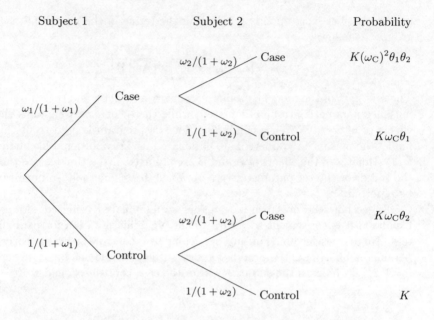

Fig. 29.1. Disease status for two subjects in a case-control study.

log likelihood for a single case-control set, and shall therefore omit the t superscript. The total log likelihood is found by adding the contributions from the single sets.

29.2   The conditional likelihood for 1:1 matched sets

First we derive the contribution for case-control studies with one case and one control in each set. The possible case or control status for any two subjects are represented as a probability tree in Fig. 29.1. Using the relationship between odds and probability, the probabilities that subject 1 is a case or a control are $\omega_1/(1+\omega_1)$ and $1/(1+\omega_1)$ respectively. Similarly, the probabilities for subject 2 are $\omega_2/(1+\omega_2)$ and $1/(1+\omega_2)$. The probabilities of the outcomes for the pair of subjects are obtained by multiplying along branches of the tree in the usual way. The last column of the figure shows such probabilities, after writing

$$\omega_1 = \omega_C\theta_1, \qquad \omega_2 = \omega_C\theta_2,$$

and

$$K = \frac{1}{1+\omega_1} \times \frac{1}{1+\omega_2}.$$

These probabilities refer to any two subjects from the study base. Conditional on the fact that one of the subjects is a case and the other is a control, the probability that subject 1 is the case is

$$\frac{K\omega_C\theta_1}{K\omega_C\theta_1 + K\omega_C\theta_2} = \frac{\theta_1}{\theta_1 + \theta_2}.$$

and the probability that subject 2 is the case is

$$\theta_2/(\theta_1 + \theta_2).$$

The contribution to the log likelihood of the case-control set is, therefore

$$\log\left(\frac{\theta_{(\text{for case})}}{\theta_{(\text{for case})} + \theta_{(\text{for control})}}\right).$$

This way of writing the log likelihood makes it clear that it does not depend on the arbitrary numbering of the subjects in the pair but only on the expressions for θ in terms of A(1), A(2) and B(1), the parameters to be estimated. The total log likelihood thus depends only on A(1), A(2), and B(1), and the nuisance parameters ω_C^t have been eliminated.

Exercise 29.1. Table 29.1 shows the data for the first two case-control sets in a 1:1 matched study. The set variable indicates which set each subject belongs to, and case or control status is indicated using a variable taking the value 1 for cases and 0 for controls. Illustrative parameter values for the multiplicative effects of the explanatory variables age and exposure, where age has three levels ($< 55, 55 - 64, 65 - 74$) and exposure has two levels, are shown below.

Parameter	Value
Age (1)	×1.5
Age (2)	×3.0
Exposure (1)	×5.0

The corner is defined as unexposed and age < 55. Calculate the values of θ predicted by the model for these four subjects. Calculate the log likelihood contributions for the two sets.

Before leaving the 1:1 case we shall verify that the method of obtaining the log likelihood described above gives the same answer as the method described in Chapter 19, for a binary exposure. The model is now

$$\text{Odds} = \boxed{\text{Corner} \times \text{Set}} \times \boxed{\text{Exposure}}$$

which has only one parameter, Exposure(1), apart from the nuisance parameters. This parameter is the multiplicative effect of exposure and we shall refer to it as ϕ. The values of θ for the case and control are determined

Table 29.1.   Data file for a 1:1 matched case-control study

Subject	Set	Case/control	Age	Exposure
1	1	1	48	1
2	1	0	64	0
3	2	1	52	1
4	2	0	70	1
...				

Table 29.2.   Likelihood contributions for the 1:1 matched study

Exposure	θ for case	θ for control	Likelihood
Neither	1	1	$1/(1+1) = 1/2$
Both	ϕ	ϕ	$\phi/(\phi+\phi) = 1/2$
Case only	ϕ	1	$\phi/(\phi+1)$
Control only	1	ϕ	$1/(1+\phi)$

by whether or not they were exposed. For example, if the case was not exposed then $\theta = 1$, while if the case was exposed then $\theta = \phi$. Similarly for the control. Table 29.2 sets out the four possible outcomes for each case-control set and the corresponding contributions to the log likelihood. The first two outcomes, in which the exposure status of case and control is the same, lead to log likelihood contributions which do not depend upon the parameter, and can be ignored. If N_1 and N_2 are the frequency of occurrence of the remaining outcomes, the total log likelihood is

$$N_1 \log \left(\frac{\phi}{1+\phi} \right) + N_2 \log \left(\frac{1}{1+\phi} \right)$$

which is the same as we obtained in Chapter 19, except that here we have called the effect ϕ rather than θ to avoid confusion.

29.3   The conditional likelihood for 1: m matched sets

We now extend the above argument to sets with one case and m controls. If the sampling had not been carried out deliberately so as to obtain a single case and m controls in the set, the probability that subject 1 is a case and the remaining m subjects are controls would be

$$\frac{\omega_1}{1+\omega_1} \times \frac{1}{1+\omega_2} \times \frac{1}{1+\omega_3} \times \cdots,$$

and making the substitutions

$$\omega_i = \omega_C \theta_i$$
$$K = \frac{1}{1+\omega_1} \times \frac{1}{1+\omega_2} \times \frac{1}{1+\omega_3} \times \cdots$$

this may be written as $K\omega_C\theta_1$. Similarly, the probability that subject 2 is a case and all other subjects controls is $K\omega_C\theta_2$, and so on. The sum of probabilities for all the outcomes in which one member of the set is a case and all other members are controls is

$$K\omega_C(\theta_1 + \theta_2 + \theta_3 + \cdots)$$

so that the conditional probability that subject 1 is the case is:

$$\frac{K\omega_C\theta_1}{K\omega_C(\theta_1 + \theta_2 + \theta_3 + \cdots)} = \frac{\theta_1}{\theta_1 + \theta_2 + \theta_3 + \cdots}.$$

The contribution of one set to the log likelihood is, therefore,

$$\log\left(\theta_{(\text{for case})} \bigg/ \sum_{\text{Case-control set}} \theta\right).$$

The total log likelihood is obtained by adding the contributions for all case-control sets.

From the form of this log likelihood it is clear that the conditional approach does not allow estimation of multiplicative effects of variables used in matching. Since all subjects in the set share the same value for such a variable its multiplicative effect will cancel out in the ratio of θ for the case to the sum of all θ's in the case-control set. However, interaction terms involving matching variables *can* be fitted. For example, for a case-control study in which sex was one of the matching variables, the sex effect cannot be estimated but the parameters for interaction between sex and exposure can be, because they will not occur in all of the θ's from the same case-control set.

29.4 Sets containing more than one case ★

The conditional argument can be generalized quite easily to allow for case-control sets containing more than one case, although the computation of the log likelihood may become rather lengthy. The idea is illustrated for a set containing two cases and one control. Fig. 29.2 shows the probability tree for case/control status of a set of three subjects. In three of the eight possible outcomes there are two cases and one control. The probabilities for these branches are written to the right of the figure, again using the

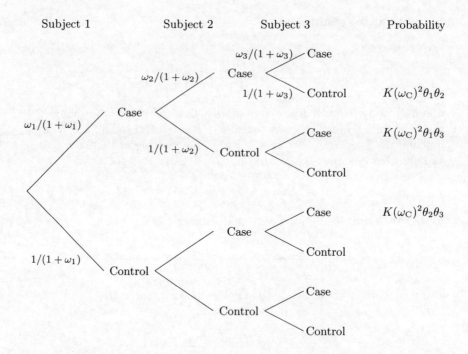

Fig. 29.2.   Sets with two cases and one control.

abbreviation
$$K = \frac{1}{1+\omega_1} \times \frac{1}{1+\omega_2} \times \frac{1}{1+\omega_3}.$$

Conditional on the observed outcome being one of the three with two cases and one control the probability that the cases are subjects 1 and 2 is

$$\frac{K(\omega_C)^2\theta_1\theta_2}{K(\omega_C)^2\theta_1\theta_2 + K(\omega_C)^2\theta_1\theta_3 + K(\omega_C)^2\theta_2\theta_3} = \frac{\theta_1\theta_2}{\theta_1\theta_2 + \theta_1\theta_3 + \theta_2\theta_3}.$$

The log of this conditional probability is the contribution of the set to the log likelihood.

It is easy to see how this argument can be extended to deal with any number of cases and controls in a set. For example, for sets of size 6 containing 3 cases, the conditional probability that subjects 1, 2, and 3 are the cases is

$$\frac{\theta_1\theta_2\theta_3}{\theta_1\theta_2\theta_3 + \theta_1\theta_2\theta_4 + \theta_1\theta_2\theta_5 + \cdots}.$$

The denominator contains a term for each of the 20 ways of selecting three subjects from 6, and does not depend on the way the subjects have been numbered.

Solutions to the exercises

29.1 The values of θ for the four subjects are:

| Subject | Corner | Multiplicative effects | | θ |
		Age	Exposure	
1	1.0		×5.0	5.0
2	1.0	×1.5		1.5
3	1.0		×5.0	5.0
4	1.0	×3.0	×5.0	15.0

Subject 1 is the case in the first set and subject 3 is the case in the second set. The log likelihood contributions are, therefore

$$\log\left(\frac{5.0}{5.0+1.5}\right) + \log\left(\frac{5.0}{5.0+15.0}\right) = -0.262 - 1.386.$$

30
Cox's method for follow-up studies

When using Poisson regression models to analyse data from follow-up studies, time is divided into fairly broad bands such as 5 or 10 years of age. Age is the most common time scale but in some applications other time scales may be more relevant. This point is discussed in more detail in the next chapter, but for the moment we refer to the time scale simply as time. Cox's method is very similar to Poisson regression but is based on a much finer subdivision of time.

30.1 Choosing parameters

When there are two explanatory variables, A and B, and the rate is allowed to vary with time, the multiplicative model for the rate takes the form

$$\text{Rate} = \text{Corner} \times \text{Time} \times \text{A} \times \text{B}.$$

Here time is a categorical variable with one level for each time band. Again we split the model into two parts, as in

$$\text{Rate} = \boxed{\text{Corner} \times \text{Time}} \times \boxed{\text{A} \times \text{B}}.$$

Algebraically this corresponds to a reparametrization of the model as

$$\lambda_i^t = \lambda_C^t \theta_i,$$

where λ_C^t is a corner parameter measuring the rate for time band t when A and B are both at level 0, and θ_i is the rate ratio which compares the rate for subject i, in time band t, to the corner rate for that time band. The parameters λ_C^t correspond to the

$$\boxed{\text{Corner} \times \text{Time}}$$

part of the model and the parameters θ_i to the

$$\boxed{\text{A} \times \text{B}}$$

part of the model.

30.2   The profile likelihood

The parameters λ_C^t are also called the *baseline* rates, and are generally nuisance parameters. The main interest is in the parameters of the second part of the model. The profile likelihood for the parameters in the second part of the model is obtained by deriving formulae for the most likely values of the nuisance parameters, λ_C^t, and substituting these into the expression for the log likelihood. The number of nuisance parameters depends upon the number of time bands into which the total study period has been partitioned. For the present we shall consider a finite number of bands, but in the next section the argument is generalized to the case where time is divided into clicks.

The contribution of subject i to the log likelihood is the sum of contributions for each time band. These have the Poisson form:

$$d_i^t \log(\lambda_i^t) - y_i^t \lambda_i^t$$

where y_i^t is the observation time in time-band t and d_i^t indicates whether the event occurred ($d = 1$) or not ($d = 0$). The total log likelihood is the sum of such terms over all subjects (i) and all time bands (t). Rewriting λ_i^t as $\lambda_C^t \theta_i$, this becomes

$$\sum_{i,t} \left[d_i^t \log(\lambda_C^t \theta_i) - y_i^t \lambda_C^t \theta_i \right].$$

The rules of calculus show that, given the θ_i, the most likely values of the baseline rates λ_C^t are

$$\frac{d^t}{\sum_i y_i^t \theta_i},$$

where d^t represents the total number of events occurring in time band t. Substituting these values into the expression for the log likelihood yields a profile log likelihood which depends only on the parameters in the second part of the model. This is

$$\sum_{j,t} d_j^t \log \left(\frac{\theta_j}{\sum_i y_i^t \theta_i} \right).$$

30.3   Time divided into clicks

The profile log likelihood derived by stratifying the follow-up interval into bands provides a satisfactory method for regression analysis of cohort studies, but although this is the approach used with frequency records it is rarely used with individual records. The reason for this is that a further generalization offers increased flexibility without seriously compromising either

statistical or computational efficiency. In this generalization the time scale
is subdivided into clicks which can contain no more than one event, thus
allowing rates to vary continuously over time.

The consequence of this generalization for the profile log likelihood are
quite minor. First consider the effect upon the observation times, y_i^t. If the
duration of the time bands is h and we allow h to become very small, almost
every y_i^t will become either zero (if subject i was not observed at click t)
or h (if subject i was observed). In these circumstances, it is convenient to
redefine y_i^t to be *at risk indicators* taking on the values 0 or 1 respectively.
The observation times then become hy_i^t and the profile log likelihood for
the rate ratio model becomes

$$\sum_{j,t} d_j^t \log \left(\frac{\theta_j}{\sum_i hy_i^t \theta_i} \right),$$

which may be further simplified to

$$\sum_{j,t} d_j^t \log \left(\frac{\theta_j}{\sum_i y_i^t \theta_i} \right) - D \log(h).$$

Since the term $D \log(h)$ does not depend upon any parameters, it may be
omitted.

Examination of the profile likelihood equation shows it to be constructed
of a sum of terms, in which d_j^t is a multiplier which takes on the value 1 for
clicks in which an event occurs, and 0 everywhere else. Thus the profile log
likelihood receives an additive contribution for every failure event. Each of
these is the log of a ratio whose numerator is the rate ratio, θ_j, predicted
by the model for subject j in whom the event occurred (the *case*), and
whose denominator,

$$\sum_i y_i^t \theta_i$$

is the sum of rate ratios, θ_i, for those subjects under observation at t, the
time of occurrence of the failure.

The collection of subjects contributing to the denominator is known
as the *risk set* for the observed failure. Using this terminology the profile
likelihood can be written

$$\sum_{\text{Failures}} \log \left(\theta_{\text{(for case)}} \bigg/ \sum_{\text{Risk set}} \theta \right).$$

The ratio in brackets is the conditional probability that, given a failure
occurred in this set of subjects, it occurred in the case rather than in
some other member of the risk set. The profile log likelihood therefore

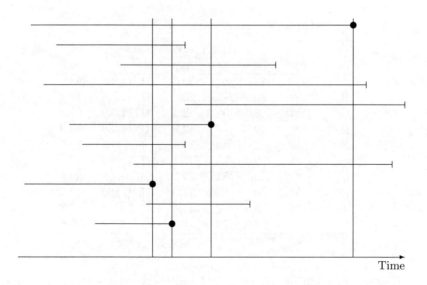

Fig. 30.1. Composition of risk sets.

corresponds exactly with the conditional log likelihood obtained for individually matched case-control studies, and analysis of a cohort study using the above profile likelihood is equivalent to its analysis as a matched case-control study in which each case is matched on time with all other members of the corresponding risk set. The composition of risk sets is illustrated by Fig. 30.1. The risk set for each failure contains all subjects whose observation lines cross the appropriate vertical, including the subject in whom the defining event occurred.

The recognition that this likelihood is a profile likelihood came some years after Cox's original proposal of the method, in which he called it the *partial likelihood*.* This name has stuck, and is in general use, so we shall continue to use it, but we emphasize that partial likelihood is the profile likelihood for the parameters in the second part of the regression model when Cox's method has been used to eliminate the parameters in the first half. Because a very large number of nuisance parameters have been eliminated — infinitely many, in fact, we have no right to expect that the partial likelihood will maintain the properties of likelihood. In the present application, however, it has been proved to behave the same way as a true

---

*Cox originally used an argument identical to that we used in Chapter 29 for individually matched case-control studies and referred to it as a *conditional* likelihood. There are, however, difficulties with this argument when applied in the present context. While each term which contributes to the log likelihood is indeed the logarithm of a conditional probability, the total is not. A later paper correcting this error introduced the term partial likelihood.

Table 30.1. A cohort of 10 subjects

Subject	Sex	Entry to Study Date	Age	End of Study Date	Age
A	F	13/ 6/65	29.3	31/12/89	53.8
B	M	23/10/72	25.2	31/12/89	42.4
C	M	3/ 3/59	22.1	31/12/89	52.8
D	F	10/10/67	32.2	31/12/89	54.4
E	M	2/ 1/60	33.1	4/ 7/79	52.6
F	M	9/ 1/75	42.1	31/12/89	57.1
G	F	5/ 8/53	35.2	3/10/68	50.4
H	M	10/10/69	27.0	31/12/89	47.2
I	M	2/ 3/72	44.8	31/12/89	62.7
J	F	1/11/70	51.5	31/12/89	70.6

likelihood as the amount of data increases.

The composition of risk sets (and hence the results of the analysis) depend upon the choice of time scale for the analysis, as is demonstrated by the following exercise.

Exercise 30.1. The data set out in Table 30.1 refer to 10 subjects from a cohort study. Subjects E and G died at the second date while the remaining eight subjects survived until the date of analysis (31/12/89). List the members of the risk sets for both deaths when the appropriate time scale is (a) calendar date (b) age (c) time since entry into the study.

The difference between these analyses is that they represent three different models. In each case the λ_C^t parameters represent variation of baseline rates along different time scales.

30.4   Choice of time scale

Our derivation of Cox's method allows for time to be interpreted in the most appropriate manner for a particular analysis. Usually this will mean the time scale with the strongest relationship to failure rate. Regrettably it is still the case that some major software packages do not allow such flexibility. This reflects the fact that the method was motivated by problems of survival following medical treatment. In such studies the appropriate time scale is time since start of follow-up so that all observation of all subjects starts at time zero. In such studies, risk sets always become smaller (as a result of failure and censoring) as time advances.

On other time scales there will be *late entry* of subjects (observation starting at time > 0) and risk sets may be supplemented by new entrants as time advances. In order to be able to select the most appropriate time scale for an analysis, the software must be capable of allowing for late entry.

30.5 Confounders other than time

The confounding effect of time is allowed for by including time in the first part of the model. For example, taking age as the time variable, the multiplicative model

$$\text{Rate} = \boxed{\text{Corner} \times \text{Age}} \times \boxed{\text{A} \times \text{B}},$$

includes the effect of age in the baseline rate parameters. The most obvious way to deal with another confounder, such as sex, is to include it in the second part of the model, as in

$$\text{Rate} = \boxed{\text{Corner} \times \text{Age}} \times \boxed{\text{Sex} \times \text{A} \times \text{B}}.$$

This model assumes that the effect of sex is constant with age so that the baseline rates for males are a constant multiple of those for females. To extend the model to allow for different patterns of baseline rates for each sex, the interaction between age and sex must be included in the model. When the age scale is divided into clicks this interaction term involves a very large number of parameters, so it is best to absorb these parameters in the baseline rate part of the model, giving

$$\text{Rate} = \boxed{\text{Corner} \times \text{Age} \times \text{Sex} \times \text{Age·Sex}} \times \boxed{\text{A} \times \text{B}}.$$

This model has the effect of allowing different sets of baseline rate parameters for males and females. If we estimate these algebraically as before, we find that the profile likelihood for the rate ratio part of the model still has the form of a partial likelihood:

$$\sum_{\text{Failures}} \log \left(\theta_{(\text{for case})} \bigg/ \sum_{\text{Risk set}} \theta \right)$$

but the risk set is now restricted to contain only those subjects who (a) were under study at the time of failure of the case, and (b) belonged to the same sex as the case. Thus the analysis simulates a matched case-control study in which controls are matched to cases with respect to sex.

This extension of Cox's method is usually referred to as a stratified analysis, although more properly it should be referred to as *doubly* stratified — Cox's method stratifies by time alone, while the extended method stratifies by both time and a further variable. In our example stratification is by age and sex.

Exercise 30.2. Repeat Exercise 30.1 for an analysis which is to be stratified by sex.

It can be seen from the last exercise that when an analysis is doubly stratified the risk sets contain fewer subjects than when it is stratified on time alone. Rather unexpectedly, therefore, the effect of adopting a more complicated model is to *reduce* the amount of computation required to estimate the parameters of interest. Further stratification can be introduced but there is a limit. If a study is overstratified, some risk sets will contain only the case, there being no other subjects matching the case in respect of all stratifying variables. Such sets make no contribution to the profile likelihood, so the information from these events is lost.

★ ## 30.6 Estimating the baseline rates

In some circumstances the dependence of rates upon time is of some interest, and we would wish to estimate the baseline rates, λ_C^t. In this section we shall show that the plot of the most likely estimate of the baseline rate against time turns out to be very similar in form to the Aalen– Nelson estimator introduced in Chapter 5.

Given the values of the parameters in the second part of the model the most likely values of the baseline rates, λ_C^t, were shown in Section 30.2 to be

$$\frac{d^t}{\sum_i y_i^t \theta_i}.$$

where θ_i is given by the second part of the model. When we divide time into clicks of duration h and redefine y_i^t to be 0 or 1 at-risk indicators, this expression becomes

$$\frac{d^t}{\sum_i h y_i^t \theta_i}.$$

In most clicks no failure occurs, $d^t = 0$, and the estimate of the rate is zero. In a click in which a failure occurs, $d^t = 1$, the estimated rate is

$$\frac{1}{h \sum_i y_i^t \theta_i},$$

which becomes very large as h becomes very small. However, the *cumulative* baseline rate increases at each click by the amounts $h\lambda_C^t$, and the estimated values of these are either zero or

$$\frac{1}{\sum_i y_i^t \theta_i}$$

when a failure occurs. Thus the cumulative baseline rate is estimated by stepped curve with jumps at the observed failure times. This is called the Aalen–Breslow estimate and is illustrated in Fig. 30.2. The height of the

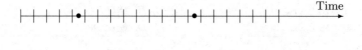

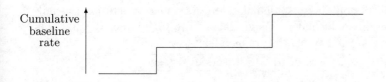

Fig. 30.2. The Aalen–Breslow estimate of the cumulative baseline rate.

jump at each failure time is now given by

$$1 \bigg/ \sum_{\text{Risk set}} \theta$$

rather than by

$$1/(\text{Number of subjects at risk})$$

as in the simpler case discussed in Chapter 5. As noted there, examination of the cumulative rate plot allows us to assess the dependence of failure rate on time.

Solutions to the exercises

30.1 When date is the time scale, membership of risk sets is determined by whether or not the subject was observed at the date of occurrence of the death. The risk sets corresponding to the two deaths are as follows:

Date of death	Subjects in risk set
3/10/68	A, C, D, E, G (case)
4/ 7/79	A, B, C, D, E (case), F, H, I, J

The risk set corresponding to the death of subject *G* contains fewer individuals since it occurred at a date earlier than some subjects had joined the cohort.

When age is the time scale, risk set membership is determined by whether the subject was observed at the age at which the death occurred. The risk sets are now as follows:

Age at death	Subjects in risk set
50.4	A, C, D, E, F, G (case),I
52.6	A, C, D, E (case), F, I, J

When time in study is the scale, the risk sets are as follows:

Time in study at death	Subjects in risk set
15.2 yrs	A, B, C, D, E, G (case), H, I, J
19.5 yrs	A, C, D, E (case), H

30.2 Since subject G is female and subject E is male, the risk set for the failure of G contains only female subjects and risk sets for the failure of E contains only males. When date is the time scale, the risk sets corresponding to the two deaths are as follows:

Date of death	Subjects in risk set
3/10/68	A, D, G (case)
4/ 7/79	B, C, E (case), H, I

When age is the time scale, the risk sets are

Age at death	Subjects in risk set
50.4	A, D, G (case)
52.6	C, E (case), F, I

When time in study is the scale, the risk sets are:

Time in study at death	Subjects in risk set
15.2 yrs	A, D, G (case), J
19.5 yrs	C, E (case), H

31
Time-varying explanatory variables

Cox's method provides a convenient way of controlling for time in the analysis of follow-up studies. In its simple form the method assumes that other explanatory variables do not change with time. In this chapter we show how the method can be extended to allow for this. We also discuss the closely related problem of analysis strategies when rates vary in relation to more than one time scale, and draw attention to some dangers and difficulties.

31.1 The model and the likelihood

We have seen that Cox's method amounts to dividing the multiplicative model for rates into two parts:

$$\text{Rate} = \boxed{\text{Corner} \times \text{Time}} \times \boxed{\text{A} \times \text{B} \times \cdots}.$$

The first part refers to the baseline rates while the second part specifies how the rate ratio

$$\theta_i = \frac{\text{Rate for subject } i \text{ at time } t}{\text{Baseline rate at time } t}$$

is related to the explanatory variables A, B, etc.. On a log scale

$$\log(\text{Rate}) = \boxed{\text{Corner} + \text{Time}} + \boxed{\text{A} + \text{B} + \cdots}.$$

In the simple form of the method θ_i is assumed to be independent of time.

The extension of Cox's method with which we are now concerned allows the relationship between θ_i and the explanatory variables to vary with time. This would be necessary, for example, when studying levels of hazardous industrial exposures in occupational studies and when studying changing treatments in long term follow-up studies of chronic disease aetiology. Indeed *most* explanatory variables of interest to epidemiologists vary with time if follow-up is over a sufficiently long period.

Allowing the rate ratio part of the model to change over time involves only a simple change to the contribution

$$\log\left(\theta_{(\text{for case})} \Big/ \sum_{\text{Risk set}} \theta\right),$$

from each risk set to the partial log likelihood. Since the model now predicts different values of θ at different times the contribution of each risk set must now be calculated using the values of θ current at the time of occurrence of the failure.

COMPUTATION

When it comes to computing the likelihood and finding the values of parameters which maximize it this simple change turns out to have major consequences, and computation times can increase by several orders of magnitude. To understand why the computation is so heavy it helps to look at the simpler version of Cox's method to see why this does *not* involve heavy computations. There are two reasons. First, for any particular set of values for the parameters, the value of θ only needs to be worked out once for each subject. Second, the value of $\sum \theta$ does not have to be calculated from scratch for each risk set because the equivalent term from the previous risk set can be updated by subtracting the values of θ for all subjects lost to follow-up in the intervening period and adding the contributions of those newly joining the cohort. Other terms needed in the computation of gradient and curvature of the log likelihood can be updated in a similar way.

When the model allows the rate ratios θ to change over time a subject who appears in several risk sets can have different values of θ in each. This means that not only must the values of θ be re-calculated for each risk set but $\sum \theta$ and other gradient and curvature terms must be calculated from scratch. The result is that the computing time rises dramatically.

Some reduction in computing time can be achieved by sampling the risk sets. The algebraic equivalence of the partial likelihood in Cox's method and the conditional likelihood for matched case-control studies means that analyzing a cohort study using Cox's method is the same as analyzing it as a case-control study in which each incident case is individually matched with a control set in which the controls are all other subjects under study at the moment of incidence. Since a case-control study which draws many controls for each case provides very little more information than one which draws only a few, we shall lose little by taking a random sample of controls drawn from each risk set rather than using the entire risk set. Sampling risk sets in this way creates what is called a *nested case-control study*. Such studies offer a number of practical advantages in addition to considerable computational savings and will be discussed further in Chapter 33.

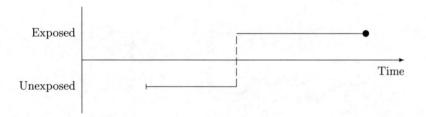

Fig. 31.1. Changing exposure group.

31.2 Changing exposure group

One simple but important way in which an explanatory variable can change
with time arises when a subject can change from being unexposed to being
exposed group (or vice versa) during the course of follow-up (see Fig. 31.1).
This is most easily dealt with by splitting the follow-up for such subjects
into an unexposed part and an exposed part, and treating the parts as
distinct subjects. The data can then be analysed using the simple form of
Cox's method in which the explanatory variables do not change with time.
The validity of the analysis depends on a relatively strong assumption concerning the *reasons* for the change of exposure group, namely that transfer
is unrelated to the subsequent probability of failure. If the transfer mechanism operates in a way that selects particularly high or low risk subjects
then subsequent comparisons will be distorted. This is another example of
selection bias. More formally, it is required that transfer must be independent of subsequent failure conditional upon the values of all other variables
in the model. If transfer and failure are both strongly related to age (say)
there will be an overall association between transfer time and outcome, but
this will not bias estimates of other effects providing there is no relationship
between transfer time and outcome *for subjects of the same age*, and providing the model takes proper account of the relationship between age and
failure rate. Similar considerations apply when there are more than two
categories of exposure or when the level of exposure varies continuously.

Exercise 31.1. Subjects enter a heart transplant programme as unexposed
on joining a waiting list for a transplant, and switch to the exposed group on
receiving the transplant. Do you think the assumptions discussed above are
likely to be met in this case?

31.3 Time scales as explanatory variables

Another very common form of time-dependent explanatory variable is an
additional time scale. For example, in a clinical study in which survival

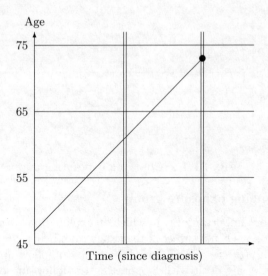

Fig. 31.2.   Follow-up by age and time.

is analysed largely in relation to time since diagnosis, it will usually be
necessary to control the comparison of different treatments for the age of
the subjects receiving them.   For short studies this can be achieved by
including age at diagnosis, which is fixed for every subject.   When follow-
up is over many years it is better to include age itself, which varies with
time. Fig. 31.2 illustrates follow-up of a subject in which observation time
is classified by time since diagnosis and age.   The risk sets are determined
by the times of occurrence of failures.   Two such times are illustrated in
the figure by narrow vertical bands.   One corresponds to the risk set for
the failure of the subject shown while the other is an earlier failure.   The
subject shown contributes to both risk sets, but is of a different age on the
two occasions.

   One possible analysis would be to include time since diagnosis in the first
part of the model, so that this is the time scale which is used to determine
the risk sets, and to include age as a time varying explanatory variable in
the second part of the model.   This could be done either by dividing the
age scale into 5- or 10-year bands and treating it as a categorical variable,
as in

$$\log(\text{Rate}) = \boxed{\text{Corner} + \text{Time}} + \boxed{\text{Age} + \text{A} + \text{B} + \cdots} \, ,$$

or by treating age as a quantitative and fitting linear effects, and possibly
quadratic effects too, as in

$$\log(\text{Rate}) = \boxed{\text{Corner} + \text{Time}} + \boxed{[\text{Age}] + [\text{Age-sq}] + \text{A} + \text{B} + \cdots} \, .$$

When the partial log likelihood is formed for either of these analyses each risk set contributes a term of the form $\log(\theta / \sum \theta)$ where the values of θ for the subjects in the risk set are determined by the relationship between $\log(\theta)$ and the parameters in the second part of the model. As an example of this computational process consider the model

$$\log(\text{Rate}) = \boxed{\text{Corner} + \text{Time}} + \boxed{\text{Age} + \text{A} + \text{B}}$$

where age has five levels, A has two levels and B has three levels. The parameters in the second part of the model are then $\text{Age}(1), \cdots, \text{Age}(4)$, $\text{A}(1)$, $\text{B}(1)$ and $\text{B}(2)$. Now consider a subject, at level 1 for A and level 2 for B, who appears as a survivor in the risk sets at two failure times, and suppose that this subject is in age band 3 at the time of the first failure, and in age band 4 at the time of the second failure.

Exercise 31.2. Write down an expression, in terms of the parameters, for the values of $\log(\theta)$ for this subject, in the two risk sets.

When there are two time scales a natural question to be considered is which should be included in the baseline rates part of the model and which should be included in the rate ratio part. The choice depends on the way that rates vary along each time scale. If this variation is to be modelled in the rate ratio part of the model then we must either divide the scale into broad bands or fit simple mathematical functions of time, such as linear or quadratic. The former strategy is adequate if the variation of rates is not too rapid, while the latter is only possible if the variation is regular enough to describe by simple mathematical functions. If variation is both rapid and irregular neither approach works very well and the variation should be modelled in the baseline rates. Thus if it is suspected that variation along one scale will be rapid and irregular this should be the scale whose effects are modelled by the baseline rates, and other scales should be treated as time varying explanatory variables. If variation is smooth along all scales it is better to use the scale with the strongest effects for the baseline rates.

Exercise 31.3. Discuss appropriate strategies for modelling the effects of age and calendar time on incidence of (a) a chronic degenerative disease, and (b) an infectious disease.

31.4 Dependencies between time scales   ⋆

Different time scales are not truly different variables but the same variable measured from different origins. It is therefore impossible for a subject to advance one year on one scale without simultaneously advancing one year on other time scales. For example, we cannot pass through a year of calendar time without advancing a year in age — would that we could! This dependency between time scales can lead to difficulties when trying to interpret the estimated effects of changes on these time scales.

As an illustration we shall return to the example of age and time since diagnosis in a clinical follow-up study. Let us first consider the model

$$\log(\text{Rate}) = \boxed{\text{Corner} + \text{Time}} + \boxed{[\text{Age-at-diagnosis}] + \cdots} \,,$$

in which the effect of time since diagnosis is the main time scale and is included in the first part of the model, while age at diagnosis is included as a linear effect in the second. The parameter [Age-at diagnosis] measures the change in the log rate per one year change in age, holding time since diagnosis constant at any arbitrary value. Fig. 31.3 shows two subjects who are diagnosed at ages 47 and 61 respectively; if we assume these subjects have the same values for any other explanatory variables the difference in log rate predicted by the model, at diagnosis, or at any value of time since diagnosis, is

$$(61 - 47) \times [\text{Age-at-diagnosis}] = 14 \times [\text{Age-at-diagnosis}].$$

Now consider the model

$$\log(\text{Rate}) = \boxed{\text{Corner} + \text{Time}} + \boxed{[\text{Age}] + \cdots}$$

in which age varies with time. The two subjects in Fig. 31.3 have a 14 year age difference at diagnosis, so this model predicts a difference in log rates between the two subjects of $14 \times [\text{Age}]$ at diagnosis. Because these two subjects have a 14 year age difference not only at diagnosis but at any time after diagnosis, the model also predicts a difference of $14 \times [\text{Age}]$ at any value of time since diagnosis. Thus both models predict a constant difference in log rate at any value of time since diagnosis. In the one case the prediction is $14 \times [\text{Age-at-diagnosis}]$, in the other the prediction is $14 \times [\text{Age}]$. This is true for any pair of subjects; the models make identical predictions and cannot be differentiated, the [Age-at-diagnosis] parameter in the first model is making the same comparison as the [Age] parameter in the second.

There may well be scientific interest in discriminating between models in which the age at diagnosis determines prognosis, and models in which age itself is the determinant, but if we were to fit the model

$$\log(\text{Rate}) = \boxed{\text{Corner} + \text{Time}} + \boxed{[\text{Age}] + [\text{Age-at-diagnosis}] + \cdots} \,,$$

in order to try and separate the linear effect of age controlled for time since diagnosis from the linear effect of age at diagnosis controlled for time since diagnosis, we would run into difficulties. When time since diagnosis and age are held constant, there can be no further variation in age at diagnosis so that the [Age-at-diagnosis] parameter cannot be estimated. Likewise,

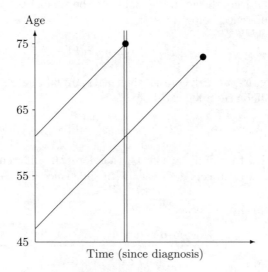

Fig. 31.3.   Observation of two subjects.

time since diagnosis and age at diagnosis uniquely determine age so that the [Age] parameter cannot be estimated. Again the two subjects shown in Fig. 31.3 demonstrate the problem. The new model also predicts that the difference in log rates remains constant at any value of time since diagnosis but this difference is now equal to

$$14 \times [\text{Age}] + 14 \times [\text{Age-at-diagnosis}] = 14 \times ([\text{Age}] + [\text{Age-at-diagnosis}]),$$

where the parameters [Age] and [Age-at-diagnosis] now refer to the new model which contains both linear effects. Because any values for the two parameters which have the same sum, make the same predictions, the parameters cannot be estimated individually. They are said to be *non-identifiable* or *aliased*.

A computer program will usually warn the user when two parameters are non-identifiable and then omit one of them from the model. This is quite useful when the object is to control for age and age at diagnosis, but if the object is to disentangle their effects, what the computer program is saying is that we are attempting the impossible.

The non-identifiability of parameters for different time scales refers to their linear effects. When we come to fit models with non-linear terms, things are not so bad. Consider for example the predictions of the model

$$\log(\text{Rate}) = \boxed{\text{Corner} + \text{Time}} + \boxed{[\text{Age}] + [\text{Age-sq}] + \cdots}$$

for the two subjects shown in Fig. 31.3. At the time of diagnosis the model predicts a difference in log rates of

$$(61 - 47) \times [\text{Age}] + (61^2 - 47^2) \times [\text{Age-sq}] = 14 \times [\text{Age}] + 1512 \times [\text{Age-sq}].$$

However, 5 years after diagnosis, their ages are 66 and 52 and the model predicts a difference in log rates of

$$(66 - 52) \times [\text{Age}] + (66^2 - 52^2) \times [\text{Age-sq}] = 14 \times [\text{Age}] + 1652 \times [\text{Age-sq}].$$

In the model with non-linear effects, therefore, the difference between log rates for the two subjects does vary with time since diagnosis. The model

$$\log(\text{Rate}) \quad = \quad \boxed{\text{Corner} + \text{Time}} \quad +$$
$$\boxed{[\text{Age-at-diagnosis}] + [\text{Age-at-diagnosis-sq}] + \cdots}$$

predicts a difference in log rates of

$$(61 - 47) \times [\text{Age-at-diagnosis}] + (61^2 - 47^2) \times [\text{Age-at-diagnosis-sq}]$$

throughout the follow-up, and this is a different prediction than the one obtained from the model with age and age-squared. The linear parts of the two predictions are still the same and cannot be separately estimated, but the non-linear parts are different and can be.

Similarly, if we were to fit the model

$$\log(\text{Rate}) \quad = \quad \boxed{\text{Corner} + \text{Time}} \quad +$$
$$\boxed{\begin{array}{l} [\text{Age}] + [\text{Age-sq}] \; + [\text{Age-at-diagnosis}]+ \\ [\text{Age-at-diagnosis-sq}] + \cdots \end{array}} \;,$$

the parameters [Age] and [Age-at-diagnosis] are not identifiable while the parameters [Age-sq] and [Age-at-diagnosis-sq] can be estimated. The same is true for any other non-linear component of the relationships.

⋆ 31.5   Discrete time bands

In the above discussion the time variables are measured exactly; when the time scales are divided into discrete bands the position is slightly more complicated. To illustrate this we shall return to the two subjects of Fig. 31.3 and imagine a model in which age has been grouped into 5-year bands but time since diagnosis is still measured exactly. At the beginning of follow-up one subject is in the 45–49 band and the other is in the 60–64 band. However, after three years the former subject has moved into the 50–54 band while the latter remains in the 60–64 band. It will appear to a computer program that the age difference between the subjects has narrowed! As a result the program will not spot the underlying non-identifiability of models such as

$$\log(\text{Rate}) = \boxed{\text{Corner} + \text{Time}} + \boxed{\text{Age} + \text{Age-diag} + \cdots}$$

and fit them without complaint. However, the linear components of the relationships with age and age at diagnosis have only become estimable because of the inaccuracy introduced by banding and the resulting parameter estimates are uninterpretable.

31.6   Modelling vital rates $\boxed{\star}$

A familiar example of these problems arises in 'age-period-cohort' modelling of mortality and other vital rates, where the aim is to disentangle the dependence of rates upon age, calendar time (period), and date of birth (birth cohort). This comparison raises exactly the same problem as above and has provoked a lot of discussion in the epidemiological literature. Much of this has been based on the misconception that the problem is a shortcoming of current statistical methods and that its solution awaits only methodological advances. This is not the case. The difficulty is inescapable and arises from the fact that subjects cannot move in one time scale without an identical move in others.

Fig. 31.4 shows a table in which both both age and calendar period have been divided into 10-year bands. Tables of rates, classified in this way, are frequently available from official published sources, and allow effects of year of birth (*birth cohort* effects) to be estimated approximately. If we remember that observation of individual subjects is represented by diagonal lines in the age and calendar time Lexis diagram (illustrated by the arrow), it is clear that diagonal groupings of cells in the table correspond *approximately* to birth cohorts. The cell labelled 0 refers to subjects born around 1870, those labelled 1 to subjects born around 1880, and so on. Although this correspondence is only approximate, the new discrete codings for age period and cohort behave very much like the underlying continuous scales. In particular, they are linearly dependent. In our example,

$$\text{Cohort} = 3 + \text{Period} - \text{Age}.$$

This means that when two are fixed the third is also fixed and in models such as

$$\log(\text{Rate}) = \text{Corner} + [\text{Age}] + [\text{Period}] + [\text{Cohort}]$$

the parameters are unidentifiable, and it is impossible to disentangle the linear effects of all three variables.

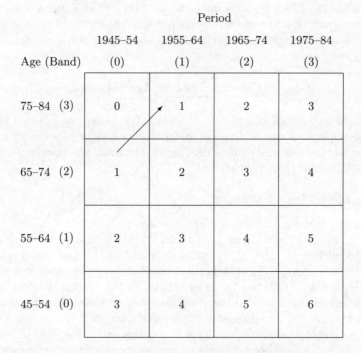

Fig. 31.4. Approximate birth cohorts.

Some investigators have returned to the raw data in order to allocate subjects to their true birth cohort. This avoids the approximation in Fig. 31.4 but leads to a serious fallacy. Fig. 31.5 shows how the exact birth cohorts move across the Lexis diagram. The cell labelled 0 refers to the 1860–69 birth cohort, those labelled 1 to the 1870–79 cohort, and so on. The discrete codings no longer behave like the underlying scales. For example, birth cohort 1 is observed in 3 cells; the transition from the first to the second involves a change of age band (from 65–74 to 75–84) without change in calendar period, while the transition from second to third corresponds to a move through calendar time without change in age! Looked at naively it would appear that, by grouping, we have created a natural experiment in which subjects can age instantaneously and travel in time without ageing. The fallacy lies in the fact that the regions are triangular and that regions shaped ▽ disproportionately represent ages towards the upper end of the 10-year band and dates towards the lower end of the period, while regions shaped △ disproportionately represent ages at the lower end of the band and periods at the upper end. Unfortunately, computer programs have no way of knowing this. They will believe that a miraculous natural experiment has been observed, and estimate separate linear effects for all

Period

	1945–54	1955–64	1965–74	1975–84
Age (Band)	(0)	(1)	(2)	(3)

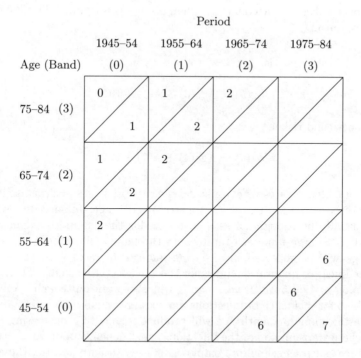

Fig. 31.5. Exact birth cohorts.

three scales without complaint. This uncritical behaviour of computer programs (which can't know better) has been hailed by some epidemiologists and statisticians (who should) as a 'solution' to the identifiability 'problem'. The reverse is the case; the computer solution is fallacious, being based entirely on grouping inaccuracies, and the resultant estimates are uninterpretable. It is worth pointing out that this pitfall is not confined to the age-period-cohort problem, but can be encountered whenever more than one time scale is involved in an analysis.

Solutions to the exercises

31.1 When a heart becomes available for transplantation and there is more than one patient eligible to receive it, there is potential selection bias. A controlled study would *randomize* such choices to exclude selection bias, but in an observational study it will always be difficult to know whether the recipient was selected because the clinician felt that this patient was most likely to benefit. Such selection would cause serious bias in a simple analysis. In theory this can be offset by including in the analysis any prognostic factors likely to have been used by the clinician making the decision, but in practice one can rarely be sure that all relevant factors have been taken into account. We shall discuss this example in more detail in Chapter 32.

31.2 For the first risk set

$$\log(\theta) = \text{Age}(3) + \text{A}(1) + \text{B}(2).$$

For the second risk set

$$\log(\theta) = \text{Age}(4) + \text{A}(1) + \text{B}(2).$$

31.3 Incidence rates of chronic degenerative diseases such as ischaemic heart disease and most cancers rise steeply with age. In such diseases age may usually be thought of as a surrogate for the cumulative damage inflicted by a large number of influences throughout life. Such cumulative damage will be reflected in a *smooth* increase of rates with age so that simple linear or quadratic models for the age effect are usually satisfactory. Grouping age by 5 or 10 year bands will also work quite well. Age relationships for incidence of infectious diseases are usually more complicated. Increasing immunity with age will produce a smoothly decreasing curve, but where transmission of the infectious agent depends upon various social influences such as schooling, employment, sexual activity etc., these may give rise to rather irregular age curves. Simple mathematical functions for age-incidence curves are therefore less likely to be useful. Grouping may also be difficult because of abrupt changes in incidence due to age related changes in social behaviour.

32
Three examples

This chapter describes three studies where the explanatory variables change with time and where the analysis has been helped by the statistical methods discussed in immediately preceding chapters. The first is a clinical follow-up study of heart transplant patients and has already been introduced in Exercise 31.1. The second is an epidemiological study into the effects of bereavement in old people. The third is concerned with the important problem of estimating the parameters of cancer screening programmes to help public health administrators in planning such services.

32.1 Mortality following heart transplantation

The first example concerns the survival of patients in the Stanford heart transplant program.* The basic nature of the data is illustrated in Fig. 32.1. The follow-up of patients starts as soon as they are enrolled in the program to await a suitable heart. In this phase of the follow-up, patients are in the *pre-transplant* state. When a heart becomes available, and if selected, transplantation takes place and the patient transfers into the *post-transplant* state. The diagram shows two patients, one of whom dies some time after transplantation while the other dies while awaiting a suitable heart.

The diagram also indicates (by the two vertical lines) a stratification by time in programme. In this time band there is some person-time pre-transplant and some post-transplant. This allows comparison of mortality in post-transplant patients with that in controls who are still awaiting transplantation. The possible biases in this comparison were the subject of Exercise 31.1. Here we are more concerned with the mechanics of the analysis. In this comparison it would be necessary to control for such variables as age (either itself, or at enrollment into the programme), date when enrolled, date when transplanted, and prognostic factors such as record of previous surgery. Multiplicative models fitted using Cox's method can be used to do this.

---

*Crowley, J. and Hu, M., *Journal of the American Statistical Association*, **72**, 27–36.

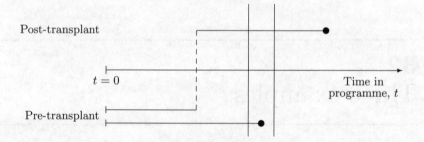

Fig. 32.1.   Mortality following heart transplant.

These models are based on the assumption that

$$\frac{\text{Mortality rate for transplanted patient}}{\text{Mortality rate for untransplanted patient}} = \text{Constant},$$

that is, the rate ratio does not vary either with time since entry into the program or with time since transplantation. The latter seems very unlikely. We might even expect an initial adverse effect of transplantation (rate ratio greater than 1) which would later be replaced by a beneficial effect (rate ratio less than 1). The assumption can be relaxed by allowing the transplantation effect to vary with time since transplantation — a variable whose evolution over time can be demonstrated by adding a further axis to the follow-up diagram, as in Fig. 32.2.

Exercise 32.1.   Time since transplant can be included in the model for the rate ratio in a number of ways. Perhaps the simplest is to include time since transplant as a quantitative variable as in

$$\log(\text{Rate}) = \text{Corner} + \text{Time} + \text{Transplant} + \text{Transplant} \cdot [\text{Time-since-transplant}] ,$$

where time is time in program. What signs would you expect for the two parameters of this model? Sketch the graph showing how the rate ratio would vary with time since transplant in this model. (You should assume that Time-since-transplant is coded zero until transplantation occurs.)

Other potential effect modifiers are age at transplantation, time spent awaiting transplantation, and closeness of matching of tissue type with the donor.

32.2   Bereavement in the elderly

The second example is drawn from a study of the effect of bereavement (death of spouse) in an elderly population.[†] There is some empirical evi-

---

[†] Jagger, C. and Sutton, C.J., *Statistics in Medicine*, **10**, 395–404.

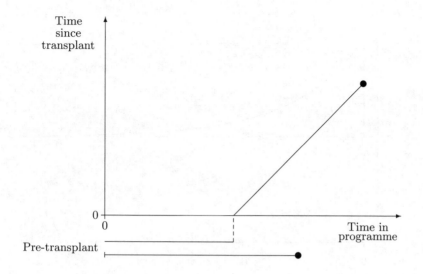

Fig. 32.2. Incorporating time since transplantation.

dence that, for a period following the death of a spouse, the mortality rate of the surviving partner is elevated. Fig. 32.3 shows a plausible relationship between mortality rate, expressed relative to mortality in persons with surviving partners, and time since death of spouse. Such a relationship can be modelled by a simple function such as

$$\text{Rate ratio} = \alpha + \beta \exp(-\gamma t),$$

where α, β, and γ are parameters. At $t = 0$ the rate ratio is $\alpha + \beta$ and, with the passage of time since bereavement, it falls away to α. The parameter γ controls how soon the rate ratio dies away.

Fig. 32.4 shows follow-up of four subjects in a cohort study by calendar time and by time since loss of spouse. Before bereavement, subjects are followed through time, thus allowing measurement of baseline mortality rates. Following death of a spouse, observation may be represented by diagonals in the Lexis diagram formed by plotting calendar time against time since bereavement. Our diagram shows the pattern of observation of two couples. For the sake of clarity, the diagram has been simplified by omitting age, although this must be included in the analysis. In a fuller representation, observation of subjects with living spouses would be represented by lines in an age by calendar time Lexis diagram, while bereaved subjects would be represented by lines in a three-dimensional diagram formed by age, calendar time and time since bereavement.

The analysis of this study must relate mortality rates to all three time

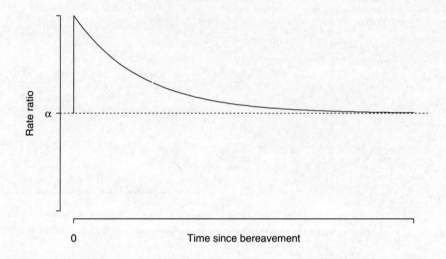

Fig. 32.3.   Mortality following bereavement.

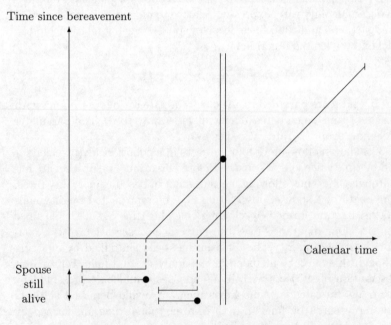

Fig. 32.4.   A study of mortality following bereavement.

scales. The effect of time since bereavement is modelled by

$$\text{Rate ratio} = \alpha + \beta \exp(-\gamma t),$$

which describes the relationship using three parameters. For modelling the effects of age and calendar time, all three possibilities discussed in Chapter 31 are open to us. A frequent recommendation is that the scale used in the construction of risk sets should be that with the strongest relationship with event occurrence, and this would argue for age being dealt with in this way. However, mortality in the elderly also varies quite markedly with calendar time, owing to climatic fluctuations, influenza epidemics, and so on. While the age relationship is a smoothly increasing function and may easily be modelled by a linear or quadratic function, the relationship with calendar time is very irregular. It follows that a better strategy is to take calendar time as the scale for definition of risk sets, and to include age in the model as a time-dependent continuous quantitative variable.

Fig. 32.4 illustrates the construction of the risk set in calendar time. The risk set corresponding to each death consists of all those subjects under study in the time slice containing it — illustrated by the vertical band in the diagram. Two of our four subjects belong to the indicated risk set — one as the case. At the relevant date, both have been bereaved and the model would assign them different values of θ (> 1.0) according to the time since their bereavement.

The analysis could also be carried out by creating a nested case-control study by sampling risk sets. This possibility also suggests the design of a *true* case-control study.

Exercise 32.2. Describe a case-control study into mortality following bereavement which mirrors the analysis described above. What sources of bias can you foresee?

32.3   Estimating the parameters of a screening test

Our final example concerns the estimation of the parameters of a cancer screening programme.[‡] The aim of such programmes is to detect cancer during the *preclinical detectable phase* (PCDP) — the period, prior to the time at which the disease would have been detected symptomatically, during which there is some possibility of detecting the disease by screening. Two parameters which it is important to know are the *sojourn time* (the name given to the duration of the PCDP) and the *sensitivity*, defined as the probability of detecting disease by screening during the PCDP. We shall denote these parameters by τ and π respectively, so that π is the probability that screening would detect the disease if applied within a period of

---

[‡]Day, N.E. and Walter, S.D., *Biometrics*, **40**, 1–14.

duration τ before the time at which the disease would have been discovered anyway.

Interpretation of these parameters and comparisons between different population groups and screening tests requires some care. In general, a better test will lead to increases in both π and τ. More rapid development of tumours will be reflected in decreased values for τ, since the disease will move through the PCDP more quickly. Finally, τ will also be affected by factors which determine rapidity of diagnosis in the absence of screening, so that populations with better access to medical services will usually have smaller values for τ.

We shall now show how these parameters may be estimated from studies of *interval tumours* — incident cases detected by normal clinical means in the intervals between screening appointments. Let us consider the expected variation of incidence following a negative screening test under our simple model, assuming first that the test is 100% sensitive (i.e. $\pi = 1.0$). In this case, there would be zero incidence of interval tumours for a period of length τ following the negative screen, since all the tumours which would have arisen in this period will have been detected at screening. Conversely, after a time τ has elapsed since screening, the rate of diagnosis of interval tumours will return to the normal incidence rate in an unscreened population, since no tumour detected in this period could possibly have been found at the screening appointment. Thus, the rate ratio

$$\frac{\text{Incidence rate of interval tumours following negative screening test}}{\text{Incidence rate in the unscreened population}}$$

will be 0 until time τ following screening, and then jump to 1. Making allowance for less than 100% sensitivity leads to the relationship shown in Fig. 32.5; the proportion of the normal incidence seen in the period after screening is contributed by those cases missed by the screening test.

This model is clearly oversimplified, and we would not expect to observe anything so clearly defined in practice. A more realistic model may be obtained either by allowing for sojourn times to vary or, alternatively, allowing the sensitivity of the test to vary smoothly throughout the PCDP from zero up to π. These models are indistinguishable and lead to a predicted incidence pattern such as is shown in Fig. 32.6. The curve shown is a simple exponential function of time elapsed since negative screen,

$$\text{Rate ratio} = 1 - \pi \exp\left(-\frac{\text{Time since screen}}{\tau}\right).$$

The parameters of this curve, π and τ, may be thought of as the sensitivity and mean sojourn time respectively.

Fig. 32.7 illustrates observation of four subjects in a follow-up study. Three of these enter the study prior to having been screened but are

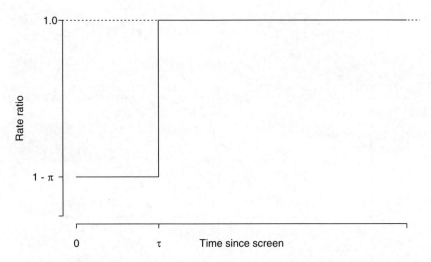

Fig. 32.5.   Incidence following a negative screen.

screened during follow-up, while the fourth enters the study some time after a negative screening test. Two of the subjects subsequently develop interval tumours. In an analysis with calendar time as the major time scale,

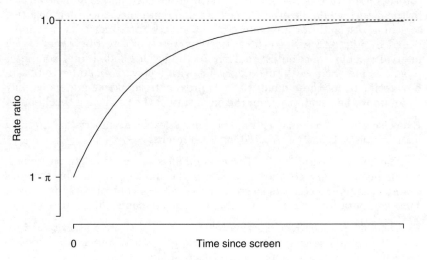

Fig. 32.6.   A more realistic evolution of incidence.

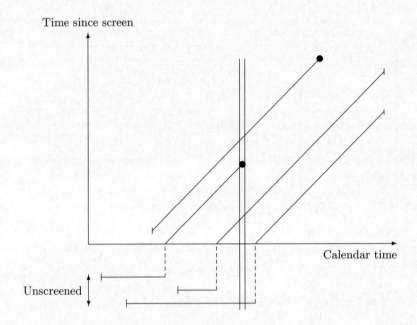

Fig. 32.7. A follow-up study of incidence following a negative screen.

these cases will be compared with risk sets comprising all individuals under study at the date of diagnosis. In the diagram this is illustrated for the first case by the vertical band. It can be seen that all four of the indicated subjects fall into this risk set; one is still unscreened and is assigned $\theta = 1$ by the model, while the other three have different times since their negative screening test and, for any values of τ and π, a model such as that illustrated by Fig. 32.6 assigns three different values of θ to the others. Each interval tumour contributes similarly to the log likelihood, and computer programs may be used to maximize this with respect to τ and π to obtain best estimates of these quantities. Approximate confidence intervals may be found in the usual way from the curvature of the profile log- likelihoods.

Exercise 32.3. What assumption concerning selection of subjects for screening must hold for this analysis to yield unbiased results?

The above discussion slightly over-simplifies the analysis. In particular, it will be necessary to allow for age in the model. As in our previous example, sampling risk sets to create a nested case-control study will avoid some computation, and also suggests a true case-control design.

Exercise 32.4. Describe a case-control study to investigate sensitivity and sojourn time of a screening test for breast cancer. Would you expect to obtain approximately the same results as in a cohort study?

Solutions to the exercises

32.1 The Transplant main effect measures the log rate ratio immediately following transplantation. We might expect this to be positive immediately after surgery, corresponding to an elevated mortality rate, but then to decrease with time, giving way eventually to a beneficial effect. In this case the interaction parameter would be negative.

The predictions of the model in terms of the log rate ratio are shown in Fig. 32.8. The parameter α is the Transplant initial effect and is shown here as positive, indicating an adverse effect. The slope of the line is the Transplant·Time interaction parameter and is shown as negative. This model predicts that transplantation will have an increasingly beneficial effect with increased time from transplantation. The horizontal dotted line represents the level of mortality in untransplanted controls. On the original scale, the rate ratio initially jumps to $\exp(\alpha)$ immediately after transplant but then falls exponentially towards zero.

32.2 The events of interest are deaths in elderly people, let us say those over 70 years of age. A geographically based case-control study would include as cases all such deaths amongst residents of a town or county. Each time such a death occurs, a set of controls would be drawn from the study base. Matching of controls to cases for age and sex would improve the efficiency of the study. Information concerning vital status of spouse and, where appropriate, date of death of spouse, would be obtained retrospectively for all cases and controls. This study would run little risk of information bias, since the relevant data are on public record. However, selection bias could be a problem. These are some of the problems:

- A suitable, accurate, sampling frame may not be available.

- Refusal to participate by potential controls could lead to 'volunteer' bias in the control group finally obtained.

- Migration away from the sampling frame as a result of bereavement is a very real possibility. A bereaved old person may not be able to care for him or herself and might be forced to go into residential care or to live with relatives.

These problems do not exist when a cohort of identified subjects is followed prospectively.

32.3 It must be assumed that individuals selected for screening would have the same subsequent incidence rates as those not selected. This assumption would not be violated by a screening policy which varies with age, providing confounding by age is dealt with in the analysis. However, if patients are referred to screening as a result of early non-specific symptoms, there would be some bias.

32.4   A population based screening programme requires a computer register to generate screening invitations, so this register can form the study base. The study would be of newly diagnosed cases who were not diagnosed as a result of routine screening and whose names could be found on the computer register. Controls for each case would then be drawn from this register. If carried out carefully, it is difficult to see any reason why such a study should give different answers from a cohort study. Indeed, the existence of the computer register means that the study is really nested within a cohort study (see Chapter 33).

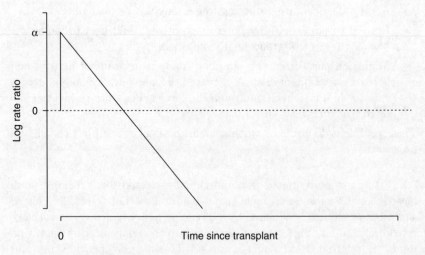

Fig. 32.8.   Log rate ratio against time since transplant.

33
Nested case-control studies

Any cohort study can be used to generate a case-control study by sampling the cohort for controls to use in place of the full cohort. The case-control study is then said to be *nested* in the cohort study. For each case the controls are chosen from those members of the cohort who are at risk at that moment, in other words from the risk set defined by the case. Although the idea of nested case-control studies predates Cox's method for the analysis of cohort studies, the design and analysis of such studies has been greatly clarified by the ideas of partial likelihood and risk sets.

33.1 Reasons for using a nested case-control study

The main reason for using a nested study is to reduce the labour and cost of data collection by collecting complete data only for those subjects who are chosen for the nested study. For example, in cardiovascular epidemiology the habitual energy expenditure of subjects has been measured using detailed diary records in which subjects record their physical activities in 15-minute blocks. Coding these diary records into energy expenditure is time consuming and expensive, but with a nested case-control design this conversion is only needed for the cases and their controls. Similar considerations apply to coding diary records in cohort studies in nutritional epidemiology, and to expensive laboratory analyses on biological specimens — these can be collected for all subjects in the cohort but "banked" and analyzed only for cases and their controls.

Another use of nested case-control studies is when an on-going cohort study is to be used to address a question about an exposure or confounder not measured in the original design. Data collection can be restricted to those subjects in a nested study. For example, suppose that routine health service monitoring data shows differences in mortality between groups of patients but, because information is not available on important confounders, it is not possible to exclude confounding as an explanation. A more detailed abstraction of medical records in a nested case-control study could make it possible to measure the confounders in the nested study and hence to control for them.

The final reason for using a nested case-control study is to avoid the computational burden associated with time-dependent explanatory vari-

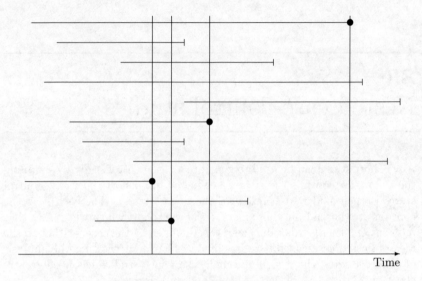

Fig. 33.1. Definition of risk sets.

ables. This problem was discussed briefly in Chapter 31, where we indicated that a natural design for such studies is to randomly sample the *risk sets* on which a full analysis by Cox's method would be based. In this chapter we discuss this suggestion in more detail.

33.2 Sampling risk sets

In nested case-control studies, controls are drawn for each case from the corresponding risk set. Fig. 33.1 shows the risk sets for a follow-up study of eleven subjects, four of whom fail. Corresponding to each of these four events is a risk set containing all those subjects under study at the moment of event occurrence — that is, all subjects whose observation lines cross the relevant vertical. To select controls we ignore the case and choose a random sample of the remaining subjects in the risk set. Sampling of a risk set must be carried out independently both of the sampling of other risk sets and of any later failure or censoring of its members.

Exercise 33.1. What are the sizes of the four risk sets? Indicate how you would select a single control for each case.

In the analysis of the full cohort study using Cox's method, each of the events contributes a term of the form

$$\log \left(\theta_{\text{(for case)}} \Big/ \sum_{\text{Risk set}} \theta \right)$$

to the log partial likelihood. When the risk sets are sampled this becomes

$$\log \left(\theta_{\text{(for case)}} \Big/ \sum_{\text{Case-control set}} \theta \right),$$

which is identical to the log likelihood contribution of a matched case-control set in a conditional logistic regression analysis.

CAN THE SAME SUBJECT BE INCLUDED MORE THAN ONCE?

In the procedure for sampling risk sets described above the same subject can be selected as a control more than once and may eventually become a case. This will not happen very often for rare events but when it does it should be permitted. Any intervention in the sampling procedure to prevent its happening violates the requirement for independent sampling of risk sets.

A second aspect of this question is illustrated by the fourth subject shown in Fig. 33.1 who belongs to all four risk sets. If this subject is drawn as a control in one of these risk sets it is tempting to use him or her as an extra control in the other sets. Including a subject in all samples for which he/she is eligible represents an extremely *interdependent* method of sampling risk sets. The result is that the successive terms which contribute to the partial likelihood are no longer independent — each term does not contribute quite as much *new* information as it appears. When this dependence is taken into account the expected gain in precision as a result of multiple use of controls largely evaporates. However, there may be other advantages. One is that, because controls are no longer tied to a particular risk set, they can be randomly selected at the time of recruitment into the cohort study. This design has been called a *case-cohort* study, and some logistic advantages have been claimed. One situation in which it might be considered is for studies in which several different types of event are of interest — for example, occurrence of several different cancers. Independent sampling of risk sets leads to a different set of controls for each type of event while the case-cohort design allows a single control sample to be used for all outcomes. Against this must be weighed the fact that a more complex analysis is required to take account of the interdependency in the sampling of controls.

HOW MANY CONTROLS?

If there are m times as many controls as cases, the precision of the case-control study compared to the cohort study is given by

$$\frac{\text{SD of estimate from case-control data}}{\text{SD of estimate from entire study base}} = \sqrt{1 + \frac{1}{m}}.$$

This formula applies to the simple situation where the exposure effect is small and there is no control for confounding, but it can also be used as a rough guide more generally. Since $\sqrt{1 + 1/m}$ is only slightly greater than 1 for $m > 5$ little accuracy is lost by taking five or at most ten controls for each case, rather than the whole risk set.

33.3   Matching

In an occupational study of lung cancer, smoking will be a strong confounder, and the comparison of occupational groups should therefore be controlled for smoking. An overall sample of (say) five controls per case could lead to a very different ratio within smokers and non- smokers. Since there will be many more cases among the smokers than among the non-smokers it is likely that there will fewer than five controls per case among smokers and many more than five per case among non-smokers. In such cases it would be better to match controls to cases with respect to smoking habits. Of course, this requires that smoking data are available for the entire cohort. The contribution to the log likelihood now becomes

$$\log \left(\theta_{(\text{for case})} \Big/ \sum \theta \right)$$

where the $\sum \theta$ denominator refers to summation over the case and the matched controls. Matching the controls to the cases on smoking does not allow estimation of the smoking effect, but when smoking is a confounder this need not concern us.

$\boxed{\star}$ 33.4   Counter-matching

In the previous section we discussed the situation where the values of the confounding variables are known for all subjects in the cohort and a nested case-control study is used to reduce the cost of measuring the exposure. Matching controls to cases on the confounding variables can improve the precision of the comparison of exposure groups although, as a side-effect, the effects of the confounding variables cannot be estimated. What about the opposite situation in which the exposure variable is measured for all subjects in the cohort and a nested case-control study is used to reduce the cost of measuring the confounding variables? In this case it would be disastrous to match the controls to the cases on exposure since we would then be unable to estimate the effect of exposure. However, the information available for the full cohort can still be used to sample controls more efficiently.

To illustrate this we consider first the case in which all subjects are classified as exposed or unexposed. For any particular risk set let the numbers of exposed and unexposed subjects be N_1 and N_0 respectively, and suppose we are to draw m controls. The nested case-control set will contain $n = m + 1$ subjects (the case plus m controls). Let the split of these n subjects between exposed and unexposed be n_1 and n_0. When controls are drawn by simple random sampling of the risk sets this can produce a very uneven split of exposed and unexposed subjects and lead to inefficiency. The efficiency of the study can be improved by fixing the split in advance — usually to be 50:50.

For example, suppose that there are 10 exposed and 100 unexposed subjects in the risk set and we wish to select a sample of 5 exposed and 5 unexposed, including the case which defines the risk set. If the case is exposed this means we need 4 exposed controls and 5 unexposed controls. If the case is unexposed we need 5 exposed controls and 4 unexposed controls. For a sample of one exposed and one unexposed an exposed case will always be paired with an unexposed control and an unexposed case with an exposed control. It is from this that the term *counter-matching* is derived.

When sampling in this way the contribution of each risk set to the partial log likelihood must be adjusted to reflect the fact that the exposure distribution in the sample is different from the exposure distribution in the risk set. The modified log partial likelihood contributions take the form

$$
\log \left((W\theta)_{\text{(for case)}} \Big/ \sum_{\text{Case-control set}} (W\theta) \right),
$$

where W are *risk weights* for each subject which compensate for the sampling. These weights take the values

$$
W = \begin{cases} N_1/n_1 & \text{for an exposed subject} \\ N_0/n_0 & \text{for an unexposed subject.} \end{cases}
$$

Note that the choice of weight depends only on exposure status and not upon whether the subject is a case or a control.

Exercise 33.2. What are the weights for exposed and unexposed subjects in a risk set with $N_1 = 10$ exposed subjects and $N_0 = 100$ unexposed subjects, in a 1:1 counter-matched study?

Exercise 33.3. For the special case where there are no confounders θ takes the value 1 for an unexposed subject and the value ϕ for an exposed subject, where ϕ is the (multiplicative) exposure effect. Show that, using the correct weights, the partial log likelihood contribution for the 1:1 sampled set is identical to the contribution of this risk set to the full cohort analysis.

The design and analysis extends readily to the case where there are more than two exposure categories. If the risk set contains N_i subjects in exposure category i and the case-control set is to contain n_i, then we draw either $n_i - 1$ or n_i controls at random according to whether or not the case falls into this category. The risk weight for subjects in this category is N_i/n_i.

The same design and analysis may be used when exposure data is difficult or expensive to collect, but in which we have a surrogate measure available for all subjects. If exposure is rare, it makes sense to use the surrogate exposure measurements to construct a more efficient nested study in which there is a more even split between exposed and unexposed subjects. In a 1:1 study, for example, a case classified as exposed by the surrogate measure would be paired with a control classified as unexposed, and a case classified as unexposed paired with a control classified as exposed. Remembering that in the 1:1 study only exposure discordant pairs are informative for the estimation of the exposure effect, this design is more efficient since it should increase the number of such pairs.

An area in which counter-matching by surrogate exposure measurement could prove particularly useful is pharmacoepidemiology. Exposure to any one drug is rare and can usually only be ascertained after detailed checking of medical records. However, a simple questionnaire might be very successful at identifying a subgroup particularly likely to have taken the drug of interest. The nested case-control study should contain all subjects in the group likely to have taken the drug, and a random sample of the remainder. With this design, the introduction of the correct risk weights into the partial likelihood analysis provides a valid estimate of the drug effect.

★ ## 33.5   Two-stage sampling of controls

Both matching and counter-matching require that some information is available for all subjects in the cohort. The general rule is that, when this concerns a confounder we should consider using it for matching controls to cases while, if it concerns an exposure of interest, we should consider counter-matching.

Similar ideas may be useful even when we have no such data for the full cohort or, indeed, in a conventional case-control study. The information to be used in the final matching or counter-matching is collected in an initial study but complete data collection is only followed through in a subsample. This is known as a *two-stage* case-control study.

Solutions to the exercises

33.1   The risk set for the first event contains 10 subjects, the others contain 9, 7, and 4 subjects respectively. A control for the first case is selected at random from the remaining 9 subjects in the risk set. Similarly the remaining controls are sampled at random from the 8, 6, and 3 eligible subjects in the remaining risk sets.

33.2   In the 1:1 counter-matched study each set contains $n = 2$ subjects,

1 exposed and 1 unexposed so that $n_1 = n_0 = 1$. The risk weights used in the analysis are therefore,

$$W = \begin{cases} 10 & \text{for an exposed subject} \\ 100 & \text{for an unexposed subject.} \end{cases}$$

33.3 Suppose the case is exposed. Using the whole risk set the contribution to the log partial likelihood is

$$\log \left(\frac{\phi}{10 \times \phi + 100 \times 1} \right).$$

Using the 1:1 counter-matched design, the contribution to the partial log likelihood is

$$\log \left(\frac{(10\phi)}{(10\phi) + (100)} \right) = \log(10) + \log \left(\frac{\phi}{10 \times \phi + 100 \times 1} \right).$$

These two expressions are the same except for a constant term, $\log(10)$, which does not depend on ϕ and can be ignored. The same is true when the case is unexposed.

34
Gaussian regression models

Most of this book has been about events such as the incidence of disease or mortality. Although events are particularly important in epidemiology, in some studies the response of interest is a quantitative measurement such as blood pressure. The most widely used probability model for such responses is the Gaussian model, described in Chapter 8. In this chapter we show how regression models are used in conjunction with the Gaussian probability model. We shall call this combination *Gaussian regression* although it is more usual for it to be called simply regression or *multiple regression* because it was developed before other regression methods.

34.1 Models for the mean

The Gaussian probability model differs from the binary model in having two parameters instead of one. These are μ, the mean, and σ, the standard deviation. In the simplest situation changing the level of an explanatory variable changes the value of μ but leaves σ unchanged. The distributions of response for a comparison of exposed and unexposed subjects predicted by such a model is illustrated in Fig. 34.1. The effect of exposure is measured by the difference between the means, $\mu_1 - \mu_0$.

To control for confounding by age, using stratification, we would stratify by age and make the assumption that $\mu_1 - \mu_0$ is constant across age groups. This is equivalent to fitting the regression model

$$\text{Mean} = \text{Corner} + \text{Age} + \text{Exposure}.$$

The effect of exposure in this model is simply the (common) difference between mean responses for exposed and unexposed subjects within age groups.

To illustrate such models we shall use some additional data from the study of diet and coronary heart disease. These concern daily intake of fibre which is the response variable. Age and occupation are the explanatory variables, both with three levels.* Table 34.1 shows a simple summary of these data in which a separate estimate of mean and standard deviation

---

*Unpublished data

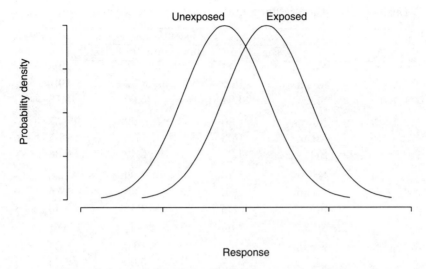

Fig. 34.1.   Effect of exposure on the mean response.

has been calculated for each of the nine age–occupation groups. The main
interest is in differences between occupations and inspection of the estimated means suggests that there is a systematic tendency for bank clerks
to eat more fibre than the drivers and conductors. There is no obvious
systematic variation in the standard deviation parameters, so the assumption that changing the levels of age and occupation does not affect σ is
reasonable.

The additive regression model relating the mean daily intake of fibre to
the effects of age and occupation is

$$\text{Mean} = \text{Corner} + \text{Age} + \text{Work}.$$

When both age and work are treated as categorical this has five parameters
in all, namely the Corner, Age(1), Age(2), Work(1), and Work(2) parameters. These are called the *regression parameters* to distinguish them from
σ, the common standard deviation, which is called the *residual standard
deviation*. The square of σ is called the *residual variance*.

34.2   Likelihood, sums of squares, and deviance

From Chapter 8, the log likelihood for a study of size N is

$$-N \log(\sigma) - \frac{1}{2} \sum_{\text{Subjects}} \left(\frac{x - \mu}{\sigma} \right)^2.$$

Table 34.1. Dietary fibre intake (gm/day) by age and occupation

Age		Occupation		
		Bus driver	Bus conductor	Bank clerk
< 45	N	23	16	38
	Mean	16.1	17.2	19.1
	SD	3.91	5.00	5.53
45 − 49	N	30	29	57
	Mean	16.3	17.0	18.5
	SD	4.22	5.42	6.88
50+	N	45	39	56
	Mean	16.6	14.8	17.6
	SD	6.28	4.48	5.43
All	N	98	84	151
	Mean	16.4	16.0	18.34
	SD	5.17	5.00	6.04

However, in contrast with Chapter 8, the mean parameter μ is not a single constant but can vary from subject to subject according to the regression model. In our example μ can take nine different values according to the combination of age and occupation. For estimating the regression parameters the $N \log(\sigma)$ term in the log likelihood can be ignored, and because σ is assumed to be the same for all subjects the parameter values which minimize the sum of squared differences,

$$\sum (x - \mu)^2,$$

will also maximize the log likelihood, regardless of the value of σ. Thus the most likely values of the regression parameters do not depend on σ. Because they minimize a sum of squared differences they are also called *least squares estimates*. The minimum value which this sum of squared differences takes is known as the *residual sum of squares*.

For example, Table 34.2 shows the parameter estimates for the model

$$\text{Mean} = \text{Corner} + \text{Work}$$

for the dietary fibre data. The table shows most likely values for the three parameters in this model, together with their standard deviations. The standard deviation of each regression parameter has been calculated from the profile log likelihood obtained by maximizing the log likelihood with respect to all the other regression parameters. Although the estimated values of these parameters do not depend on σ their standard deviations do, and in constructing the table σ has been taken equal to 5.5401 (we

Table 34.2. Effects of work on fibre intake (gm/day)

Parameter	Estimate	SD
Corner	16.425	0.560
Work(1)	−0.402	0.824
Work(2)	1.911	0.719

shall see where this value comes from later in the chapter).

Exercise 34.1. Use the results in Table 34.2 to find the 90% confidence interval for the Work(1) parameter.

34.3   Analysis of deviance

The deviance for any fitted model is defined as minus twice the log likelihood ratio, when this compares the fitted model with a *saturated* model which has a parameter for each record. When the records refer to individual subjects the saturated model has $\mu = x$ so the deviance is

$$\sum \left(\frac{x - \mu}{\sigma}\right)^2.$$

This is proportional to the residual sum of squares for that model.[†] As before, the degrees of freedom for the deviance are equal to the the number of parameters in the saturated regression model, which is equal to the number of subjects N, less the number of parameters in the regression model which has been fitted. These are also the degrees of freedom for the residual sums of squares.

The deviance can be used to compare models in the same way as in Chapter 24, but all calculations are first done in terms of residual sums of squares and later converted to deviances by dividing by a suitable estimate of the square of σ. The residual sums of squares are obtained from the *analysis of variance* table which is usually in the output when a Gaussian regression model is fitted. For example, the analysis of variance table produced when fitting the model

$$\text{Mean} = \text{Corner} + \text{Age} + \text{Work}$$

to the data in Table 34.1 would look something like Table 34.3. The most important line in this table is the middle one labelled 'Error' which gives

---

[†]In the original definition of the idea of deviance, this was called the *scaled* deviance because of its dependence on the unknown scale parameter σ and the word deviance was reserved for its value when σ is taken as 1. However, this usage has not received widespread acceptance.

Table 34.3. Analysis of variance for the variable work

Source	DF	SSq
Model	2	369.891
Error	330	10128.636
Total	332	10498.527

the residual sum of squares for the model which has been fitted and its degrees of freedom. Since the number of subjects is $N = 333$ and the regression model has three parameters, the degrees of freedom here are $333 - 3 = 330$. The last line of the table, headed 'Total' gives the same information for the degenerate model

$$\text{Mean} = \text{Corner}$$

in which the mean response is the same for all subjects. This regression model has only one parameter so the degrees of freedom for its residual sum of squares and deviance are 332. The line labelled 'Model' is obtained by subtracting the degrees of freedom and the residual sum of squares for the error and total lines. When this difference in residual sum of squares is converted to a difference in deviance by division by the square of a suitable estimate of σ, it provides us with a test of the null hypothesis that all parameters in the model, other than the corner parameter, are zero. In this case this would be a test of the difference between occupations.

With more than one explanatory variable, testing the hypothesis that all the parameters in the model are zero is rarely of any interest. The only use of analysis of variance tables for such models is to obtain the residual sum of squared deviations from the second line. By fitting a series of models a more useful table can be constructed, as follows. Table 34.4 shows the residual sums of squares extracted from the analysis of variance tables for five models fitted to the fibre data. Changes in residual sums of squares from one model to another can be converted to deviances and used to test a variety of hypotheses. For example, the effects of work controlled for age can be tested by using the change in residual sum of squares between models 3 and 4.

ESTIMATING σ

Using the joint likelihood for the regression parameters and σ it can be shown, using calculus, that the most likely value of σ is

$$\sqrt{\frac{\text{Residual sum of squares}}{N}}.$$

Table 34.4.   Analysis of deviance ($\sigma = 5.5445$)

Mean = Corner + $\cdots$	DF	SSq	Deviance
1. –	332	10498.527	341.510
2. Work	330	10128.636	329.478
3. Age	330	10384.702	337.807
4. Age + Work	328	10048.456	326.870
5. Age + Work + Age·Work	324	9960.268	324.000

This is the value of σ which maximizes the total likelihood and it therefore also maximizes the profile likelihood for σ. When the number of regression parameters is large compared with the number of subjects, it is preferable to use a conditional likelihood which depends only on σ, rather than the profile likelihood. The most likely value of σ is then equal to the residual sum of squares divided by its degrees of freedom. For example, the value of σ used throughout Table 34.4 was

$$\sigma = \sqrt{9960.268/324} = 5.5445$$

which is the conditional estimate obtained from model 5, although the overall most likely value is

$$\sigma = \sqrt{9960.268/333} = 5.4691$$

It can be seen that the use of the degrees of freedom in place of N has a negligible effect for a study of this size. The reason why σ is generally estimated from the conditional likelihood can be illustrated by a simple argument. If we imagine a study of 10 subjects and fit a regression model with 10 parameters it will fit the observations exactly. The overall most likely value of σ would be zero but the reality is that we have no data for estimating σ. Only when we add an eleventh subject to our study do we start collecting information about σ. It follows that the *effective* size of the study for the purposes of estimating σ is given by the N minus the number of regression parameters — the degrees of freedom — and the estimated value of σ should be

$$\sqrt{\frac{\text{Residual sum of squares}}{\text{Degrees of freedom}}}.$$

One consequence of using this estimate is that the deviance for the model used to estimate σ is equal to its degrees of freedom.

A test for interaction between work and age may be obtained by comparing the deviances for models 4 and 5. The difference in deviance is $326.870 - 324.000 = 2.870$ with $326 - 324 = 2$ degrees of freedom. Referring this to the chi-squared distribution shows this to be clearly non-

Table 34.5.   Effects of age and work on fibre intake (gm/day)

Parameter	Estimate	SD
Corner	16.430	0.560
Age(1)	−0.223	0.814
Age(2)	−1.118	0.788
Work(1)	−0.387	0.824
Work(2)	1.828	0.720

significant so that we are reassured concerning our assumption of constant occupational effects over age groups.

The parameter estimates for model 4 are shown in Table 34.5. Note, however, that the value of σ used to calculate the standard deviations of the parameters is slightly different from that used in Table 34.4. This is because, whereas the estimate of σ used in Table 34.4 was obtained from model 5, Table 34.5 refers to model 4 and it is therefore logical to estimate σ using this model, that is by

$$\sigma = \sqrt{10048.456/328} = 5.5349.$$

The significance of the occupational effect, controlled for age, can be tested by comparing the deviances for models 4 and 3. However, since this test only makes sense when there is no interaction, deviances should properly be calculated using the model 4 estimate of σ rather than that used in Table 34.4.

Exercise 34.2. Carry out the test for the effect of occupation controlled for age.

Similarly, the value of σ used to calculate standard deviations of parameter estimates in Table 34.2 is obtained from model 2,

$$\sigma = \sqrt{10128.636/330} = 5.5401$$

and this is the value which would be used if we wished to compare models 1 and 2. In practice the difference between the possible estimates of σ are usually inconsequential except in very small studies.

F RATIO TESTS

The tests discussed above refer changes in deviance to the appropriate chi-squared distribution. If the value of σ were a known constant, these would be *exact tests*. However, when σ is estimated they are only approximate. Exact tests which take account of the fact that σ is estimated may be carried out using *F distributions*, tables of which are readily available. Instead of referring the change in deviance to the chi-square distribution, we divide it by the corresponding degrees of freedom to obtain the *F ratio*. For example, the change in deviance for the test for interaction was 2.870, with two degrees of freedom, so the corresponding F ratio is 1.435. To obtain the exact p-value, the F ratio is referred to the correct F distribution. However, to select the correct F distribution, we must specify two different numbers of degrees of freedom. The first, called the *numerator* degrees of freedom, is the same as the degrees of freedom for the approximate chi-squared test while the second, called the *denominator* degrees of freedom, is the number of degrees of freedom used to estimate σ. In our example these are 2 and 334 respectively.

In practice there is only a noticeable difference between F ratio tests and the approximate chi-squared test in small studies. In our example, the p-value obtained from the chi-squared distribution is 0.2381 while that obtained from the F distribution is 0.2396. Since the F ratio test is only exact if the assumptions of Gaussian distribution shape and constancy of σ are true, they are not usually worth the (admittedly slight) extra trouble.

34.4 Multiplicative models $\boxed{\star}$

A basic assumption in the Gaussian regression model is that changes in the explanatory variables affect the mean level of response but not the variability. However, it is commonly the case that as the level of response goes up, so does its variability. A simple multiplicative model acting at the individual level would explain this, for if the effect of changing the level of work is to double the values of the individual responses, then the standard deviation of these individual values will also get doubled. On a log scale, however, the effect of doubling the response will be to add log(2) to the log response, leaving the standard deviation of the log responses unchanged. This suggests that when the effects appear to act multiplicatively at an individual level, the log response should be analysed in place of the response.

There is some suggestion in Table 34.1 that standard deviation of fibre intake goes up with the mean, so that a multiplicative model may be more appropriate. This suggests analysing log fibre intakes rather than fibre intakes themselves. Inspection of the data suggests that the distribution of log fibre intake is closer to the Gaussian shape than the distribution of fibre intake, and this is another point in favour of analysing log fibre intakes. When the Gaussian regression model

$$\text{Mean} = \text{Corner} + \text{Age} + \text{Work}.$$

is fitted to the logs of the fibre intakes we obtain the parameter estimates shown in Table 34.6.

The effect parameters shown in this table are additive effects upon log fibre intake and these should be exponentiated to express them as multi-

Table 34.6.　Effects of age and work on log fibre intake

Parameter	Estimate	SD
Corner	2.8039	0.0430
Age(1)	−0.0253	0.0445
Age(2)	−0.0800	0.0431
Work(1)	−0.0345	0.0451
Work(2)	0.0962	0.0394

plicative effects on fibre intake. The error factor method can be used to calculate confidence intervals for the multiplicative effects.

Exercise 34.3. Express the estimates of the Work parameters as multiplicative effects, and calculate 90% confidence intervals.

Apart from this change in the way the parameter estimates are interpreted the use of the log response in place of the response does not affect matters. Models are compared using residual sums of squares in the same way as before.

If the effect of the explanatory variables is multiplicative at a group level, but not at an individual level, so that σ is constant, a multiplicative model such as

$$\text{Mean} = \text{Corner} \times \text{Age} \times \text{Work},$$

can be fitted to the data on the original scale. Computer programs are available for fitting such models but the need for them rarely arises because the idea of an explanatory variable acting multiplicatively at a group level but not at an individual level is rather implausible.

Solutions to the exercises

34.1　The 90% confidence interval is from $-0.402 - 1.645 \times 0.824 = -1.757$ to $-0.402 + 1.645 \times 0.824 = 0.953$. The lower limit is a reduction of 1.757 gm, the upper limit is an increase of 0.953 gm.

34.2　The appropriate value for σ is 5.5349, taken from the model which includes both age and work. The deviance for this model is then 328.000, and the deviance for the model which includes age alone is

$$10384.702/5.5349^2 = 338.982.$$

The change in deviances is $338.982 - 328.000 = 10.982$ on 2 degrees of freedom, for which $p = 0.004$ (from the chi-squared distribution on two degrees of freedom.

34.3   The Work(1) parameter is estimated as -0.0345, and since

$$\exp(-0.0345) = 0.966,$$

the fibre intakes of conductors are 0.966 times those of drivers. The 90% confidence interval for this ratio is found from the error factor

$$\exp(1.645 \times 0.0451) = 1.077,$$

to be from $0.966/1.077 = 0.897$ to $0.966 \times 1.077 = 1.04$. Similarly, the multiplicative effect of Work(2) is 1.101 with 90% confidence interval from 1.032 to 1.175.

35
Postscript

No scientific methodology stands still and statistical modelling is no exception. In this book we have deliberately restricted our attention to well-established methods which have become a routine part of modern epidemiology, and omitted newer developments, even though some of these will undoubtedly make important contributions to epidemiology in the future. Two areas in particular are worth mentioning. The first is the extension of the models discussed in this book to deal with errors of measurement of explanatory variables (see Chapter 27). The second concerns the extension of these models to *longitudinal studies* in which the response is measured on several different occasions for each subject.

The methods we have described concentrate on the analysis of response at the level of the individual subject. Even when these analyses have been carried out using frequency records this has been purely for computational convenience and parameters still refer to the effects upon the response for an individual subject. However, some epidemiological research is based upon the behaviour of aggregated groups of individuals, for example the inhabitants of a country, region, or town. Statistical analysis then concentrates on description and 'explanation' of differences in the aggregate responses of such groups in time and space. By analogy with the discipline of economics, such activity could be termed *macro-epidemiology*. We have not dealt with it in this book, firstly because this field is currently undergoing active development, and secondly because new likelihoods and fitting procedures become necessary as a result of the more complicated probability models which are a necessary response to lack of data at the subject level.

Some further reading

A good elementary introduction to statistical modelling using the computer program GLIM is:

Healy, M. (1988) *GLIM. An Introduction.* Oxford Science Publications, Oxford University Press, Oxford.

The reader who requires more mathematical details can find them in a number of statistical texts. General treatments of regression model, including Poisson and logistic regression, are given by the following authors.

Aitkin, M., Anderson, D., Francis, B., and Hinde, J. (1989) *Statistical modelling in GLIM*. Oxford Science Publications, Oxford University Press, Oxford.

McCullagh, M. and Nelder, J.A. (1989) *Generalized linear models* (2nd edn). Chapman and Hall, London.

Descriptions of modern statistical approaches to the analysis of life tables and survival data are given by the following authors.

Cox, D.R. and Oakes, D. (1984) *The analysis of survival data*. Chapman and Hall, London.

Kalbfleisch, J.D. and Prentice, R.L. (1980) *The statistical analysis of failure time data*. Wiley, New York.

A detailed exposition of a more general mathematical approach to modelling event occurrence in time is to be found in:

Andersen, P.K., Borgan, Ø., Gill, R.D., and Keiding, N. (1993) *Statistical models based on counting processes*. Springer, New York.

Intermediate in technical level between these purely statistical texts and this book are:

Breslow, N.E. and Day, N. (1980) *Statistical methods in cancer epidemiology. Vol. I – The analysis of case-control studies*. IARC Scientific Publications No. 32. International Agency for Research on Cancer, Lyon.

Breslow, N.E. and Day, N. (1987) *Statistical methods in cancer epidemiology. Vol. II – The design and analysis of cohort studies*. IARC Scientific Publications No. 82. International Agency for Research on Cancer, Lyon.

A collection of papers dealing with very recent research in epidemiological modelling is:

Moolgavkar, S.H. and Prentice, R.L. (ed.) (1986) *Modern statistical methods in chronic disease epidemiology*. Wiley, New York.

An extensive review of the more recent statistical literature is:

Gail, M.H. (1991) A bibliography and comments on the use of statistical models in epidemiology in the 1980s. *Statistics in Medicine*, **10**, 1819–95.

Part III

Appendices

Appendix A
Exponentials and logarithms

Raising 10 to different powers is a familiar operation. For example,

$$10^1 = 10, \ 10^2 = 100, \ 10^3 = 1000, \ \cdots$$

Mathematically this is regarded as a rule for getting from the power (1, 2, 3, etc.) to the value of 10 raised to that power (10, 100, 1000, etc.). The power is often referred to as the *exponent* and 10 raised to a power is called an *exponential* with base 10.

Raising 10 to a power can be extended to cover fractional powers using the convention that $10^{\frac{1}{2}}$ stands for the square root of 10, $10^{\frac{1}{3}}$ stands for the cube root of 10, and so on. The rule can also be extended to cover negative powers using the convention that 10^{-1} stands for $1/10 = 0.1$. Table A.1 shows the rule for obtaining 10^x from x for a variety of values of x.

Now suppose that we wish to go the other way and, starting with a value of 10^x, find the value of x. For example, starting with 1000 gives $x = 3$, while starting with 0.1 gives $x = -1$. Starting with any positive number y, the value of x which makes $10^x = y$ is called the *logarithm* of y with the base 10 and is written $\log_{10}(y)$. Taking logarithms with base 10 is the inverse operation to exponentiation with base 10. Thus $10^3 = 1000$ and $\log_{10}(1000) = 3$.

Table A.1. Rules for finding 10^x from x

x	$y = 10^x$
0	1
1	10
2	100
3	1000
-1	0.1
-2	0.01
-3	0.001
$\frac{1}{2}$	$\sqrt{10}$
$\frac{1}{3}$	$\sqrt[3]{10}$

Table A.2.   Multiplication using logarithms

Number		Logarithm
7.2	$\longrightarrow$	0.8573
16.9	$\longrightarrow$	1.2279
121.7	$\longleftarrow$	2.0852

Logarithms were introduced as a computational device in the seventeenth century to avoid multiplication and division. Tables were prepared so that the logarithm of any number could be looked up. Similarly, tables of exponentials were prepared so that logarithms could be converted back to the original numbers. These tables of exponentials were called *antilogarithms*. The use of logarithms to multiply 7.2 by 16.9 is shown in Table A.2. Arrows from left to right refer to looking up logarithms while arrows from right to left refer to looking up antilogarithms (exponentiation). The result line follows from addition on the logarithmic (right-hand) side or multiplication on the exponential (left-hand) side. The widespread availability of cheap electronic calculators means that nobody now uses logarithms for multiplication or division. However, their mathematical property of converting multiplication to addition, embodied in

$$\log(7.2 \times 16.9) = \log(7.2) + \log(16.9)$$

is still very useful. Another useful property which follows from this is that

$$\log(7.2^2) = 2 \times \log(7.2)$$

$$\log(7.2^3) = 3 \times \log(7.2)$$

and so on.

Raising 2 to a power is called exponentiation with base 2. The inverse process produces logarithms to the base 2 and these are written $\log_2(y)$. Both exponentials and logarithms can be defined with respect to any base. Fig. A.1 shows plots of the exponential functions 10^x, 3^x, e^x, and 2^x, where the symbol e represents the number 2.71828183. The number e is chosen so that the tangent to the plot of e^x versus x drawn at $x = 0$ has a slope of exactly 1 (shown by the broken line). It follows that *when x is very small,*

$$e^x \approx 1 + x.$$

and, therefore,

$$\log_e(1 + x) \approx x.$$

Logarithms to the base e are referred to as *natural* logarithms, and it is the above property that makes them 'natural'. The natural logarithm

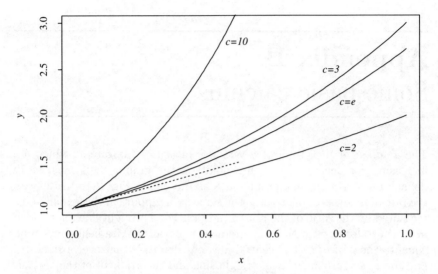

Fig. A.1.   Plots of the function $y = c^x$

function is sometimes written as $\ln(y)$, but in this book we shall *always* use logarithms to the base e, and write them simply as $\log(y)$. We also write the exponential function with base e as $\exp(x)$. Note, however, that many electronic calculators assign an entirely different meaning to a key marked *exp*.

The logarithms of the same number, using different bases, are related by a simple constant multiplier. For example

$$\log_e(y) = \log_{10}(y) \times 2.3026$$

where $2.3026 = \log_e(10)$. Similarly

$$\log_2(y) = \log_{10}(y) \times 3.3219$$

where $3.3219 = \log_2(10)$.

Appendix B
★ Some basic calculus

The *gradient* of the graph of y versus x measures the rate at which y is increasing (or decreasing) at any point on the graph. It is most easily defined for a straight line graph, such as the one in Fig. B.1. In this case the rate of increase or decrease is the same at any point on the graph, and is measured by the ratio of the *rise* to the *run*. For a straight line relationship in which y *decreases* with x the gradient is negative. Gradients have units equal to those of y/x. The central idea of calculus is that over a small run any curve is approximately a straight line and the gradient of the curve at any point in the run is approximately equal to the gradient of this line.

Differential calculus consists of a number of simple rules which are used to evaluate gradients of curves for which the y co-ordinate of any point on the curve is given by some function of the x co-ordinate. The most useful of these are shown in Table B.1. A further very important rule is that the gradient of a function constructed as the *sum* of two simpler functions is

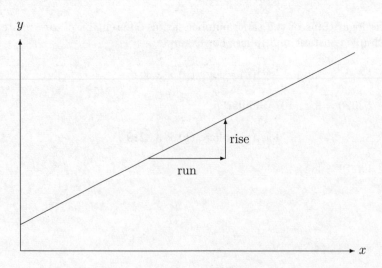

Fig. B.1. Gradient of a straight line graph

Table B.1.   Gradients of some simple functions of x

Function	Gradient
c (constant)	0
x	1
$-x$	-1
cx	c
$(x)^2$	$2x$
$(x)^m$	$m(x)^{m-1}$
$\frac{1}{x} = (x)^{-1}$	$-(x)^{-2} = -\frac{1}{(x)^2}$
$\exp(x)$	$\exp(x)$
$\log(x)$	$\frac{1}{x}$
$(c+x)^2$	$2(c+x)$
$(c-x)^2$	$-2(c-x)$
$\log(c+x)$	$\frac{1}{c+x}$
$\log(c-x)$	$-\frac{1}{c-x}$

the sum of the gradients of the constituent functions so that, for example, the gradient of $x + \log(x)$ is $1 + 1/x$.

The use of these rules is now illustrated by finding the gradient of the log likelihood for a rate λ, based on D cases and Y person years. The log likelihood for λ is

$$D \log(\lambda) - \lambda Y.$$

From Table B.1 the gradient of $\log(\lambda)$ is $1/\lambda$ and the gradient of λ is 1. Hence the gradient of the log likelihood is

$$\frac{D}{\lambda} - Y.$$

The maximum value of the log likelihood occurs when the gradient is zero, that is, when $\lambda = D/Y$, so the most likely value of λ is D/Y.

The curvature of the log likelihood curve at the peak is important in determining the range of supported values. A highly curved peak corresponds to a narrow range. The curvature at a point on a curve is a measure of how fast the gradient is changing from one value of x to the next; if the gradient is changing quickly then the curvature is high, while if the gradient is changing slowly the curvature is low. For log likelihood curves the gradient changes from a positive quantity (on the left) to a negative quantity (on the right) so the gradient decreases as x increases and the curvature is negative.

The curvature of a curve, at a point, is defined to be the rate of change of the gradient of the curve at that point. The way that Table B.1 can be used to find curvature is now illustrated using the log likelihood for λ

again. The gradient of the log likelihood at any value of λ has been shown to be

$$\frac{D}{\lambda} - Y.$$

From Table B.1 the gradient of a constant is zero and the gradient of $1/\lambda$ is $-1/(\lambda)^2$, so the curvature of the log likelihood at any value of λ is

$$-\frac{D}{(\lambda)^2}.$$

Appendix C
Approximate profile likelihoods

★

This appendix describes the mathematics underlying Gaussian approximation of profile log likelihoods.

C.1 The difference between two parameters

We shall start with an important special case. Consider a model with two parameters, β_1 and β_0, and suppose that our main interest is in the *difference*

$$\gamma = \beta_1 - \beta_0.$$

We shall further assume that the log likelihoods for β_1 and β_0 are based on two independent sets of data so that the total log likelihood is the sum of the two separate log likelihoods.

Fig. C.1 illustrates the construction of the profile likelihood for γ. The upper panel of the figure shows the total log likelihood obtained by adding the log likelihoods for β_1 and β_0. Contours are shown for log likelihood ratios of $-5, -4, \ldots, -1$. The four diagonal lines correspond to different values of γ. For example, the top leftmost line represents values of β_1, β_0 satisfying

$$\beta_1 - \beta_0 = 0$$

so that this line corresponds to $\gamma = 0$. Similarly, the remaining lines correspond to values of γ of 0.5, 1.0, and 1.5 respectively. To find the profile likelihood for γ, we find the maximum value of the log likelihood along each of these lines. This maximum is plotted against γ in the lower panel of the figure.

The Gaussian approximation of the profile log likelihood can be obtained from making use of the relationship between gradients and curvatures of the total log likelihood (upper panel), and the gradient and curvature of the profile log likelihood (lower panel). These relationships can be derived using the laws of calculus but are only quoted here.

If, at the maximum of the log likelihood along the line $\beta_1 - \beta_0 = \gamma$, the gradient is G_1 with respect to β_1 and G_0 with respect to β_0 the gradient

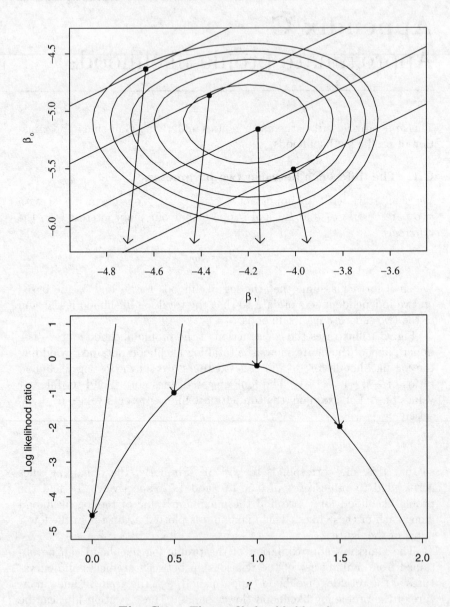

Fig. C.1.   The profile log likelihood

of the profile log likelihood at γ is G, where

$$G = G_1 = -G_0.$$

If C_1, C_0 are the corresponding curvatures with respect to β_1 and β_0, then the curvature of the profile log likelihood at γ is C, where

$$\frac{1}{C} = \frac{1}{C_1} + \frac{1}{C_0}.$$

From these results it follows directly that, if the most likely values of β_1 and β_0 are M_1 and M_0 respectively, and the corresponding standard deviations of the estimates are S_1 and S_0, then the most likely value of γ is

$$M = M_1 - M_0,$$

and the standard deviation of the estimate is

$$S = \sqrt{(S_1)^2 + (S_0)^2}.$$

THE RATE RATIO REVISITED

As an example, we shall apply use these general rules to the problem of estimating and testing the logarithm of the rate ratio. Let λ_0 and λ_1 be the two rate parameters and define

$$\beta_1 = \log(\lambda_1), \qquad \beta_0 = \log(\lambda_0)$$

then

$$\begin{aligned}
\gamma &= \beta_1 - \beta_0 \\
&= \log\left(\frac{\lambda_1}{\lambda_0}\right) \\
&= \log(\theta),
\end{aligned}$$

the log of the rate ratio.

If, in the exposed group, D_1 cases are observed in Y_1 person-years, and in the unexposed group D_0 cases are observed in Y_0 person-years, the total log likelihood is

$$D_1 \log(\lambda_1) - \lambda_1 Y_1 \quad + \quad D_0 \log(\lambda_0) - \lambda_0 Y_1.$$

The gradients of this with respect to β_1 and β_0 are

$$G_1 = D_1 - \lambda_1 Y_1 \qquad G_0 = D_0 - \lambda_0 Y_0,$$

and the curvatures are

$$C_1 = -\lambda_1 Y_1 \qquad C_0 = -\lambda_0 Y_0.$$

The most likely values for β_1 and β_0 are

$$M_1 = \log(D_1/Y_1), \qquad M_0 = \log(D_0/Y_0)$$

and the corresponding standard deviations are

$$S_1 = \sqrt{1/D_1}, \qquad S_0 = \sqrt{1/D_0}.$$

Using the rules given at the end of the last section, the Gaussian approximation for the profile log likelihood for $\gamma = \log(\theta)$ has

$$
\begin{aligned}
M &= \log(D_1/Y_1) - \log(D_0/Y_0) \\
&= \log\left(\frac{D_1/Y_1}{D_0/Y_0}\right),
\end{aligned}
$$

and

$$S = \sqrt{\frac{1}{D_1} + \frac{1}{D_0}}.$$

These expressions are identical to those obtained in Chapter 13.

The Wald test is also based on the Gaussian approximation shown above. The score test is obtained from the gradient and curvature of the profile log likelihood at the null value of the parameter, $\gamma = 0$. Here λ_1 and λ_0 are equal and their most likely common value is D/Y so that the gradients and curvatures are

$$
\begin{aligned}
G_1 &= D_1 - E_1 & G_0 &= D_0 - E_0 \\
C_1 &= -E_1 & C_0 &= -E_0
\end{aligned}
$$

where $E_1 = (D/Y)Y_1$ and $E_0 = (D/Y)Y_0$ represent 'expected' numbers of failures in the two groups under the null hypothesis. The score, U, is given by either G_1 or $-G_0$ (it can easily be verified that these are identical). The score variance is minus the curvature of the profile log likelihood and, using the relationship

$$\frac{1}{C} = \frac{1}{C_1} + \frac{1}{C_0}.$$

this is

$$V = \left(\frac{1}{E_1} + \frac{1}{E_0}\right)^{-1}$$

$$= \frac{E_1 E_0}{E}$$

Since $D = E$, this can also be written

$$V = D\frac{E_1}{E}\frac{E_0}{E}$$

$$= D\frac{E_1}{E}\left(1 - \frac{E_1}{E}\right)$$

and this agrees with the expression given in Chapter 13.

THE DIFFERENCE BETWEEN TWO MEANS

A second example is the difference between two mean parameters in a Gaussian model for responses measured on a continuous metric scale. For example, we might wish to compare blood pressure in two groups of subjects. We shall let μ_1 and μ_0 represent the mean parameters for the two groups and assume that the standard deviation of responses about the mean is the same in both groups, σ let us say. As in Chapter 8 we shall assume σ to be a known constant although, in practice, it would also have to be estimated from the data.

Exercise C.1. Derive expressions for the most likely value and for the standard deviation of the estimate of the parameter

$$\gamma = \mu_1 - \mu_0.$$

C.2 Weighted sums

Similar results hold for more general problems. For example, the parameter of interest may be defined as

$$\gamma = W_1\beta_1 + W_0\beta_0$$

where W_1 and W_0 are known constants. In this case the same argument illustrated in Fig. C.1 may be applied, but the parallel lines corresponding to fixed values of γ now have different slopes. The relationship between gradients in the total log likelihood and the gradient of the profile likelihood is now

$$G = \frac{G_1}{W_1} = \frac{G_0}{W_0}.$$

and for the curvatures we have

$$\frac{1}{C} = \frac{(W_1)^2}{C_1} + \frac{(W_0)^2}{C_0}.$$

These results generalize in an obvious way to a function of more than two parameters, of the form

$$\gamma = W_1\beta_1 + W_2\beta_2 + W_3\beta_3 + \cdots \ ,$$

the gradient of the profile log likelihood now being

$$G = \frac{G_1}{W_1} = \frac{G_2}{W_2} = \frac{G_3}{W_3} = \cdots$$

and its curvature

$$\frac{1}{C} = \frac{(W_1)^2}{C_1} + \frac{(W_2)^2}{C_2} + \frac{(W_3)^2}{C_3} + \cdots \ .$$

If the most likely values of $\beta_1, \beta_2, \ldots$ are $M_1, M_2, \ldots$ with standard deviations $S_1, S_2, \ldots$, then the most likely value of γ is

$$M = W_1M_1 + W_2M_2 + W_3M_3 + \cdots$$

with standard deviation

$$S = \sqrt{(W_1S_1)^2 + (W_2S_2)^2 + (W_3S_3)^2 + \cdots} \ .$$

Solutions to the exercises

C.1 The log likelihoods for μ_1 and μ_0 are Gaussian with most likely values M_1 and M_0 — the arithmetic means of the N_1 observations in the first group and the N_0 observations in the second. The corresponding standard deviations are

$$S_1 = \frac{\sigma}{\sqrt{N_1}}, \qquad S_0 = \frac{\sigma}{\sqrt{N_0}}.$$

It follows from the results of this section that the profile log likelihood for $\mu_1 - \mu_0$ has most likely value $M_1 - M_0$ and standard deviation

$$\sqrt{\frac{(\sigma)^2}{N_1} + \frac{(\sigma)^2}{N_0}} = \sigma\sqrt{\frac{1}{N_1} + \frac{1}{N_0}}.$$

Appendix D
Table of the chi-squared distribution

Probability	Degrees of freedom, ν				
p	1	2	3	4	5
0.50	0.455	1.386	2.366	3.357	4.351
0.25	1.323	2.773	4.108	5.385	6.626
0.10	2.706	4.605	6.251	7.779	9.2367
0.075	3.170	5.181	6.905	8.496	10.008
0.050	3.841	5.991	7.815	9.488	11.070
0.025	5.024	7.378	9.348	11.143	12.833
0.0100	6.635	9.210	11.345	13.277	15.086
0.0075	7.149	9.786	11.966	13.937	15.780
0.0050	7.879	10.597	12.838	14.860	16.750
0.0025	9.141	11.983	14.320	16.424	18.386
0.0010	10.828	13.816	16.266	18.467	20.515

Probability	Degrees of freedom, ν				
p	6	7	8	9	10
0.50	5.348	6.346	7.344	8.343	9.342
0.25	7.841	9.037	10.219	11.389	12.549
0.10	10.645	12.017	13.362	14.684	15.987
0.075	11.466	12.883	14.270	15.631	16.971
0.050	12.592	14.067	15.507	16.919	18.307
0.025	14.449	16.013	17.535	19.023	20.483
0.0100	16.812	18.475	20.090	21.666	23.209
0.0075	17.537	19.229	20.870	22.471	24.038
0.0050	18.548	20.278	21.955	23.589	25.188
0.0025	20.249	22.040	23.774	25.462	27.112
0.0010	22.458	24.322	26.124	27.877	29.588

The above tables give the value that a variable, distributed according to the chi-squared distribution with ν degrees of freedom, will exceed with probability p. For example, a variable distributed according to the chi-squared distribution with one degree of freedom has a probability of $p = 0.1$ of exceeding the value 2.706.

Index